T0293399

Endometriosis: Pathogenesis, Diagnosis and Management

Endometriosis: Pathogenesis, Diagnosis and Management

Editor: Chris Flagstad

AMERICAN
MEDICAL PUBLISHERS
www.americanmedicalpublishers.com

AMERICAN
MEDICAL PUBLISHERS
www.americanmedicalpublishers.com

Cataloging-in-Publication Data

Endometriosis : pathogenesis, diagnosis and management / edited by Chris Flagstad.
  p. cm.
Includes bibliographical references and index.
ISBN 978-1-63927-667-7
1. Endometriosis. 2. Endometriosis--Pathogenesis. 3. Endometriosis--Diagnosis.
4. Endometriosis--Treatment. 5. Generative organs, Female--Diseases. 6. Endometrium.
I. Flagstad, Chris.
RG483.E53 E53 2023
618.1--dc23

American Medical Publishers,
41 Flatbush Avenue,
1st Floor, New York,
NY 11217, USA

ISBN 978-1-63927-667-7 (Hardback)

Contents

Preface.. VII

Chapter 1 **Does Endometriosis Influence the Embryo Quality and/or Development? Insights from a Large Retrospective Matched Cohort Study**..........................1
Ana M. Sanchez, Luca Pagliardini, Greta C. Cermisoni, Laura Privitera, Sofia Makieva, Alessandra Alteri, Laura Corti, Elisa Rabellotti, Massimo Candiani and Paola Viganò

Chapter 2 **Biomarkers for the Noninvasive Diagnosis of Endometriosis: State of the Art and Future Perspectives**..........................11
Costin Vlad Anastasiu, Marius Alexandru Moga, Andrea Elena Neculau, Andreea Bălan, Ioan Scârneciu, Roxana Maria Dragomir, Ana-Maria Dull and Liana-Maria Chicea

Chapter 3 ***BIRC5*/Survivin Expression as a Non-Invasive Biomarker of Endometriosis**..........................35
Carolina Filipchiuk, Antonio Simone Laganà, Rubia Beteli, Tatiana Guida Ponce, Denise Maria Christofolini, Camila Martins Trevisan, Fernando Luiz Affonso Fonseca, Caio Parente Barbosa and Bianca Bianco

Chapter 4 **Genetic Characterization of Endometriosis Patients: Review of the Literature and a Prospective Cohort Study on a Mediterranean Population**..........................45
Stefano Angioni, Maurizio Nicola D'Alterio, Alessandra Coiana, Franco Anni, Stefano Gessa and Danilo Deiana

Chapter 5 **Differential Diagnosis of Endometriosis by Ultrasound: A Rising Challenge**..........................68
Marco Scioscia, Bruna A. Virgilio, Antonio Simone Laganà, Tommaso Bernardini, Nicola Fattizzi, Manuela Neri and Stefano Guerriero

Chapter 6 **Microbiome Profile of Deep Endometriosis Patients: Comparison of Vaginal Fluid, Endometrium and Lesion**..........................82
Camila Hernandes, Paola Silveira, Aline Fernanda Rodrigues Sereia, Ana Paula Christoff, Helen Mendes, Luiz Felipe Valter de Oliveira and Sergio Podgaec

Chapter 7 **Peritoneal Fluid Cytokines Reveal New Insights of Endometriosis Subphenotypes**..........................93
Jieliang Zhou, Bernard Su Min Chern, Peter Barton-Smith, Jessie Wai Leng Phoon, Tse Yeun Tan, Veronique Viardot-Foucault, Chee Wai Ku, Heng Hao Tan, Jerry Kok Yen Chan and Yie Hou Lee

Chapter 8 **A Prospective Study Comparing Three Dimensional Rectal Water Contrast Transvaginal Ultrasonography and Computed Tomographic Colonography in the Diagnosis of Rectosigmoid Endometriosis**..........................109
Fabio Barra, Ennio Biscaldi, Carolina Scala, Antonio Simone Laganà, Valerio Gaetano Vellone, Cesare Stabilini, Fabio Ghezzi and Simone Ferrero

Chapter 9   **Impaired Expression of Ectonucleotidases in Ectopic and Eutopic Endometrial Tissue is in Favor of ATP Accumulation in the Tissue Microenvironment in Endometriosis**..**124**
Carla Trapero, August Vidal, Maria Eulàlia Fernández-Montolí, Buenaventura Coroleu, Francesc Tresserra, Pere Barri, Inmaculada Gómez de Aranda, Jean Sévigny, Jordi Ponce, Xavier Matias-Guiu and Mireia Martín-Satué

Chapter 10   **Uncovering Potential Roles of Differentially Expressed Genes, Upstream Regulators and Canonical Pathways in Endometriosis Using an In Silico Genomics Approach**..**143**
Zeenat Mirza and Umama A. Abdel-dayem

Chapter 11   **Assessment of Coagulation Parameters in Women Affected by Endometriosis: Validation Study and Systematic Review of the Literature**..........................**159**
Jessica Ottolina, Ludovica Bartiromo, Carolina Dolci, Noemi Salmeri, Matteo Schimberni, Roberta Villanacci, Paola Viganò and Massimo Candiani

Chapter 12   **Role of B-Cell Translocation Gene 1 in the Pathogenesis of Endometriosis**...........................**177**
Jeong Sook Kim, Young Sik Choi, Ji Hyun Park, Jisun Yun, Soohyun Kim, Jae Hoon Lee, Bo Hyon Yun, Joo Hyun Park, Seok Kyo Seo, SiHyun Cho, Hyun-Soo Kim and Byung Seok Lee

Chapter 13   **Endometriosis in Menopause—Renewed Attention on a Controversial Disease**................................**190**
Cristina Secosan, Ligia Balulescu, Simona Brasoveanu, Oana Balint, Paul Pirtea, Grigoraş Dorin and Laurentiu Pirtea

Chapter 14   **The Pathogenesis of Endometriosis: Molecular and Cell Biology Insights**...........................**202**
Antonio Simone Laganà, Simone Garzon, Martin Götte, Paola Viganò, Massimo Franchi, Fabio Ghezzi and Dan C. Martin

Permissions

List of Contributors

Index

Preface

Endometriosis occurs when the tissue outlining the uterus from inside happens to grow outside the uterus. It affects the fallopian tubes, ovaries and the tissue lining the pelvis. The tissue similar to endometrial solidifies, breaks down and then bleeds with every menstrual cycle. However, in this condition there is no space for this tissue to exit the body and it gets trapped. Consequently, when this condition occurs in the ovaries, it creates cysts known as endometriomas. Pelvic pain often linked to mensuration is the primary indicator of endometriosis. Other symptoms and signs involve painful mensuration, painful intercourse, pain while urination or bowel movements, and infertility. Its diagnosis involves pelvic exam, ultrasound, magnetic resonance imaging (MRI) and laparoscopy. Endometriosis is generally treated through medicines, surgery or hormonal therapy, and it depends on the severity of symptoms. This book explores all the important aspects of endometriosis in the present day scenario. It will serve as a valuable source of reference for those interested in the pathogenesis, diagnosis and management of this disease.

This book is a result of research of several months to collate the most relevant data in the field.

When I was approached with the idea of this book and the proposal to edit it, I was overwhelmed. It gave me an opportunity to reach out to all those who share a common interest with me in this field. I had 3 main parameters for editing this text:

1. Accuracy – The data and information provided in this book should be up-to-date and valuable to the readers.

2. Structure – The data must be presented in a structured format for easy understanding and better grasping of the readers

3. Universal Approach – This book not only targets students but also experts and innovators in the field, thus my aim was to present topics which are of use to all

Thus, it took me a couple of months to finish the editing of this book.

I would like to make a special mention of my publisher who considered me worthy of this opportunity and also supported me throughout the editing process. I would also like to thank the editing team at the back-end who extended their help whenever required.

Editor

Does Endometriosis Influence the Embryo Quality and/or Development? Insights from a Large Retrospective Matched Cohort Study

Ana M. Sanchez [1], Luca Pagliardini [1,*]⊙, Greta C. Cermisoni [2], Laura Privitera [2], Sofia Makieva [1], Alessandra Alteri [2]⊙, Laura Corti [2], Elisa Rabellotti [2], Massimo Candiani [2] and Paola Viganò [1]

[1] Reproductive Sciences Laboratory, Division of Genetics and Cell Biology, IRCCS San Raffaele Scientific Institute, 20132 Milano, Italy; asg.alcala@gmail.com (A.M.S.); makieva.sofia@hsr.it (S.M.); vigano.paola@hsr.it (P.V.)

[2] IRCCS San Raffaele Scientific Institute, Obstetrics and Gynecology Unit, 20132 Milano, Italy; cermisoni.greta@hsr.it (G.C.C.); privitera.laura@hsr.it (L.P.); alteri.alessandra@hsr.it (A.A.); corti.laura@hsr.it (L.C.); rabellotti.elisa@hsr.it (E.R.); candiani.massimo@hsr.it (M.C.)

* Correspondence: pagliardini.luca@hsr.it

Abstract: In vitro fertilization can be an effective tool to manage the endometriosis-associated infertility, which accounts for 10% of the strategy indications. Nevertheless, a negative effect of endometriosis on IVF outcomes has been suggested. The aim of this study was to evaluate the potential effect of endometriosis in the development of embryos at cleavege stage in assisted reproduction treatment cycles. A total of 429 cycles from women previously operated for moderate/severe endometriosis were compared with 851 cycles from non-affected women. Patients were matched by age, number of oocyte retrieved and study period. A total of 3818 embryos in cleavage stage have been analyzed retrospectively. Overall, no difference was found between women with and without endometriosis regarding the number of cleavage stage embryos obtained as well as the percentage of good/fair quality embryos. Excluding cycles in which no transfers were performed or where embryos were frozen in day three, no difference was observed for blastulation rate or the percentage of good/fair blastocysts obtained. Despite similar fertilization rate and number/quality of embryos, a reduction in ongoing pregnancy rate was observed in patients affected, possibly due to an altered endometrial receptivity or to the limited value of the conventional morphological evaluation of the embryo.

Keywords: embryo quality; endometriosis; blastulation rate; ongoing pregnancy

1. Introduction

Endometriosis affects from 10% to 15% of reproductive aged women and around 30% of women suffering from infertility, which is up to 10-fold more frequent than in the general population (0.5–5%) [1,2]. Mechanisms that have been postulated to explain the low fecundity of women with endometriosis include altered folliculogenesis, reduced quality and cytoplasmic mitochondrial content of oocytes, oocyte/embryo exposure to a hostile inflammatory environment (macrophages, cytokines and vasoactive substances in the peritoneal fluid), anatomical dysfunctions of the tubes and/or ovary and reduced endometrial receptivity [3].

Assisted Reproduction Technology (ART) can be an effective tool to manage the endometriosis-associated infertility, which indeed accounts for 10% of the strategy indications. Nevertheless, a negative effect of endometriosis on ART outcomes has been suggested [4–6], albeit not consistently [7–9]. Both oocyte/embryo number and quality have been claimed to be affected by the disease [3]. Lower implantation rates have been as well postulated. However, the reasons to explain the suboptimal performance of ART in endometriosis patients are still poorly understood and can only be hypothesized.

Data from meta-analyses are only partially informative in this regard. The meta-analysis from Barnhart et al. [4] including data from 22 studies, found a reduction in fertilization and implantation rates in women with endometriosis when compared with non-affected women or with women that underwent ART for tubal-factor infertility only [4]. Harb and colleagues, including 27 studies, reported a reduction in clinical pregnancy rate in women with stage III/IV endometriosis compared to controls, but not a reduction in live births [10]. No differences in reproductive outcomes were found by Barbosa and colleagues between women with and without endometriosis. Only the number of oocytes at the time of retrieval was found to be lower in women affected [11].

Unfortunately, few studies have considered the consequence of endometriosis on the embryological outcomes. This aspect is important considering that in recent years the reproductive medicine laboratories are trying to optimize embryo transfer strategies, e.g., by transferring the embryo later in development instead of transfer at an early stage. Additionally, single blastocyst transfer has been preferred to a simultaneous transfer of multiple early stage embryos.

In association with the importance of the embryonic developmental stage for an optimal uterine transfer, it is critical to elucidate factors that can threaten embryonic competence to progress in a healthy pregnancy. In this context, Freis and colleagues have recently reported that the relative morphokinetic profiles of embryos from patients with endometriosis are altered, indicating a negative impact of the disease independently from the stage on the embryo quality [12]. Herein, we have scrutinized the plausible negative impact of endometriosis on embryonic parameters in a retrospective non-interventional analysis of ART cycles in our center.

The aim of the study was to investigate whether endometriosis affects embryo development and/or quality. The primary outcome of the study was the quality of cleavage stage (day 3) embryo in terms of number of cells, cell fragmentation and symmetry. Secondary outcome measures were (1) fertilization rate, (2) number of good/fair embryos at cleavage stage, (3) blastulation rate (defined as percentage of total blastocyst obtained per number of fertilized eggs, excluding cycles in which embryos were transferred or frozen in day 3, (4) good/fair blastocyst formation rate, and (5) ongoing pregnancy rate (defined when the pregnancy had completed ≥20 weeks of gestation per transfer).

2. Results

The baseline characteristics of the cycles for the two study groups are presented in Table 1: the maternal age, Body Mass Index (BMI), antral follicle count and Anti-Müllerian hormone (AMH) levels were significantly different between the two groups.

Table 1. Basal characteristics of the analyzed cycles.

Parameters	Controls $n = 851$	Endometriosis $n = 429$	p-Value
Age (years)	37.5 ± 3.6	36.9 ± 3.6	0.003
BMI (kg/m^2)	22.4 ± 3.6	21.6 ± 2.9	0.004
Antral follicle count	8.0 ± 4.7	6.3 ± 3.2	<0.001
AMH (ng/mL)	1.9 ± 2.5	1.5 ± 1.9	<0.001
Total dose FSH administered (IU)	3112 ± 1600	3419 ± 1641	0.003
E2 at the time of hCG administration (pg/mL)	1635 ± 1084	1562 ± 1057	0.18
Number of oocytes retrieved	5.8 ± 4.4	5.9 ± 4.6	0.90
Number of oocytes retrieved/1000 IU of FSH	2.8 ± 4.1	2.2 ± 2.6	0.09
Percentage of mature oocytes	75 (50–100)	71 (50–100)	0.25
Sperm Count (×10^6/mL)	31.2 ± 28.2	37.5 ± 26.9	<0.001
% Motility (a + b)	35 (20–50)	40 (30–50)	<0.001

Data are presented as mean ± standard deviation or median (interquartile range). IU: International Units; BMI: Body Mass Index; AMH: Anti-Müllerian Hormone; FSH: Follicle-Stimulating Hormone; hCG: Human Chorionic Gonadotropin.

Age was used as a variable to match cases and controls and a significant difference was observed between the two groups, that was however limited as an absolute value and for which the subsequent results were adjusted. The semen characteristics of the endometriosis and non-endometriosis groups are shown in Table 1. Sperm concentration and motility were significantly different between the groups. No differences were found in the levels of estrogen at the time of hCG administration and in the number of oocytes retrieved per 1000U of FSH (2.8 ± 4.1 controls vs 2.2 ± 2.6 endometriosis patients, $p = 0.09$).

The number of oocytes retrieved in both groups was similar (5.8 ± 4.4 non-endometriosis vs 5.8 ± 4.6 endometriosis patients, $p = 0.9$). We did not find any statistically significant differences in the percentage of MII oocytes (75% (50–100%) controls vs. 71% (50–100%) endometriosis patients, $p = 0.25$) and in fertilization rate (75% (50–100%) controls vs. 75% (50–100%) endometriosis patients, adjusted $p = 0.85$) (Table 2).

Table 2. ART outcomes in the two studied groups.

Header Parameters	Controls $n = 851$	Endometriosis $n = 429$	Estimated Difference	95% CI Lower Limit	95% CI Upper Limit	p-Value	corrected p-Value *
Fertilization rate, median (IQR)	75 (50–100)	75 (50–100)	0.0	−4.5	4.5	0.29	0.85
Cleavage rate, median (IQR)	100 (100–100)	100 (100–100)	0.0	0.0	0.0	0.33	0.83
Clevage stage embryos (n), mean ± SD	3.5 ± 2.6	3.7 ± 2.6	0.1	−0.2	0.5	0.42	0.77
Number of cells of the embryos, mean ± SD	7.0 ± 1.4	6.9 ± 1.5	−0.1	-0.3	0.1	0.22	0.42
Percentage of good/fair embryos, median (IQR)	56 (25–100)	50 (17–88)	−5.6	−15.0	4.0	0.20	0.36
Blastulation rate, median (IQR)	50 (25–67)	50 (25–67)	0.0	−6.0	6.0	0.68	0.22
Percentage of good/fair blastocysts, median (IQR)	50 (33–80)	50 (25–75)	0.0	−7.0	7.0	0.43	0.88

Data are presented as mean ± standard deviation or median (IQR: interquartile range). * Adjusted for age, BMI, semen parameters and percentage of mature oocytes.

Overall, we did not find any difference regarding the number of cleavage stage embryos obtained (3.5 ± 2.6 non-endometriosis vs. 3.7 ± 2.6 endometriosis patients, adjusted $p = 0.77$) and the mean number of blastomers of the embryos (7.0 ± 1.4 controls vs 6.9 ± 1.5 endometriosis patients, adjusted $p = 0.42$) between endometriosis women and controls. In addition, the percentage of good/fair quality embryos was similar (56% (25–100%) controls vs. 50% (17–88%) endometriosis patients, adjusted $p = 0.36$). Excluding cycles whereby embryos were transferred or frozen in day 3, no difference was found in blastulation rate between the two groups (50% (25–67%) controls vs. 50% (25–67%) endometriosis patients, adjusted $p = 0.22$). Finally, we calculated the percentage of good/fair blastocysts obtained and we did not find any difference (50% (33–80%) controls vs. 50% (25–75%) endometriosis patients, adjusted $p = 0.88$) (Table 2). No differences in terms of the number of cancelled cycles and/or freeze-all cycles were found between both groups (Supplementary Table S1).

Despite similar fertilization rate and number/quality of embryos obtained, we found a reduction in ongoing pregnancy after adjusting for the number of transferred embryos and the day of transfer (cleavage or blastocyst stage) (24.2% in controls vs. 17.8% in endometriosis group, adjusted OR = 0.62; 95% CI 0.40–0.94, $p = 0.02$) (Table 3).

A similar reduction was observed when considering transfers at day 3 or day 5, separately. Similar results were observed in terms on ongoing pregnancy rate considering frozen embryo transfers (Supplementary Table S2).

Table 3. Embryo transfer details and ongoing pregnancy rate.

Header Parameters	Controls $n = 516$	Endometriosis $n = 253$	p-Value
Number of transferred embryos, mean ± SD	1.6 ± 0.7	1.7 ± 0.7	0.10
Day 3 transfers	1.7 ± 0.7	1.8 ± 0.7	0.16
Day 5 transfers	1.3 ± 0.5	1.4 ± 0.5	0.20
Number of transfers (%)			
Day 3 transfers	396 (76.7)	192 (75.9)	
Day 5 transfers	120 (23.3)	61 (24.1)	0.86
Ongoing pregnancy rate (95% CI)			
All transfers	24.2 (20.7–28.1)	17.8 (13.5–22.9)	0.05
Day 3 transfers	21.7 (17.9–26.0)	15.1 (10.7–20.9)	0.07
Day 5 transfers	32.5 (24.8–41.3)	26.2 (16.8–38.4)	0.49
Adjusted Odds Ratios for ongoing pregnancy rate, (95% CI)			
All transfers *	-	0.62 (0.40–0.94)	0.02
Day 3 transfers **	-	0.58 (0.35–0.97)	0.04
Day 5 transfers **	-	0.76 (0.35–1.64)	0.49

* Adjusted for age, BMI, semen parameters, percentage of mature oocytes, day of the transfer and number of transferred embryos. ** Adjusted for age, BMI, semen parameters, percentage of mature oocytes and number of transferred embryos.

3. Discussion

This is, at least to the best of our knowledge, the largest study that analyzed the potentially deleterious effect of endometriosis on the in vitro development of embryos in ART cycles. We were unable to demonstrate an impact of endometriosis on day three embryo quality and developmental potential. The fertilization rates and percentage of good/fair quality embryos from endometriosis patients and controls were also similar. Moreover, in patients who did not perform a fresh transfer and/or freeze embryos at day three, we did not find any statistical difference in blastulation rate and/or the percentage of good/fair quality blastocyst obtained. Therefore, in the light of the results obtained, women with endometriosis may as well opt for the blastocyst culture in the presence of good quality embryo at day three in order to improve the reproductive outcomes after ART [13].

A limited number of studies have been published in relation to the in vitro development of embryos obtained from women with endometriosis. Coccia and colleagues published one of the first studies in 2011. In contrast to our results, the total number of embryos obtained in their ART cycles was significantly different between the endometriosis and the control group represented by women with tubal factor infertility. This discrepancy may be explained by methodological differences: firstly, they did not match for age, number of oocytes retrieved and/or study period. Secondly, only 3 oocytes were used for conventional IVF (under Italian law 40/2004 for ART) [5]. Finally, in endometriosis patients they notably observed a decrease in the number of oocytes retrieved, which could have impacted the number of embryos obtained. The reduction in the number of oocytes retrieved demonstrated in several studies may be ascribed to the detrimental effect of previous surgical treatments rather than to the disease itself. It is for this reason that we have decided to match our population for this parameter in order to avoid this bias. More recently, two studies have been performed using the time-lapse technology for the assessment of embryo morphokinetics in endometriosis patients [12,14]. In the study by Demirel and colleagues, the endometriosis population was constituted only by patients with a diagnosis of endometrioma. Specifically, the authors compared embryos derived from oocytes collected from an ovary affected by an endometrioma to embryos developed from oocytes from the contralateral healthy ovary failing to find differences in terms of morphokinetic parameters [14]. In contrast, Freis and colleagues compared embryo morphokinetics between women with and without endometriosis (tubal factor) showing a poorer relative kinetics in embryos from affected patients [12].

The group of Song and colleagues have demonstrated that the number of mature follicles and good embryos, and fertilization and blastulation rates were reduced in women with endometriosis compared with women with a male factor indication [15]. In line with our results, Benaglia and colleagues found that, in women with bilateral endometriomas, despite the lower number of oocytes retrieved, no differences could be observed in terms of fertilization rate, number of embryos obtained and rate of top-quality embryos per oocyte used compared to controls without the disease [16]. Finally, in a recent work of Muteshi and colleagues they demonstrated that endometriosis may affect embryo development due to a reduction in the percentage of women with endometriosis that reach blastocyst transfer compare with women with unexplain infertility [17]. Therefore, overall, data from the literature addressing the embryological parameters in ART cycles of women with endometriosis are very controversial.

Unfortunately, some of these previous studies are characterized by important limitations: firstly, the small sample size resulting in lack of statistical power and secondly, the lack of matching for age or number of collected oocytes or of corrections for confounders. These limitations of others have been addressed in the present study and represent the main strength of our work. Based on our results, at present, there are no strong evidence to set up a different culture or transfer strategy or to change the conventional embryological practice in ART cycles performed in patients with endometriosis.

In terms of IVF clinical outcomes, despite a similar number of transferred embryos and no differences in the day of transfer between women with and without the disease, we found a reduction in the ongoing pregnancy rates in the affected women. Several meta-analyses describing the effect of endometriosis on IVF outcomes have been published, again with contradictory results [4,6,10,11]. The inclusion of studies with very heterogeneous populations both for endometriosis and control group represents the main problem of these meta-analyses. The presence of side causes of infertility other than endometriosis are also rarely considered in the meta-analyses [18]. It should be considered that our endometriosis population consists of all operated women for a stage III/IV disease and that we have corrected for confounders potentially affecting fertility such as BMI and sperm motility/concentration.

In terms of ongoing pregnancy rate we found a similarly reduction of ongoing pregnancy rate in the endometriosis group compared to the control one in the freeze all cycles, consequently we cannot conclude that endometriosis women have better ART outcome after freeze all cycle. This data is supported by the recent study of Roque and colleagues [19], that reported that even if initial studies showed that the freeze-all strategy could be beneficial for certain groups of infertility including endometriosis patients [20], there is still lack of evidence to support its routine use not only for indications as endometriosis but also for implantation failure. In conclusion the data published until now is very controversial about better ART outcomes after freeze all cycles in endometriosis patients [19].

Two hypotheses can be put forward to explain our overall findings. The first is that, given the lack of differences in terms of embryo development/quality and blastulation rate in the endometriosis group, one might wonder whether an altered endometrial receptivity may explain the reduced chance of an ongoing pregnancy in affected women. Inflammatory-related changes in gene expression and/or a progesterone resistance in the endometrium of women with endometriosis might have a role [21,22]. This again represents a critical point. Some endometrial receptivity defects have been detected in these women [23]. However, data from clinical IVF egg donation program do not support this idea [24].

The second explanation is that the conventional morphological evaluation of the embryos, even at day 3 of development, may scarcely predict the embryo competence in these patients. Embryo grade has some value in predicting implantation [25] but, certainly, the embryo selection based on morphologic criteria could be imprecise [26] and may be even more imprecise in women with endometriosis. Indeed, oocytes have been demonstrated to more likely fail in vitro maturation and to have lower cytoplasmic mitochondrial content in women affected compared to women with other causes of infertility [3]. The time-lapse technology might be of value in this context.

The main limitation of our study is its retrospective design; however, for the calculation of the main outcome, no clinical decision/intervention has been done between the time of fertilization and day three of culture. The majority of the women from control group did not undergo laparoscopy prior to ART, therefore we cannot totally exclude the possibility that we incorrectly selected some affected women. This possibility could have influenced the study power to detect differences between the two groups. Similarly to the study of Barbosa and colleages, we have considered to include in the control group all the other women (without the diagnosis of endometriosis), because applying any other selection criterion would be arbitrary and might introduce biases [11]. Finally, the heterogeneity of the control group in terms of cause of infertility represents another bias that should be considered. Indeed, the different prevalence of causes underlying infertility could significantly impact on the quality of the embryos analyzed. This problem may be one of the reasons for the disagreements in terms of ART outcomes in the different studies already published and might have impacted the outcomes related to the blastulation rate and pregnancies. Similarly, although all cases were post-surgical, parameters such as moderate/severe disease, the different intervals from surgical management of endometriosis and ART treatment may have affected the results. In fact, based on a recent study of AlKudmani and collaborators [27], significant higher IVF ongoing pregnancy rates were observed in women with endometriosis after 6–25 months from the surgery compared with women with endometriosis undergoing IVF after 25 months from surgery [27]. In addition, another limitation of the study is the lack of information about the location of endometriosis lesions (superficial endometriosis, deep infiltrating endometriosis, endometriomas). At this regard, in a recent study of Ashrafi and colleagues [28], they demonstrated that the presence of deep infiltration endometriosis in the presence or not of endometrioma was associated with an 80% decrease in the probability of live births in comparison with that of a control group, but no information concerning the performance in the laboratory has been published.

In conclusion, we report that endometriosis does not compromise fertilization rate, the quality of cleavage stage embryos, of the blastocysts and blastulation rates. Thus, this study does not support the need to tailor embryo transfer strategy to the incidence of endometriosis. On the other hand, we found a reduction in ongoing pregnancy in patients affected, but an explanation for this observation warrants certainty. These results can help in understanding the mechanisms by which endometriosis impacts fertility.

4. Materials and Methods

4.1. Patients

This is a single center retrospective study matched cohort study, non-interventional, including patients who underwent ART cycles at the San Raffaele Hospital (Milan, Italy) from 2013 to 2017.

We performed a matched cohort study of the variables believed to be confounding (in order to avoid confounding) in our study design and to ensure an equal distribution among affected and non-affected.

Endometriosis was laparoscopically diagnosed in all the patients before ART treatment and classified according to the American Society for Reproductive Medicine ASRM criteria into stage III-IV (moderate/severe) [29], all women received a complete surgical treatment for endometriosis and all the lesions were removed. A total of 309 women were included in the study with a total of 429 ART cycles performed.

The control group were patients without a laparoscopic diagnosis or a history of endometriosis and did not have any ultrasonographic evidence of endometriotic ovarian cyst at the time of the cycle, including patients with tubal factor (female infertility caused by diseases, obstructions, damage, scarring, congenital malformations or other factors that impede the descent of a fertilized or unfertilized ovum into the uterus through the Fallopian tubes), male factor (patients that underwent at least two consecutive semen analyses, both showing below-standard values for normal semen parameters according to the World Health Organization (WHO) criteria), poor ovarian reserve (Bologna criteria definition [30]), idiopatic or patients that underwent PGT-M cycles for monogenic diseases (diseases that not affect the fertility of the couple, excluding genetic causes of male infertility) (Supplementary Table S3). Controls were matched to cases on a ratio 2:1 by age (± 1 year), number of oocytes retrieved (± 1 oocyte) and study period (± 4 months). A total of 851 cycles from control women were included in the analysis (from 766 patients). A total of 3818 cleavage stage embryos (day 3) have been analyzed.

Data collection followed the principles defined in the Declaration of Helsinki; all women undergoing ART in San Raffaele Hospital routinely provide informed consent for their clinical data and anonymized records to be used for research purposes in general. Women who denied this consent were excluded. Local Institutional Review Board approval (ID: BC-GINEOS, date of approval: 09/02/2012, San Raffaele Hospital Ethics Committee) for the use of clinical data for research studies was obtained.

4.2. Controlled Ovarian Stimulation, In Vitro Fertilization, Embryo Culture and Grading

All patients were treated with a GnRH antagonist protocol as previously descrived [31]. Oocyte collection was performed 36 h after triggering of ovulation. In both groups, in order to avoid biases in the evaluation of the number of MII oocytes and in the fertilization rate, only ICSI cycles were considered for analysis (that represents the 91% of the study group before matching). ICSI cycles were performed as previously descrived [32]. Sixteen-eighteen hours after ICSI, oocytes were checked for fertilization and transfer to 10% of Serum substitute supplement (SSS, Irvine, CA, USA)-supplemented Cleavage medium (REF ART-1026, Sage In-Vitro Fertilization, inc. Trumbull, CT, USA) under oil. Embryos were checked at 68 ± 1 after ICSI, and an embryo evaluation was performed according to the Istanbul consensus [33]. Briefly, the embryo quality was calculated in terms of number of blastomers, cell fragmentation and symmetry. A good/fair-quality embryo was considered that with ≥7 cells on day 3, with a fragmentation rate lower than 10% and a stage-specific cell size for majority of cells [33].

For evaluation of blastocyst data [cultured into 10% of Serum substitute supplement (SSS, Irvine, CA, USA)-supplemented Blastocyst medium (REF ART-1029, Sage In-Vitro Fertilization, inc. Trumbull, CT, USA)], only patients who did not perform transfer or freezing of day 3 embryos were included, hence patients who underwent prolonged culture of the whole cohort of embryos formed.

Blastocyst evaluation was performed according to the Istanbul Consensus (116 ± 2 h post insemination) [33] as previously described [31]. Based on the rating, a good/fair blastocyst was defined as expanded or hatched blastocyst with both an inner cell mass and multicellular trophectoderm scored good or fair or at least one of them scored as good or fair. Blastocysts were never frozen before the expanded stage.

All embryo transfers were scheduled in day 3 (at cleavage stage). The decision to transfer in day 3 or delay the embryo culture to day 5 (blastocyst stage) depends on the evaluation of the quality and the number of cleave stage embryos at day 3 and woman's age. Criteria for blastocyst culture were the presence at day 3 of 4 or more embryos and at least 2 good/fair embryos in women younger than 38 years old and three good/fair embryos for women aged 38 years and older [34].

In our laboratory, an embryo quality control is performed with a biannual frequency, together with other subjective evaluations (i.e., oocyte quality control, preimplantation diagnosis biopsy control) among the embryologists as previously described [31,35]. In any case, for this specific study, we choose to enroll in the study only cycles in which the quality of the embryos was evaluated every day by the same embryologist (P.V.) who is assigned to this specific task most of the time. To prove the reliability of the evaluations, we have measured the ability of conventional morphological analysis of the embryo to predict ART outcomes. An odds ratio of 5.7 (95% confidence interval 1.7–19.5, $p = 0.006$) for ongoing pregnancy was found after a single embryo transfer of day 3 good/fair embryos compared to poor quality embryos.

4.3. Statistical Methods

All continuous variables are presented as mean ± standard deviation (SD) or median with interquartile range (IQR). Normality of variables distributions were checked using the Kolmogorov–Smirnoff test. Student's *t*-test, Mann–Whitney U test and chi-squared test were used as appropriate. Multivariate analysis was conducted using the generalized estimating equation (GEE) approach, thus making it possible to use multiple cycles of the same patient and at the same time allow the analysis of variables with non-normal distribution. Age, BMI, concentration and motility of sperm and percentage of mature oocytes were used as predictors in the GEE model in order to obtain adjusted estimation for the differences between cases and controls. The ongoing pregnancy rate was adjusted for day of transfer and also for the number of transferred embryos and the adjusted estimate was reported as odds ratio (OR) with 95% confidence interval (95% CI). Differences were considered statistically significant if $p < 0.05$. Data were analyzed using the SPSS software 17.0 (SPSS, Inc., Chicago, IL, USA).

Author Contributions: Conceptualization, A.M.S., L.P. and G.C.C.; methodology, A.M.S., L.P., G.C.C. and L.C.; data curation, A.M.S., G.C.C., L.P., A.A, L.C. and E.R.; statistical analysis, A.M.S. and L.P.; writing—original draft preparation, A.M.S., L.P., S.M. and P.V.; writing—review and editing, A.M.S., L.P., G.C.C., L.P., S.M., A.A., L.C., E.R., M.C. and P.V. All authors have read and agreed to the published version of the manuscript.

Abbreviations

ART	Assisted Reproduction Technology
BMI	Body Mass Index
AMH	Anti-Müllerian Hormone
IU	International Unit
FSH	Follicle-Stimulating Hormone
IQR	Interquantile Range
SD	Standard Deviation
IVF	In Vitro Fertilization
GnRH	Gonadotropin-Releasing Hormone
hCG	human Chorionic Gonadotropin
PGT-M	Preimplantation Genetic Testing for Monogenic/single gene diseases.

References

1.   Somigliana, E.; Vigano, P.; Benaglia, L.; Busnelli, A.; Berlanda, N.; Vercellini, P. Management of Endometriosis in the Infertile Patient. *Semin. Reprod. Med.* **2017**, *35*, 31–37. [PubMed]
2.   Zondervan, K.T.; Becker, C.M.; Koga, K.; Missmer, S.A.; Taylor, R.N.; Viganò, P. Endometriosis. *Nat. Rev. Dis. Primers.* **2018**, *4*, 9. [CrossRef] [PubMed]
3.   Sanchez, A.M.; Vanni, V.S.; Bartiromo, L.; Papaleo, E.; Zilberberg, E.; Candiani, M.; Orvieto, R.; Viganò, P. Is the oocyte quality affected by endometriosis? A review of the literature. *J. Ovarian Res.* **2017**, *10*, 43. [CrossRef] [PubMed]
4.   Barnhart, K.; Dunsmoor-Su, R.; Coutifaris, C. Effect of endometriosis on in vitro fertilization. *Fertil. Steril.* **2002**, *77*, 1148–1155. [CrossRef]
5.   Coccia, M.E.; Rizzello, F.; Mariani, G.; Bulletti, C.; Palagiano, A.; Scarselli, G. Impact of endometriosis on in vitro fertilization and embryo transfer cycles in young women: A stage-dependent interference. *Acta Obs. Gynecol. Scand.* **2011**, *90*, 1232–1238. [CrossRef]
6.   Hamdan, M.; Omar, S.Z.; Dunselman, G.; Cheong, Y. Influence of endometriosis on assisted reproductive technology outcomes: A systematic review and meta-analysis. *Obs. Gynecol.* **2015**, *125*, 79–88. [CrossRef]

7. Bukulmez, O.; Yarali, H.; Gurgan, T. The presence and extent of endometriosis do not effect clinical pregnancy and implantation rates in patients undergoing intracytoplasmic sperm injection. *Eur. J. Obs. Gynecol. Reprod. Biol.* **2001**, *96*, 102–107. [CrossRef]

8. Al-Fadhli, R.; Kelly, S.M.; Tulandi, T.; Lin Tan, S. Effects of different stages of endometriosis on the outcome of in vitro fertilization. *J. Obs. Gynaecol. Can.* **2006**, *28*, 888–891. [CrossRef]

9. Opøien, H.K.; Fedorcsak, P.; Byholm, T.; Tanbo, T. Complete surgical removal of minimal and mild endometriosis improves outcome of subsequent IVF/ICSI treatment. *Reprod. Biomed. Online.* **2011**, *23*, 389–395. [CrossRef]

10. Harb, H.M.; Gallos, I.D.; Chu, J.; Harb, M.; Coomarasamy, A. The effect of endometriosis on in vitro fertilisation outcome: A systematic review and meta-analysis. *BJOG* **2013**, *120*, 1308–1320. [CrossRef]

11. Barbosa, M.A.; Teixeira, D.M.; Navarro, P.A.; Ferriani, R.A.; Nastri, C.O.; Martins, W.P. Impact of endometriosis and its staging on assisted reproduction outcome: Systematic review and meta-analysis. *Ultrasound Obs. Gynecol.* **2014**, *44*, 261–278. [CrossRef] [PubMed]

12. Freis, A.; Dietrich, J.E.; Binder, M.; Holschbach, V.; Strowitzki, T.; Germeyer, A. Relative Morphokinetics Assessed by Time-Lapse Imaging Are Altered in Embryos From Patients With Endometriosis. *Reprod. Sci.* **2018**, *25*, 1279–1285. [CrossRef] [PubMed]

13. Glujovsky, D.; Farquhar, C.; Quinteiro Retamar, A.M.; Alvarez Sedo, C.R.; Blake, D. Cleavage stage versus blastocyst stage embryo transfer in assisted reproductive technology. *Cochrane Database Syst. Rev.* **2016**, *6*, CD002118. [CrossRef] [PubMed]

14. Demirel, C.; Bastu, E.; Aydogdu, S.; Donmez, E.; Benli, H.; Tuysuz, G.; Keskin, G.; Buyru, F. The Presence of Endometrioma Does Not Impair Time-Lapse Morphokinetic Parameters and Quality of Embryos: A Study On Sibling Oocytes. *Reprod. Sci.* **2016**, *23*, 1053–1057. [CrossRef]

15. Song, Y.; Liu, J.; Qiu, Z.; Chen, D.; Luo C1 Liu, X.; Hua, R.; Zhu, X.; Lin, Y.; Li, L.; Liu, W.; et al. Advanced oxidation protein products from the follicular microenvironment and their role in infertile women with endometriosis. *Exp. Med.* **2018**, *15*, 479–486. [CrossRef]

16. Benaglia, L.; Bermejo, A.; Somigliana, E.; Faulisi, S.; Ragni, G.; Fedele, L.; Garcia-Velasco, J.A. In vitro fertilization outcome in women with unoperated bilateral endometriomas. *Fertil. Steril.* **2013**, *99*, 1714–1719. [CrossRef]

17. Muteshi, C.M.; Ohuma, E.O.; Child, T.; Becker, C.M. The effect of endometriosis on live birth rate and other reproductive outcomes in ART cycles: A cohort study. *Hum. Reprod. Open.* **2018**, *2018*, hoy016. [CrossRef]

18. Senapati, S.; Sammel, M.D.; Morse, C.; Barnhart, K.T. Impact of endometriosis on in vitro fertilization outcomes: An evaluation of the Society for Assisted Reproductive Technologies Database. *Fertil. Steril.* **2016**, *106*, 164–171. [CrossRef]

19. Roque, M.; Nuto Nóbrega, B.; Valle, M.; Sampaio, M.; Geber, S.; Haahr, T.; Humaidan, P.; Esteves, S.C. Freeze-all strategy in IVF/ICSI cycles: An update on clinical utility. *Panminerva Med.* **2019**, *61*, 52–57. [CrossRef]

20. Bourdon, M.; Santulli, P.; Maignien, C.; Gayet, V.; Pocate-Cheriet, K.; Marcellin, L.; Chapron, C. The deferred embryo transfer strategy improves cumulative pregnancy rates in endometriosis-related infertility: A retrospective matched cohort study. *PLoS ONE.* **2018**, *13*, e0194800. [CrossRef]

21. Patel, B.G.; Rudnicki, M.; Yu, J.; Shu, Y.; Taylor, R.N. Progesterone resistance in endometriosis: Origins, consequences and interventions. *Acta. Obs. Gynecol. Scand.* **2017**, *96*, 623–632. [CrossRef]

22. Makieva, S.; Giacomini, E.; Ottolina, J.; Sanchez, A.M.; Papaleo, E.; Viganò, P. Inside the endometrial cell signaling subway: Mind the gap(s). *Int. J. Mol. Sci.* **2018**, *21*, 19. [CrossRef] [PubMed]

23. Lessey, B.A.; Kim, J.J. Endometrial receptivity in the eutopic endometrium of women with endometriosis: It is affected, and let me show you why. *Fertil. Steril.* **2017**, *108*, 19–27. [CrossRef] [PubMed]

24. Miravet-Valenciano, J.; Ruiz-Alonso, M.; Gómez, E.; Garcia-Velasco, J.A. Endometrial receptivity in eutopic endometrium in patients with endometriosis: It is not affected, and let me show you why. *Fertil. Steril.* **2017**, *108*, 28–31. [CrossRef] [PubMed]

25. Weitzman, V.N.; Schnee-Riesz, J.; Benadiva, C.; Nulsen, J.; Siano, L.; Maier, D. Predictive value of embryo grading for embryos with known outcomes. *Fertil. Steril.* **2010**, *93*, 658–662. [CrossRef] [PubMed]

26. Ebner, T.; Moser, M.; Sommergruber, M.; Tews, G. Selection based on morphological assessment of oocytes and embryos at different stages of preimplantation development: A review. *Hum. Reprod. Update.* **2003**, *9*, 251–262. [CrossRef]

27. AlKudmani, B.; Gat, I.; Buell, D.; Salman, J.; Zohni, K.; Librach, C.; Sharma, P. In Vitro Fertilization Success Rates after Surgically Treated Endometriosis and Effect of Time Interval between Surgery and In Vitro Fertilization. *J Minim Invasive Gynecol.* **2018**, *25*, 99–104. [CrossRef]

28. Ashrafi, M.; Arabipoor, A.; Hemat, M.; Salman-Yazdi, R. The impact of the localisation of endometriosis lesions on ovarian reserve and assisted reproduction techniques outcomes. *J. Obs. Gynaecol.* **2019**, *39*, 91–97. [CrossRef]

29. American Society for Reproductive Medicine—ASRM. Revised American Society for Reproductive Medicine classification of endometriosis. *Fertil. Steril.* **1996**, *67*, 817–882. [CrossRef]

30. Ferraretti, A.P.; La Marca, A.; Fauser, B.C.; Tarlatzis, B.; Nargund, G.; Gianaroli, L.; ESHRE working group on Poor Ovarian Response Definition. ESHRE consensus on the definition of 'poor response' to ovarian stimulation for in vitro fertilization: The Bologna criteria. *Hum. Reprod.* **2011**, *26*, 1616–1624. [CrossRef]

31. Vanni, V.S.; Somigliana, E.; Reschini, M.; Pagliardini, L.; Marotta, E.; Faulisi, S.; Paffoni, A.; Vigano', P.; Vegetti, W.; Candiani, M.; et al. Top quality blastocyst formation rates in relation to progesterone levels on the day of oocyte maturation in GnRH antagonist IVF/ICSI cycles. *PLoS ONE.* **2017**, *12*, e0176482. [CrossRef] [PubMed]

32. Rubino, P.; Viganò, P.; Luddi, A.; Piomboni, P. The ICSI procedure from past to future: A systematic review of the more controversial aspects. *Hum. Reprod. Update.* **2016**, *22*, 194–227. [CrossRef] [PubMed]

33. ALPHA Scientists In Reproductive Medicine; ESHRE Special Interest Group Embryology. Istanbul consensus workshop on embryo assessment: Proceedings of an expert meeting. *Reprod. Biomed. Online.* **2011**, *22*, 632–646. [CrossRef] [PubMed]

34. Cutting, R.; Morroll, D.; Roberts, S.A.; Pickering, S.; Rutherford, A.; BFS; ACE. Elective single embryo transfer: Guidelines for practice British Fertility Society and Association of Clinical Embryologists. *Hum. Fertil.* **2008**, *11*, 131–146. [CrossRef] [PubMed]

35. Gentilini, D.; Somigliana, E.; Pagliardini, L.; Rabellotti, E.; Garagnani, P.; Bernardinelli, L.; Papaleo, E.; Candiani, M.; Di Blasio, A.M.; Viganò, P. Multifactorial analysis of the stochastic epigenetic variability in cord blood confirmed an impact of common behavioral and environmental factors but not of in vitro conception. *Clin. Epigenetics.* **2018**, *10*, 77. [CrossRef] [PubMed]

2

Biomarkers for the Noninvasive Diagnosis of Endometriosis: State of the Art and Future Perspectives

Costin Vlad Anastasiu [1][ORCID], Marius Alexandru Moga [1], Andrea Elena Neculau [2,*], Andreea Bălan [1,*], Ioan Scârneciu [1], Roxana Maria Dragomir [1], Ana-Maria Dull [3] and Liana-Maria Chicea [4]

[1] Department of Medical and Surgical Specialties, Faculty of Medicine, Transilvania University of Brasov, 500019 Brasov, Romania; canastasiu@gmail.com (C.V.A.); moga.og@gmail.com (M.A.M.); urologie_scarneciu@yahoo.com (I.S.); roxana.gidinceanu@unitbv.ro (R.M.D.)
[2] Department of Fundamental, Prophylactic and Clinical Sciences, Faculty of Medicine, University Transilvania Brasov, 500019 Brasov, Romania
[3] Regina Maria Hospital, 500091 Brasov, Romania; dullana2005@yahoo.com
[4] "Victor Papilian" Medical School, University "Lucian Blaga" of Sibiu, 550024 Sibiu, Romania; liana.chicea@gmail.com
* Correspondence: andrea.neculau@unitbv.ro (A.E.N.); dr.andreeabalan@gmail.com (A.B.)

Abstract: Background: Early and accurate diagnosis of endometriosis is crucial for the management of this benign, yet debilitating pathology. Despite the advances of modern medicine, there is no common ground regarding the pathophysiology of this disease as it continues to affect the quality of life of millions of women of reproductive age. The lack of specific symptoms often determines a belated diagnosis. The gold standard remains invasive, surgery followed by a histopathological exam. A biomarker or a panel of biomarkers is easy to measure, usually noninvasive, and could benefit the clinician in both diagnosing and monitoring the treatment response. Several studies have advanced the idea of biomarkers for endometriosis, thereby circumventing unnecessary invasive techniques. Our paper aims at harmonizing the results of these studies in the search of promising perspectives on early diagnosis. Methods: We selected the papers from Google Academic, PubMed, and CrossRef and reviewed recent articles from the literature, aiming to evaluate the effectiveness of various putative serum and urinary biomarkers for endometriosis. Results: The majority of studies focused on a panel of biomarkers, rather than a single biomarker and were unable to identify a single biomolecule or a panel of biomarkers with sufficient specificity and sensitivity in endometriosis. Conclusion: Noninvasive biomarkers, proteomics, genomics, and miRNA microarray may aid the diagnosis, but further research on larger datasets along with a better understanding of the pathophysiologic mechanisms are needed.

Keywords: biomarker; angiogenesis; cytokines; urinary biomarkers; endometriosis

1. Introduction

Endometriosis is considered a debilitating gynecological pathology with a high prevalence among young women [1]. The incidence of the disease varies between 6–10% [2]. Various sources indicate a constant increase in the number of cases, reaching almost 15% worldwide [3]. Endometriosis is characterized by the migration of endometrial-like cells in ectopic places outside the uterus. The clinical manifestations thereof consist of chronic pelvic pain, dysmenorrhea, and infertility, the latter being reported in 30–50% of cases, while 20–25% of patients remain asymptomatic [4].

Given the nonspecific symptoms of this disease that can usually mimic those associated with pelvic inflammatory disease or other conditions associated with chronic pelvic pain, the gold standard for a definitive diagnosis consists of surgical procedures, followed by histopathological exams [5]. Under these circumstances, a considerable diagnostic delay is explicable [6,7], leading to 8–12 years of belated appropriate treatment [8]. As of yet, reliable laboratory biomarkers for this gynecological pathology remain elusive. The increased incidence of this pathology in women with early menarche compels the development of novel noninvasive diagnostic biomarkers for faster diagnosis, appropriate treatment, and for triaging potential patients for surgery [9,10]. A biomarker is a biological molecule that can be "objectively measured and evaluated as an indicator of normal biological processes, pathogenic processes, or pharmacological responses to a therapeutic intervention" [11]. Therefore, a biomarker or a panel of biomarkers found in the biological fluids of the affected women could be an expedient diagnostic tool for endometriosis as well as an objective assessment of the effectiveness of the treatment [12].

The pathophysiology of this disease is not thoroughly understood. Sampson's theory of retrograde menstruation is still viewed as the principal etiopathogenic factor of endometriosis. However, approximately 90% of non-affected women undergo retrograde menstruation [13]. Novel pieces of evidence support the hypothesis that endometriosis development is caused by the occurrence of primitive endometrial cells outside the uterus, during organogenesis. Following puberty, these cells differentiate into functional endometriotic implants [14]. Other authors suggested that the principal source of extrapelvic endometriosis is represented by bone marrow-derived stem cells, which are able to migrate through the peripheral circulation and induce endometriosis in remote sites [15].

According to the "embryonic theory" or epigenetic theory, during organogenesis, the genes of the Homeobox and Wingless family are essential for the differentiation of the anatomical structures of the urogenital tract. Any dysregulation of these genes through the Wnt/b-catenin signaling pathway will lead to various anomalies and may cause aberrant placement of the stem cells. The abnormal placement of these cells, associated with immune alterations and the pro-inflammatory peritoneal environment, will determine the progression towards endometriosis [14]. An ectopic endometrium displays a distinctive epigenetic expression profile, which involves homeobox A (HOXA) clusters and Wnt signaling pathway genes [16]. Furthermore, miRNAs dysregulations were found to modulate the proliferation and invasiveness of ectopic endometrial cells. Eggers et al. [17] pointed out that dysregulation of miR-200b family affects the differentiation of ectopic cells by regulating epithelial-to-mesenchymal transition. Moreover, epigenetics plays an important indirect role in the recruitment and differentiation of bone marrow-derived stem cells by modulating the relationship between the inflammatory microenvironment and steroid action. This interaction represents the trigger for the recruitment of bone marrow-derived stem cells, and it is highly influenced by the epigenetic expression profile [16].

Endometriosis is considered an inflammatory disease, due to increased levels of activated macrophages and cytokines such as interleukins (IL-6, IL-8, IIL-1β), tumor necrosis factor-alpha (TNF-α), and macrophage migration inhibitory factor (MIF), in the peritoneal fluid of affected women [2]. Furthermore, several inflammatory biomarkers registered increased levels in the serum of endometriotic women: C-reactive protein (CRP), IL-4, TNF-α, monocyte chemoattractant protein-1 (MCP-1), IL-6, IL-8, and regulated on activation, normal T cell expressed and secreted (RANTES) [13].

Recently, a wide range of papers revealed the importance and effectiveness of various putative biomarkers from the biological fluids of affected patients. Despite considerable research on this topic, noninvasive biomarkers of endometriosis have eluded the transition from bench to bedside. Some of the limitations of biomarker studies consist of reduced datasets, methodological flaws (the variability of biomarkers under physiological conditions such as menstrual phases), the lack of reproducibility across multiple studies, and, last but not least, high costs of the complex assays.

This paper aims to synthesize the expanding body of knowledge regarding the putative noninvasive biomarkers (Figure 1) of endometriosis. Furthermore, it presents the opportunities offered by the newest technologies such as proteomics, genomics, and miRNA microarray, which may represent the future perspective of diagnosis.

2. Material and Methods

This study is a synthesis of noninvasive biomarkers of endometriosis, based on literature review, highlighting their possible use for early and precise diagnosis while emphasizing the newest perspectives and opportunities in the diagnostic field.

Our research included all the publications in Google Scholar, PubMed and Cross Ref related to noninvasive biomarkers for endometriosis, during the period January 2000 to December 2019, using the following Medical Subject Headings (MeSH) keywords: biomarker, angiogenesis, cytokine, urinary biomarkers, and endometriosis. Two authors independently identified and selected relevant articles based on the following inclusion criteria: full-text articles, written in English, human-based studies, biomarkers retrieved from serum, plasma, or urine. All the studies included patients and controls that have either tested positive or negative for endometriosis. The exclusion criteria were, as follows: studies on animals or involving cell cultures, biomarkers retrieved from any invasive procedure (endometriotic tissue, endometriomas content or peritoneal fluid), papers written in other languages than English, duplicate papers, abstracts and papers that only compared biomarker levels between affected women with different stages of endometriosis, without the inclusion of healthy controls. A total number of 55 studies met our criteria.

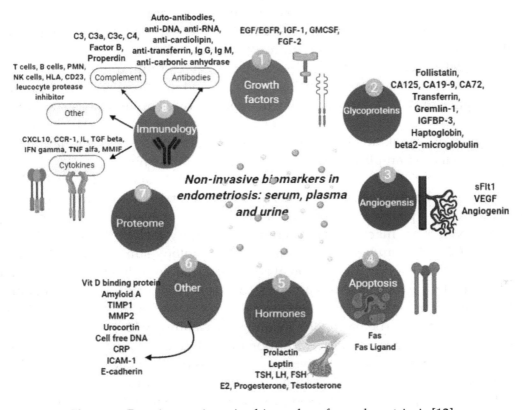

Figure 1. Putative noninvasive biomarkers for endometriosis [12].

3. Endometriosis—An Inflammatory Disease

A thorough understanding of the pathogenic and molecular mechanisms of endometriosis represents the springboard in finding various molecules that could serve as noninvasive biomarkers for early diagnosis.

Endometriosis is characterized by chronic abdominal pain, infertility, dysmenorrhea, and sometimes anxiety, related to the degree of the pelvic pain [18,19]. This pathology is the result of interactions between various hormonal, immunological, and genetic factors, and it is characterized by an increased expression of inflammatory factors and angiogenesis [20].

The central role in endometriosis belongs to local inflammation, which triggers the development of the disease and induces pain and infertility [21]. In support of this statement, a wide range of studies reported that the peritoneal fluid of endometriotic patients contained high levels of macrophages and immune cells, which secrete cytokines, angiogenic factors, and growth factors [22]. A further factor influencing the expression of these cytokines and of other cell adhesion molecules is represented by oxidative stress, thought to be an associated compound of endometriosis-related inflammation [23].

Normally, the peritoneal fluid contains 85% macrophages, as well as mast cells, lymphocytes, and mesothelial cells [24]. During menstruation and in endometriosis, this percentage is increased, and macrophages are more able to release prostaglandins (PG), cytokines, complement components, hydrolytic enzymes, and growth factors, which are central contributors to the endometriosis pathogenesis [25], and thus, possible biomarkers for the early diagnosis of this pathology. Since elevated values of PGs have been discovered in the peritoneal fluid of affected women, it is considered that PGs can trigger the progression of the disease by their inhibitory action through macrophage function, and their capacity to increase cellular proliferation and angiogenesis rate [25].

The inflammatory environment of this disease points out an increased production of estrogens, which in turn will raise the production of PGs through the activation of both NF-kB and cyclooxygenase-2 (COX-2) [26]. A paper by Banu et al. highlighted the influence of COX-2 and prostaglangin E2 (PGE2) on the migration and invasion of endometrial cells. Furthermore, the inhibition of COX-2 was able to decrease the invasion of epithelial and stromal cells in endometriosis [27].

COX-2 usually presents high values in ectopic endometrioid implants. Some studies found increased COX-2 expression and increased COX-2-derived PGE2 production in ectopic implants [27]. PGE2 and other proinflammatory cytokines induce increased values of COX-2 in normal and ectopic endometrial cells [28]. In ectopic endometriotic stromal cells, proinflammatory cytokines, such as interleukine-1β (IL-1β), are able to increase mRNA stability and to upregulate COX-2 promoter activity. This positive regulation of COX-2 is achieved via mitogen-activated protein kinase (MAPK)-dependent signaling pathways, which facilitate the binding of COX-2 promoter to the cAMP-responding element site. The subsequent dysregulation of MAPK signaling pathways increases inflammation, thereby recruiting immune cells and amplifying the inflammatory response [29].

Human endometrial cells have been shown to express NF-kappa B subunits [30,31], which are activated during normal menstruation [32]. In vitro, the activation of NF-kappa B in endometriotic stromal cells has proven a positive modulation of the proinflammatory cytokines, interleukins (IL-8, IL-6), RANTES, TNF-alpha, macrophage migration inhibitory factor (MIF), MCP-1, intercellular adhesion molecule (ICAM)-1, and granulocyte-macrophage colony-stimulating factor (GM-CSF) [33]. Alternatively, in vivo, the integrative activation of NF-kappa B subunits has been highlighted in ectopic areas of endometrial tissue [34]. The researcher's common point of view is that in endometriosis, NF-kappa B activated macrophages release IL-1, 6, 8, COX-2, TNF-alpha, and vascular endothelial growth factor (VEGF); thus, perpetuating the inflammatory pathway [21].

Several studies also suggested the contribution of oxidative stress in endometriosis-associated inflammation. Increased production of reactive oxygen species (ROS) inside the peritoneal environment may promote the inflammatory process through the positive regulation of several proinflammatory genes [35]. Zeller et al. [36] reported increased production of ROS into the peritoneal fluid of affected women. Portz and collab. [37] suggested that injecting antioxidant enzymes into the peritoneal cavity of endometriotic subjects could prevent the formation of intraperitoneal adhesions. However, other researchers, which directly measured the production of ROS in the peritoneal cavity of the affected patients did not find any obvious oxidant or antioxidant imbalance [38,39]

4. Immunological Aspects of Endometriosis

Immune dysfunction characterized by hyperactive peritoneal macrophages with altered phagocytic ability represents another key-point in endometriosis development and progression. The phagocytic ability of macrophages is mediated by matrix metalloproteinases (MMP), enzymes capable of destroying the structure of the extracellular matrix, and by the expression of several macrophage surface receptors, that can promote the dissolution of cellular debris [40]. Lagana et al. [41] suggested that macrophages are classified into M1 macrophages, and M2 macrophages, which display anti-inflammatory and pro-fibrotic activities. Moreover, these molecules are able to induce immunotolerance. In their study, Lagana and coworkers collected tissues from the ovarian endometriomas of women at different stages of endometriosis and measured M1 and M2 macrophage levels. They observed that the number of both M1 and M2 macrophages was significantly higher in the endometriosis group compared to controls. Furthermore, a progressive decrease of M1 macrophages and an increase of M2 macrophages from stage I to stage IV endometriosis was also noted [41].

Tie-2-expressing macrophages is a subset of macrophages that have been proved to promote tumor growth and angiogenesis. Using a murine model, these molecules were observed surrounding recently developed endometriotic blood vessels [42]. Should this hypothesis be proven accurate, it would infer the progression from endometriosis to ovarian cancer, thus explaining the increased risk of ovarian cancer in women affected by endometriosis [43].

Natural Killer cells (NK) activity is usually significantly decreased in endometriosis patients. This immunosuppressive effect, which consists of the reduction of T cell-mediated cytotoxicity, is not related to steroid hormone levels or to the day of the menstrual period. Wu et al. [44] explained this low activity of NK cells through highly increased levels of killer cell inhibitory receptors (KIRs) on NK cells of women with stage III-IV endometriosis. Recently, a new subset of T cells was identified, Invariant Natural Killer T cells (iNKT). They combine both classically innate and adaptive immunologic characteristics. These molecules are able to secrete both Th1 and Th2 cytokine patterns, and their actions in the eutopic and ectopic endometrium are subject to further research [45].

The contribution of IL-10 to endometriosis has also been suggested. Elevated levels of this cytokine-induced a decreased activity of cytotoxic T lymphocytes and CD+ helper cells into the peritoneal fluid of affected patients [46]. Furthermore, M1 to M2 macrophage polarization is promoted by the increased expression of IL-10 [47].

Several studies were conducted on transgenic mice in order to asses the levels of mucin 1 (MUC1) and Foxp3+ CD4 lymphocytes (Tregs). Under normal conditions, MUC1 is present on eutopic endometrial glands but is overexpressed in ectopic lesions. Preclinical investigations have revealed that upon disease development, endometriotic mice displayed high titers of anti-MUC1 antibodies and increased levels of Tregs [48]. These findings suggest that Treg lymphocytes could represent a promising venue for additional research.

Further immunological factors involved in the development of endometriosis are represented by T helper cells (Th), IL-17A and IL-4, as showed by Osuga et al. [49]. They observed increased levels of Th2 and Th17 cells in endometriotic tissues. IL-4 stimulates the proliferation of endometriotic stromal cells and IL-17A induces neutrophil migration in endometriotic tissues. Moreover, IL-17A, combined with TNFα, enhances the secretion of IL-8 and CCL-20, suggesting the cooperation of inflammation and Th17 immune response. Given the body of scientific proof, these molecules could be the focus of further reasearch for endometriosis treatment as well as potentially viable biomarkers for the disease development.

Since endometriosis is now considered an immune dysregulation with profound changes in the activities of various cells involved in immune reactions, further studies might offer novel therapeutic targets as well as biomarkers for early detection of endometriosis.

5. Angiogenesis in Endometriosis

Endometriosis is a polygenic and multifactorial disease, and increased angiogenesis and proteolysis may trigger its development and progression [50]. Studies have shown an essential involvement of several angiogenesis-related factors in endometriosis, such as the Delta-like 4 (Dll4)-Notch signal pathways, angiopoietin, vascular endothelial growth factor (VEGF), and vascular endothelial growth factor receptor (VEGFR) [51].

Vascular endothelial growth factor (VEGF), and vascular endothelial growth factor receptor (VEGFR) are the most well-known molecules involved in the angiogenesis process. They are able to regulate the proliferation, migration, and permeability of the cells. A study by Ahn et al. [52] pointed out that IL-17A is emerging as a potent angiogenic factor, and it can upregulate VEGF and IL-8. This mechanism promotes intraperitoneal angiogenesis in order to maintain the ectopic foci and to facilitate the development of new ones. Furthermore, plasmatic concentrations of IL-17A displayed a significant decrease following surgical removal of ectopic endometrial tissue.

The expression of VEGF microRNA (mRNA) is more increased in hypoxic areas. The growth of endometriotic cells creates hypoxia, enhancing the production of several molecules with pro-angiogenic potentials, such as TNF-α, VEGF, IL-8, bFGF, and TGF-β. All these factors trigger vessel hyperpermeability, release plasmatic proteins, induce the formation of fibrin, endothelial cells proliferation, and promote angiogenesis and fibrinolysis [53].

Several studies reported that interleukins also display a pro-angiogenic effect. Interleukins with a Glutamic Acid-Leucine-Arginine-amino-terminal site, such as IL-8, increase the angiogenesis rate, while those lacking this sequence, such as IL-4, impede this process [54]. Volpert et al. [55] highlighted that in vivo, IL-4 inhibits the vessel's neoformation induced by bFGF, while in vitro, it impedes the transmigration of endothelial cells towards bFGF. Another interleukin involved in endometriosis-related angiogenesis is IL-1α, which promotes this process through the augmented expression of various angiogenic factors such as VEGF, IL-8, and bFGF, according to the results published by Torisu and collab [56].

Donnez et al. [57] highlighted that red and white endometriosis foci exhibit different degrees of expression of pro-angiogenic factors. Consequently, they have shown that red endometriosis lesions display a more pronounced vascularization and a higher cell proliferative activity.

Figure 2 is a schematic representation of the mechanism of development and progression of endometriosis, illustrating the inflammatory and angiogenetic pathways.

Figure 2. Angiogenesis process—In endometriosis, the central role in pathophysiological mechanisms is attributed to macrophages. These cells increase the intranuclear expression of vascular endothelial growth factor (VEGF) and cyclooxigenase 2 (COX-2) genes, leading to increased angiogenesis and an inflammatory environment [58].

6. Studies of New Noninvasive Biomarkers in Endometriosis

A noninvasive biomolecule for endometriosis diagnosis could be extracted and quantified from serum, plasma, or urine and would be beneficial for patients with chronic pelvic pain, infertility, and dysmenorrhea, in the context of a regular ultrasound.

Blood and urine make for excellent sources of biomarkers due to their reproducibility, ease of access, and measurement [59]. Promising potential endometriosis biomarkers that underwent testing were: glycoproteins, growth factors, miRNAs, lncRNAs, as well as proteins related to the angiogenesis process or immunology [12]. Despite extensive research, neither a single biomarker nor a panel of biomolecules has been considered sufficiently specific and sensitive to be used as a diagnostic test for endometriosis [12].

6.1. Serum/Plasma Biomarkers of Endometriosis

6.1.1. Glycoproteins

Although lacking both specificity and sensitivity for this pathology, the most representative glycoprotein used as a biomarker for endometriosis is CA-125 [60]. However, the simultaneous measurement of CA-125 with other molecules and their combination showed different sensitivities and specificities for endometriosis. For example, Mihalyi et al. combined CA-125 with IL-8 and TNF-α during the secretory phase of the menstrual cycle and observed that this combination gives a sensitivity of 89.7% and specificity of 71.1% for endometriosis [61]. Furthermore, the combination of CA-125, chemokine receptor (CCR) type1, mRNA, and MCP1 proved to be efficient as a biomarker panel, with a sensitivity of 92.2% and specificity of 81.6%, according to Agic et al. [62]. Vodolazkaia combined four biomarkers, namely: VEGF, CA-125, Annexin V, and glycodelin resulting in a sensitivity and a specificity of 74–94% and 55–75%, respectively [63].

Another tumor marker, CA-19-9, was investigated as a possible biomarker for endometriosis diagnosis. Elevated values of this glycoprotein were detected in endometriotic women in comparison to healthy patients, but the sensitivity of this molecule was significantly lower when compared to CA-125 [12]. It is worthwhile mentioning that CA-19-9 has shown a positive correlation with the severity of the disease [64].

Glycodelin is a glycoprotein that promotes cell proliferation and neovascularization. Serum levels of this molecule have been found higher in endometriotic women when compared to non-affected patients. Mosbah et al. conducted a study that included women 21–48 years old with endometriosis and measured the levels of intercellular adhesion molecule 2 (ICAM-2), IL-6, and glycodelin A in their serum samples. Their results showed that IL-6 and glycodelin A displayed higher serum as well as peritoneal fluid levels in affected subjects compared to controls, with a sensitivity and specificity of 91.7% and 75.0% for serum glycodelin A, 93.8% and 80.0% for serum IL-6, 58.3%, and 60.0%, respectively for ICAM-1 [65]. Kocbek et al. [66] also identified significantly increased concentrations of glycodelin-A in the serum of cases compared to controls. Furthermore, combinations that included leptin/glycodelin-A ratio and ficolin 2/glycodelin-A ratio displayed a sensitivity and specificity of 72.5% to 84.2% and 78.4% to 91.2%, respectively.

Prentice Crapper [67] analyzed eight putative serum biomarkers for endometriosis, and they observed a significant elevation of only two of these molecules. Its results indicated that glycodelin has a sensitivity and specificity of 81.6% and 69.6%, respectively, for disease diagnosis. Zinc alpha 2-glycoprotein also registered increased values in affected women, with a sensitivity of 46% and a specificity of 100%. The combination of these two markers showed a greater specificity and sensitivity for the detection of this gynecological disorder (65% and 90%, respectively).

Follistatin is an inhibitor of activin, produced by the endometrium. It is increased in endometriosis, and thus, it could be used as a noninvasive biomarker for endometriosis diagnosis. Reis et al. simultaneously evaluated the levels of serum activin A and follistatin in healthy and affected subjects (with ovarian endometrioma, peritoneal endometriosis, and deep infiltrating endometriosis). Their study concluded that follistatin and activin A are not significantly modified in peritoneal or deep infiltrating endometriosis, but their serum concentrations in ovarian endometrioma were slightly higher [68].

Intercellular adhesion molecule-1 (ICAM-1) is a glycoprotein that seems to be involved in the development and promotion of endometriosis. It plays an essential role in the promotion of the inflammatory and immunological reactions, and recent studies associated the polymorphism of the ICAM-1 gene with the severity of this gynecological disorder. Vigano et al. [69] analyzed two polymorphic sites of the ICAM-1 gene, known as G/R241 and E/K469, using a cohort of 188 women with confirmed endometriosis and 175 controls. They observed that the frequency of the R241 allele was slightly higher in the endometriosis cohort than in the control group, while the frequency of the second allele was approximately the same in both groups. In conclusion, genetic polymorphism in the ICAM-1 gene domain G/R241 offers a promising perspective in the field of noninvasive biomarkers. Furthermore, concomitantly with the development of genomics, this glycoprotein could prove conducive in diagnosing endometriosis, as well as in predicting the degree of severity of this pathology.

6.1.2. Inflammatory Cytokines and Immunological Molecules

In the last decades, immunological molecules and inflammatory cytokines have been extensively studied for their potential as noninvasive biomarkers for endometriosis, with the most representative being IL-1, IL-6, IL-8, interferon-γ (IFN-γ), MCP-1, and TNF-α. Othman et al. tested three serum cytokines, both separately and in various combinations. They collected blood samples and measured cytokines levels with the Bio-Plex Protein Array System. The final results concluded that Il-6, MCP-1, and IFN-γ were significantly increased in the serum of affected women, in comparison with non-affected subjects. No difference has been found between serum concentration levels of tumor necrosis factor-alpha (TNF-α), or granulocyte macrophage colony-stimulating factor (GM-CSF). IL-2, IL-8 and, IL-15 were undetectable both in endometriosis and healthy group [70]. Borrelli et al. determined increased levels of IL-8, MCP-1, and RANTES in the peripheral blood of affected patients vs. controls, in 46.1%, 50%, and 75%, of the assessed cases, suggesting their potential use as noninvasive biomarkers for endometriosis [71].

Interleukin 6 is a proinflammatory cytokine that has shown increased serum levels in affected women. A study of Martinez et al. [72] pointed out that patients with Stage I-II endometriosis had increased levels of IL-6, with a sensitivity of approximately 75% and a specificity of 83.3%. In 2010, Socolov et al. [73] included 24 cases of endometriosis and 24 controls in a study and investigated their serum levels of IL-6, IL-8, IL-1, CA-125, and TNF. Their results indicated that IL-6 was above the cut-off threshold of 2 pg/mL in 71% of the cases and 87% of controls, with a sensitivity and specificity of 71% and 12%, respectively. They concluded that the difference between the two groups was not statistically significant.

Interleukin-8 is a chemokine derived from monocyte/macrophage that has also been considered for the noninvasive diagnosis of endometriosis. While some studies found no differences between cases and controls in terms of IL-8 levels [74]. Pizzo et al. [75] pointed out that this interleukin has increased levels in affected women with Stage I–II endometriosis and even higher levels in endometriomas [76].

Tumor necrosis factor alpha (TNF-α) is a proinflammatory cytokine with pro-angiogenic potential. Its role as a biomarker for endometriosis is controversial; while several studies proved increased serum levels of TNF-α in women with endometriosis [77–79], others showed no difference between affected patients and healthy controls [70,80]. Cho et al. [79] concluded that TNF-α increases only in the serum of endometriotic women, while urinary levels remain unchanged. The severity of endometriosis has also been associated with elevated serum TNF-α levels [75]. A recent study conducted by Steff et al. [81] revealed that the level of soluble TNF receptor in affected patients registered a significant increase during the follicular phase of the menstrual cycle.

Choi et al. [82] collected serum samples from 50 patients with endometriosis and 35 healthy individuals and used enzyme-linked immunosorbent assay (ELISA) in order to measure the levels of IL-32, 6, 10, 1β, TNF-α, and CA-125. Only IL-32 displayed significantly higher levels in patients compared to controls. When IL-32 was associated with CA-125, the specificity and sensitivity of this combination reached 60% and 82.9%, respectively, thereby suggesting IL-32 as a potential biomarker for endometriosis diagnosis.

Several studies have also assessed Natural killer (NK) cells as potentially viable biomarkers. Kikuchi et al. [83] reported declining levels in the subset of NK cells (CD57 + CD16) in endometriosis, followed by significantly elevated levels of these cells one month following surgery.

Copeptin is a molecule that has augmented values in inflammatory conditions. Tuten et al. [84] determined the serum levels of copeptin, CA-125, C-reactive protein, CA-15-3, and CA-19-9 in a study on 50 women laparoscopically diagnosed with endometriosis and 36 controls. Their results indicated that the level of copeptin was significantly higher in affected women in comparison to controls. Furthermore, these levels were positively correlated with the stage of the disease. However, there is no consensus indicating that cytokines are suitable for early-stage detection of endometriosis, or discriminating patients with endometriosis from patients with other pelvic pathologies.

6.1.3. Oxidative Stress Markers

Despite being still inconclusive, the pathophysiology of endometriosis seems to be based on several theories, including the imbalance between reactive oxygen species (ROS) and antioxidants [85]. This causes an inflammatory response in the peritoneal cavity and ROS to modulate the proliferation of the endometriotic cells [86].

Malondialdehyde (MDA) is a lipid peroxidase which can be considered an oxidative stress marker. A study conducted by Nasiri et al. [87] concluded that, in the serum of endometriotic patients, there are higher values of MDA in comparison with healthy individuals. Furthermore, women with endometriosis have higher levels of lipid hydroperoxides [88], vitamin E [89], and catalase [90], without any conclusive explanation yet.

Superoxide dismutase (SOD) is an enzyme involved in oxidative stress. It registered diminished activity in the plasma of affected patients, supporting the theory of a decreased antioxidant capacity in endometriosis [91]. Andrisani and coworkers [92] studied the activity of carbonic anhydrase in endometriotic women, in comparison to healthy controls. They observed increased enzymatic activity in response to oxidative stress, along with a cytosolic decrease of glutathione content in affected patients.

The major limitations of all the above-mentioned research papers consist of interlaboratory variations. As such, in order to compare the results across different studies, an all-encompassing methodology is needed.

6.1.4. Growth Factors and Peptides

Our research revealed a scarce number of studies conducted on growth factors and peptides, with a large body of uncertainty and controversy regarding their possible use as biomarkers.

Insulin-like growth factor-1 (IGF-1) has been increased in stages III–IV of endometriosis, but not in stages I–II [93]. However, Steff et al. [94] revealed no statistically significant difference between patients and controls in terms of IGF-1. IGFBP3 is a protein that ensures the transport of IGF-1 and is involved in endometrial cell growth. There are two studies that have proven no difference between serum levels of IGFBP3 in healthy women compared to endometriotic patients [93,95].

Nesfatin-1 was initially described as a hypothalamic neuropeptide, with the ability to lower the intake of food [96]. Sengul et al. [97] investigated the level of serum nesfatin-1 in women with endometriosis, before and after the adjustment for body mass index (BMI). At the end of the study, their results indicated that serum nesfatin-1 levels were significantly decreased in the group of subjects, compared to healthy controls, with unchanged results following BMI adjustment.

Urocortin is a neuropeptide that can be found in both endometrium and ovary, and several research papers highlighted the similarity of serum urocortin levels in endometriotic subjects and healthy controls [98,99]. A further study indicated that serum levels of urocortin were significantly increased in women with ovarian endometriosis in comparison to women with other benign ovarian cysts with a sensitivity of 88% and specificity of 90% [100].

Leptin is a helical cytokine that regulates the process of steroidogenesis as well as the decidual transformation of the endometrium. Chmaj-Wierzchowska et al. [99] revealed that the serum level of this molecule was slightly lower in women with ovarian endometriomas compared to control. However, these differences were not statistically significant.

6.1.5. Angiogenesis Molecules

While some studies suggested that VEGF-A levels following laparoscopic excision of endometriosis foci are reduced [101,102], Szubert et al. [103] concluded that following danazol treatment, plasmatic VEGF concentrations were significantly increased, therefore implying that this molecule could not be associated with the disease.

Pigment epithelium-derived factor (PEDF) is an inhibitor of angiogenesis with neurotrophic and anti-inflammatory properties, and modified values of this molecule have been found in endometriotic patients. Chen et al. [104] analyzed the serum levels of PEDF in 43 women with laparoscopically confirmed endometriosis and 28 controls, using the enzyme-linked immunosorbent assay. The results of their study indicated that PEDF was significantly decreased (16.3 ± 6.6 ng/mL) in cases compared to controls (24.5 ± 7.3 ng/mL) and was correlated with the severity of the symptoms.

While elevated values of serum fibroblast growth factor-2 (FGF-2), and angiogenin have also been recorded in the quest for viable biomarkers, soluble endothelial growth factor (EGF) and platelet-derived growth factor (PDGF) revealed no sizable differences between cases and controls; therefore, being sidelined as potential candidates [12].

6.1.6. Autoantibodies

In the last years, several authors focused on the role of circulating antibodies that could be involved in the pathogenesis of endometriosis. The close interrelation of the endometrium with the immune system justifies and partly explains the mechanism of development, as well as the progression of endometriosis.

Anti-endometrial antibodies and total immunoglobulin have also been considered as noninvasive biomarkers for endometriosis. The antibodies with the highest potential as biomarkers for this pelvic pathology were antibodies against α2-HS glycoprotein, malondialdehyde-modified low-density lipoprotein, laminin-I, lipid peroxide, modified rabbit serum albumin, cardiolipin, and specific antibodies against carbonic anhydrase and transferrin [12]. Ozhan et al. [105] researched serum syntaxin-5, anti-endometrial antibody, and other molecules as noninvasive biomarkers. They concluded that the blood serum levels of syntaxin-5 were significantly increased in the endometriosis group, compared to the control group. Furthermore, serum levels of syntaxin-5 in stage I and II endometriosis were found to have different levels compared to controls.

Gajbhiye et al. [106] included 40 endometriosis patients in their study and noted higher serum levels of autoantibodies compared to tropomodulin 3 (TMOD3), tropomyosin 3 (TPM3), and stomatin-like protein 2 (SLP2) in contrast to control's serum samples. Elevated values were associated with both minimal to mild and moderate to severe disease. Additionally, in women with endometriomas, autoantibodies against IGF-2 mRNA-binding protein 1 (IMP1) were identified by Yi et al. to be significantly elevated compared to healthy controls [107].

Anti-α-enolase antibodies in endometriotic subjects were significantly elevated compared to non-affected subjects. The sensitivity and specificity of serum Anti-α-enolase antibodies were comparable to CA125 values, and the combination of these molecules revealed potentially high diagnostic utility [108].

Anti-laminin-1 antibodies were associated with recurrent miscarriage, and increased levels were described in infertile women, as well as in patients with endometriosis. However, this biomarker has not yet passed a diagnostic threshold in current medical practice [109,110].

Two studies conducted by Mathur et al. [111] and Odukoya et al. [112] identified a potential correlation between IgG and endometriosis. IgG antibodies were identified in 56% of affected women and 5% of healthy controls. Another investigation highlighted the presence of IgG in 33% of cases, and of IgM in 27% of them [113].

Given the results of these studies, some autoantibodies could be considered as noninvasive biomarkers for the diagnosis of endometriosis, but further research is necessary.

6.1.7. Proteomics, Metabolomics, and Genomics: The Novel Perspectives of Noninvasive Biomarkers

Proteomics is a new and challenging perspective in the field of noninvasive biomarkers for early detection of endometriosis, which includes all the protein "fingerprints" used for endometriosis diagnosis. Despite promising results, these technologies need better standardization and are cost and time-intensive [12].

Long et al. [113] collected serum samples from several affected women and compared them to controls, in order to detect different protein fingerprints of this disease, by using MALDI-TOF–MS. Their results indicated that 13 protein peaks were over-expressed, and five protein peaks were down-regulated in the affected group compared to healthy subjects.

A further study analyzed distinct patterns of serum proteins in 90 endometriotic women, using SELDI-TOF MS. Following surgical intervention, 51 out of 90 patients were diagnosed with endometriosis, while 39 were unaffected. The researchers concluded that a unique combination of proteins, with molecular weights ranging between 2000 and 20,000 Da made a difference between affected women and controls. The sensitivity of this technique was 81.3%, with a specificity of 60.3% [114]. According to Zheng et al. [115], a proteomic fingerprint model including three peptide peaks showed a sensitivity and specificity of 91.4% and 95%, respectively, for the detection of endometriosis, when compared to controls. In an independent cohort, this combination of peptides revealed a sensitivity of 89.3% and a specificity of 90%.

Wang and collab. [116] illustrated a panel of five protein peaks with a specificity of 90% and a sensitivity of 91.7% for endometriosis, and Jing et al. [117] highlighted two protein peaks with specificity and sensitivity of 97% and 87%, respectively.

Given the inflammatory nature of the disease, inflammation-related proteins have also been investigated for their utility as noninvasive biomarkers. Plasma levels of AXIN1 and ST1A1 were analyzed using ELISA in both affected subjects and healthy controls. AXIN1 and ST1A1 had higher values in endometriosis when compared to healthy controls, regardless of the anatomical location of the lesions [118]. AXIN1 is a promising protein that should be further investigated as a biomarker for endometriosis diagnosis.

Signorile and coworkers [119] used 2D gel analysis in order to describe the potential of two proteins (serum albumin and complement C3 precursor) as diagnostic markers for endometriosis. Their technique was easily reproducible, and their results indicated a sensitivity/specificity for albumin and the complement C3 of 83.3%/83.3% and 58.1%/100%, respectively. In conclusion, this study confirmed the statistical significance of the differential expression for these two proteins in endometriotic women with respect to unaffected individuals. The same authors conducted, in the year 2014, a study comprising 120 women with endometriosis and 20 healthy controls, in order to highlight their serum levels of Zn-alpha2-glycoprotein. After performing ELISA, they observed that the serum levels of this protein were significantly increased in the endometriosis group than in healthy women [120]. In the issue of this observation, the analysis of Zn-alpha2-glycoprotein levels in the serum could become an innovative noninvasive diagnostic test for endometriosis.

Additionally, several studies regarding the metabolome of endometriotic patients have been conducted. Dutta et al. [121] included 22 endometriotic patients and 23 healthy women. They revealed elevated values of Lactate, 3-Hydroxybutyrate, Alanine, Glycerophosphatidylcholine, Valine, Leucine, Threonine, 2-Hydroxybutyrate, Lysine, and Succinic acid in the serum samples of affected women. Furthermore, lower values of glucose, L-Isoleucine, and L-Arginine were discovered in the endometriosis group.

Another study, conducted by Vouk et al. [122] analyzed plasma samples from 40 women with ovarian endometriosis and 52 controls, who underwent laparoscopy. The researchers used electrospray ionization tandem mass spectrometry for more than 140 targeted analytes, including sphingolipids, glycerophospholipids, and acylcarnitines. The results concluded that a model containing hydroxysphingomyelin C16:1 and the ratio between phosphatidylcholine PCaa C36:2 to ether-phospholipid PCae C34:2, had a sensitivity and specificity of 90% and 84.3%, respectively.

In order to establish if the metabolomic profile of affected patients could serve as a noninvasive biomarker for the diagnosis of this pathology, further thorough research is needed.

Genomics may prove an untapped biomarker source with a promising perspective in early diagnosis of endometriosis. Gene-based technologies include cDNA microarray techniques and cDNA hybridization. Recent studies suggested higher plasma concentrations of circulating cell-free cDNA in women with endometriosis [123], in comparison to healthy individuals.

The mitochondrial genome represents another unexplored and potentially promising biomarker pool [108]. Creed et al. [124], highlighted two Mitochondrial DNA (mtDNA) deletions (1.2 and 3.7 kb) which could serve as noninvasive biomarkers.

6.1.8. miRNAs

MicroRNAs (miRNA) are non-coding RNAs with approximately 21–25 nucleotides and represent major modulators of gene expression in a wide range of pathologies, including endometriosis [125]. miRNA profiling is usually achieved by microarray, followed by qRT-PCR validation. Due to their high stability in the biological fluids and tissue specificity, miRNAs might prove desirable molecules for the diagnosis of endometriosis and other pathologies [126], giving a whole new dimension to the noninvasive diagnosis of endometriosis [127].

Despite several studies on miRNA in endometriosis, the results are still equivocal, with no single miRNA or panel of biomarkers showing enough specificity and sensitivity for this pathology, but with promising results.

MiR-200 is a miRNAs family consisting of three members: miR-200a, miR-200b, and miR-141, which have been thoroughly studied for their dysregulations associated with endometriosis. A study performed by Ohlsson et al. [127] revealed a sensitivity of 84.4% and a specificity of 66.7% in endometriotic patients.

Although not highly specific, miR-20 can be potentially used as a biomarker in early diagnosis of endometriosis. Furthermore, it has been proven that miR-20a targets TGF-β and Il-8, and its down-regulation leads to increased concentrations of these pro-inflammatory molecules [128].

MiR-199a revealed a specificity and sensitivity of 78.33% and 76%, respectively, for endometriosis, according to the results of Wang and collab. [129]. Furthermore, this molecule targets CLIC4 and VCL, inducing a high infiltration proclivity of endometrial cells [129]. Kozomara et al. [130] quantified miR-145 in the peripheral blood of endometriotic patients and compared the values with those from healthy controls. They observed that miR-145 is up-regulated in advanced stages of endometriosis, but in early stages, its down-regulated values are not suitable for diagnosis.

Wang and collab [129] analyzed various miRNAs in 765 serum samples from both cases and healthy controls. Their results showed that miR-199a and miR-122 were up-regulated in affected women in comparison to controls, while miR-9, mi-R-141, mi-R-145, miR-542-3p registered decreased values in endometriosis.

miRNA-200 family is one of the most studied groups of miRNAs molecules, and Rekker et al. [131] concluded that miR-200a-3p and miR-141-3p are more sensitive and specific for endometriosis and that these members of miR-200 family are down-regulated in endometriosis, in comparison with the control group.

As previously mentioned, the results regarding the role of miRNAs as a diagnostic tool in endometriosis are controversial and still equivocal. While several studies support the considerable potential of miRNAs as biomarkers for early stages diagnosis, others revealed a modest specificity of these molecules. Nisenblat et al. [132] determined 49 miRNAs, differentially expressed in endometriotic women. A panel formed by miR-155, miR574-3p, and miR139-3p revealed a sensitivity of 83% and a specificity of only 51%.

Vanhie et al. [133] considered 42 miRNAs, out of which only one panel, namely: hsa-miR-125b-5p, hsa-miR-28-5p and hsa-miR-29a-3p revealed a moderate sensitivity and modest specificity of 78% and 37%, respectively.

In Table 1, we summarized the previous studies illustrating the sensitivity and specificity of different dysregulated miRNAs in endometriosis.

Table 1. Studies reporting the sensitivity and specificity of dysregulated miRNAs in endometriosis.

Author, Reference	Dysregulated miRNA	Specificity	Sensitivity
Ohlsson et al., 2009 [127]	miR-200a, miR-200b, and miR-141	66,7%	84,4%
	miR-22	90%	90%
Jia et al., 2013 [134]	miR-17-5p	80%	60%
	miR-20a	90%	60%
	miR-145	96%	70%
Wang et al., 2013 [129]	miR-122	76%	80%
	miR-199a	76%	78,3%
	miR-141-5p	96%	71,7%
Suryavanshi et al., 2013 [135]	miR-195, miR-16, miR-191	60%	88%
	miR-200a-3p	70.8%	71.9%
Rekker et al., 2015 [131]	miR-200b-3p	90.6%	70.8%
	miR-141-3p	70.8%	71.9%
Cosar et al., 2016 [136]	miR-125b	96%	100%
Nisenblat et al., 2019 [132]	miR-155, miR574-3p and miR139-3p	51%	83%
Vanhie et al., 2019 [133]	hsa-miR-125b-5p, hsa-miR-28-5p and hsa-miR-29a-3p	37%	78%

Long non-coding RNAs (lncRNAs) represent a class of molecules with a length of more than 200 nucleotides. They lack the ability of protein-coding [137]. Wang W. et al. [138] applied genome-wide profiling in order to investigate serum lncRNAs differentially expressed in endometriosis women in comparison to healthy controls. They concluded that these molecules presented significant deregulated expressions. Using the PCR quantification method, the authors revealed that 16 lncRNAs were clearly able to distinguish endometriosis from healthy patients—the levels of NR_038452 and ENST00000393610 lncRNA molecules were significantly higher in the serum of affected women, while ENST00000529000, ENST00000482343, ENST00000544649, NR_038395, NR_033688, and ENST00000465368 were decreased in endometriosis. Furthermore, they highlighted an optimal panel of lncRNAs (NR_038395, NR_038452, ENST00000482343, ENST00000544649, and ENST00000393610) able to differentiate between affected and healthy patients. This study concluded that the lncRNAs panel with the highest potential for early detection of endometriosis contains five molecules, namely: NR_038395, NR_038452, ENST00000482343, ENST00000544649, and ENST00000393610.

TC0101441 is a lncRNA molecule with high potential as a biomarker for endometriosis diagnosis, severity, and recurrence prediction. A recent study [139] analyzed the expression of TC0101441 in the serum of affected women versus healthy controls. The authors observed increased TC0101441 levels in the exosomes derived from the serum of endometriotic patients, and a positive and statistically significant correlation between these levels and infertility, chronic pelvic pain, and recurrence of the disease.

6.2. Urinary Biomarkers in Endometriosis

Given its ease of access and fluid composition, urine is one of the most widely used biological samples. As such, the increased accuracy of a urinary test could ideally establish the diagnosis of endometriosis without the need for undergoing invasive surgical interventions. Similar to serum, urinary biomarkers have been measured by a wide range of protein detection methods and have been reported both alone and in combinations [7].

Several urinary peptides and proteins were analyzed for their potential as biomarkers, but further studies are required, with larger sample sizes, in a more diverse population [140]. Creatinine-corrected soluble fms-like tyrosine kinase (sFlt-1) is one of these promising urinary biomarkers for endometriosis.

Cho et al. [79] described increased urinary sFlt-1 levels in endometriotic patients. Furthermore, serum sFlt-1 and urinary sFlt-1 levels, corrected for creatinine, were increased in women with endometriosis stage I and II.

Cytokeratin-19 (CK19) is another molecule that could be used in the detection of endometriosis. Kuessel et al. [141] measured urinary levels of CK19 by ELISA on a cohort of 76 women. The study concluded that there was no significant correlation between urinary levels of CK19 and endometriosis. Tokushige et al. [142] used an immunoblot technique to prove that CK19 is expressed only in the urine of women with confirmed endometriosis while absent in the urine of healthy women.

Matrix metalloproteinases (MMP) have been proven to be involved in the pathophysiology of endometriosis, and thus, several authors studied their level in affected women. A panel composed of MMP-2, MMP-9, and MMP-9/neutrophil gelatinase-associated lipocalin was found to increase in 33 subjects with confirmed endometriosis when compared to controls [143].

Using MALDI-TOF MS (matrix-assisted laser desorption/ionization mass spectrometry (MALDI MS) and time-of-flight analyzer (TOF)), differential peptide profiles have been described in the urine of endometriotic women, compared to healthy subjects. Tokushige and colleagues [144], revealed a 12-fold higher expression of five proteins in affected women by combining MALDI-TOF with two-dimensional polyacrylamide gel electrophoresis and El-Kasti et al. [145] highlighted a 3280.9 Da periovulatory peptide that differentiates women with all stages of endometriosis from healthy subjects (sensitivity 82% and specificity 88%).

Cho et al. [146] used western blot and ELISA to investigate urinary proteins of patients with endometriosis. They concluded that 22 protein spots were differentially expressed in the urine of endometriotic women, and one of them was urinary vitamin D-binding protein (VDBP). The conclusion was that urinary VDBP corrected for creatinine (VDBP-Cr) was significantly elevated in patients with endometriosis. The sensitivity of this biomarker was 58%, and the specificity, 76%. When combined with serum CA-125 levels, the authors observed that the positive predictive value was not significantly increased compared to CA-125 alone.

Potlog-Nahari et al. [147] included 40 affected women, with histologically confirmed endometriosis, and 22 healthy controls. They measured the urinary level of VEGF corrected for creatinine. The results of this study revealed no significant difference between urinary levels of VEGF in women with and without endometriosis. Furthermore, these values have not significantly varied between groups according to the phase of the menstrual cycle, hence the unlikeliness that urinary VEGF could serve as a biomarker for endometriosis. No other authors investigated this molecule with respect to endometriosis.

Chen and coworkers [148] were the first to identify histone 4 as a potential urinary biomarker in endometriosis. The authors observed an elevated level of histone 4 in the urine of endometriotic women with a sensitivity and specificity of 70% and 80%, respectively. Considering this research as a key stone, further studies could be conducted in order to validate and strengthen the hypothesis of Chen et al.

In Table 2, we summarize the studies illustrating the main noninvasive biomarkers assessed for endometriosis.

Table 2. Studies assessing the main noninvasive biomarkers for endometriosis.

Author, Reference	Source	Investigated Biomarkers
Agic et al, 2008 [62]	Serum	CA-125, CCR-1, miRNA, MCP-1
Borrelli et al., 2014 [71]	Serum	IL-8, MCP-1, RANTES
Chen et al., 2012 [104]	Serum	Serum pigment epithelium-derived factor
Chen et al., 2019 [148]	Urine	Histone 4
Chmaj-Wierzchowska et al., 2015 [99]	Serum	Urocortin, ghrelin, leptin
Cho et al., 2007 [79]	Serum, Urine	TNF-α, urinary sFlt-1

Table 2. *Cont.*

Author, Reference	Source	Investigated Biomarkers
Cho et al., 2012 [146]	Urine	Vitamin D-binding protein
Choi et al., 2019 [82]	Serum	IL-32, IL-6, IL-10, IL-1β, TNF-α, CA-125
Cosar et al., 2016 [136]	Serum	miR-125b
Creed et al., 2019 [124]	Serum	mtDNA
Darai et al., 2003 [77]	Serum	IL-6, IL-8, TNF-α
Dutta et al., 2012 [91]	Serum	Lactate, 3-Hydroxybutyrate, Alanine, Glycerophosphatidylcholine, Valine, Leucine, Threonine, 2-Hydroxybutyrate, Lysine, Succinic acid
Gajbhiye et al., 2012 [106]	Serum	Autoantibodies against tropomodulin 3 (TMOD3), tropomyosin 3 (TPM3), stomatin-like protein 2 (SLP2)
Gmyrek et al., 2005 [149]	Serum	MCP-1
Gungor et al., 2009 [150]	Serum	Leptin
Huang et al., 2004 [151]	Serum	MMP2
Jia et al., 2013 [134]	Serum	miR-22 miR-17-5p miR-20a
Jing et al., 2008 [117]	Plasma	Proteomics-mass spectrometry
Kocbek et al., 2015 [66]	Serum	Glycodelin-A
Kuessel et al., 2014 [141]	Urine	CK19
Liu et al., 2007 [139]	Plasma	Proteomics – mass spectrometry
Malin et al., 2019 [118]	Serum	AXIN1
Martinez et al., 2007 [70]	Serum	IL-6
May et al., 2010 [12]	Serum	FGF-2, angiogenin
Mihalyi et al., 2010 [61]	Serum	CA-125, IL-8, TNF-α
Morin et al., 2005 [152]	Peripheral blood	Macrophage migration inhibitory factor
Mosbah et al., 2016 [65]	Serum	ICAM-1, glycodelin
Nabeta et al., 2009 [108]	Serum	Anti-α-enolase antibodies
Nasiri et al., 2017 [87]	Serum	Malondialdehyde (MDA)
Nisenblat et al., 2019 [132]	Serum	miR-155, miR574-3p, and miR139-3p
Ohata et al., 2008 [76]	Seum	IL-8
Ohlsson et al., 2009 [127]	Serum	miR-200a, miR-200b, and miR-141
Othman et al., 2008 [70]	Serum	Il-6, MCP-1, IFN-γ IL-2, IL-8, IL-15
Ozhan et al., 2014 [105]	Serum	Syntaxin-5, anti-endometrial antibody
Philippoussis et al., 2004 [95]	Serum	IGFBP3, EGF
Pizzo et al., 2002 [75]	Serum	IL-8
Potlog-Nahar.i, 2004 [147]	Urine	VEGF
Qui et al., 2019 [139]	Serum	lncRNA
Reis et al., 2012 [68]	Serum	Activin A, follistatin
Rekker et al., 2015 [125]	Serum	miR-200a-3p miR-200b-3p miR-141-3p
Seeber et al., 2008 [80]	Serum	TNF-α
Sengul et al., 2014 [97]	Serum	Nesfatin-1
Socolov et al., 2010 [73]	Serum	IL-6, IL-8, IL-1, CA-125, TNF
Steff et al., 2004 [94]	Serum	IGF-1, IGFBP3
Suryavanshi et al., 2013 [135]	Serum	miR-195, miR-16, miR-191
Tokmak et al., 2011 [98]	Serum	Urocortin
Tokushige et al., 2011 [144]	Urine	CK19
Becker et al., 2010 [143]	Urine	MMP-2, MMP-9
Tuten et al., 2014 [64]	Serum	Copeptin, CA-125, C-reactive protein, CA-15-3, CA-19-9
Vanhie et al., 2019 [133]	Serum	hsa-miR125b-5p, hsa-miR-28-5p and hsa-miR-29a-3p
Vigano et al., 2003 [69]	Serum	ICAM-1
Vodolazkaia et al., 2012 [63]	Serum	VEGF, CA-125, Annexin V, glycodelin
Wang et al., 2013 [129]	Serum	miR-145 miR-122 miR-199a miR-141-5p
Wang et al., 2016 [138]	Serum	lncRNA
Xavier et al., 2006 [78]	Serum	TNF-α, VEGF

7. Conclusions

Despite its benign character, endometriosis remains a debilitating disease that interferes with the quality of life of millions of women. The main symptoms: pelvic pain, infertility, and severe dysmenorrhea are nonspecific, and thus, invariably lead to a long-term delay in establishing the appropriate diagnosis. An invasive procedure, surgery, followed by a histopathological exam, represents the gold standard for diagnosis. As such, literature review proved to be a saga of noninvasive biomarkers, with researchers focusing their efforts into developing noninvasive putative biomarkers for this pathology in hope for promising perspectives on early diagnosis.

Various lines of evidence support the potential role of many biomolecules or panels of biomolecules, but, as of yet, none of them have the test proof sensitivity and specificity. Therefore, they can only complement the diagnosis of this pathology, in conjunction with imaging techniques or laparoscopic surgery.

Inflammatory cytokines proved to be the most non-suitable candidates for noninvasive diagnosis of endometriosis, despite the ability of several panels of cytokines to discriminate between affected and non-affected patients. Similarly, no single miRNA or lncRNA was considered as a sole noninvasive biomarker. According to various authors, a panel of miRNAs or lncRNAs could be more conducive indicators of this gynecological pathology.

The latest technologies consisting of proteomics, metabolomics, and genomics that investigate a complete panel of molecules or a profile of genes could evolve into the gold standard diagnostic tool and thus eliminate invasive laparoscopies.

Furthermore, increased knowledge of the pathophysiologic mechanisms of endometriosis is crucial for a more expedient and accurate diagnosis, improving the overall health-related quality of life.

Author Contributions: C.V.A., M.A.M., I.S.: conceptualization, formal analysis, investigation, A.B., A.E.N., A.-M.D.: writing original draft, editing, drawing figures. R.M.D., L.-M.C.: methodology, supervision, validation. All authors read and approved the final manuscript.

Abbreviations

BMI	Body mass index
C3	Complement
CK 19	Cytokeratin 19
COX-2	Cyclooxygenase 2
CRP	C-reactive protein
DNA	Deoxiribonucleic acid
EGF	Endothelial growth factor
EGFR	Endothelial growth factor receptor
ELISA	Enzyme-linked immunosorbent assay
FGF	Fibroblast growth factor
GM-CSF	Granulocyte macrophage colony-stimulating factor
HOXA	Homebox A
ICAM	Intercellular adhesion molecule
IFN	Interferon
IGF	Insulin-like growth factor
Il	Interleukin
iNKT	Invariant natural killer T cells
lncRNA	Long non-coding ribonucleic acid
MCP-1	Monocyte chemoattractant protein 1
MIF	Macrophage inhibitory factor
MMP	Matrix metalloproteinase
miRNA	Micro ribonucleic acid

mtDNA	Mitochondrial DNA
NK	Natural killer
NF-KB	Nuclear factor-kappa beta
PDGF	Platelet-derived growth factor
PG	Prostaglandins
PGE2	Prostaglandin E2
PK-1	Prokinetitsin 1
RANTES	Regulated on Activation, Normal T Cell Expressed and Secreted
ROS	Reactive oxygen species
SOD	Superoxide dismutase
sFlt1	Soluble fms-like tyrosine kinase
TNF	Tumor-necrosis factor
TSP-1	Thrombospondin 1
VDBP	Urinary vitamin D binding protein
VEGF	Vascular endothelial growth factor
VEGFR	Vascular endothelial growth factor receptor
Wnt/b-catenin	Wingless-type mouse mammary tumor virus integration site family

References

1. Bratila, E.; Comandasu, D.-E.; Coreleuca, C.; Cirstoiu, M.; Bohiltea, R.; Mehedintu, C.; Vladareanu, S.; Berceanu, C. Gatrointestinal Symptoms in Endometriosis Correlated With the Disease Stage. 2016. Available online: https://www.researchgate.net/publication/312552546_Gastrointestinal_symptoms_in_endometriosis_correlated_with_the_disease_stage (accessed on 27 October 2019).

2. Giudice, L.C.; Kao, L.C. Endometriosis. *Lancet* **2004**, *364*, 1789–1799. [CrossRef]

3. Moga, M.A.; Balan, A.; Dimienescu, O.G.; Burtea, V.; Dragomir, R.M.; Anastasiu, V.C. Circulating miRNAs as biomarkers for endometriosis and endometriosis-related ovarian cancer—An overview. *J. Clin. Med.* **2019**, *8*, 735. [CrossRef]

4. Bulletti, C.; Coccia, M.E.; Battistoni, S.; Borini, A. Endometriosis and infertility. *J. Assist. Reprod. Genet.* **2010**, *27*, 441–447. [CrossRef]

5. Argawal, S.K.; Chapron, C.; Giudice, L.C.; Laufer, M.R.; Lyland, N.; Missmer, S.A.; Singh, S.S.; Taylor, H.S. Clinical diagnosis of endometriosis: A call to action. *Am. J. Obstet. Gynecol.* **2019**, *220*, 354.e1–354.e12. [CrossRef]

6. Nnoaham, K.E.; Hummelshoj, L.; Webster, P.; D'Hooghe, T.; de Cicco Nardone, F.; de Cicco Nardone, C.; de Cicco Nardone, C.; Jerkinson, C.; Kennedy, S.H.; Zondervan, K.T.; et al. Impact of endometriosis on quality of life and work productivity: A multicenter study across ten countries. *Fertil. Steril.* **2011**, *96*, 366–373. [CrossRef]

7. Fassbender, A.; Burney, R.O.; D'Hooghe, T.; Giudice, L. Update on biomarkers for the detection of endometriosis. *BioMed Res. Int.* **2015**, *2015*, 130854. [CrossRef]

8. Hadfield, R.; Mardon, H.; Barlow, D.; Kennedy, S. Delay in the diagnosis of endometriosis: A survey of women from the USA and the UK. *Hum. Reprod.* **1996**, *11*, 878–880. [CrossRef]

9. Ahn, S.H.; Singh, V.; Tayade, C. Biomarkers in endometriosis: Challenges and opportunities. *Fertil. Steril.* **2017**, *107*, 523–532. [CrossRef] [PubMed]

10. Irungu, S.; Mavrelos, D.; Worthington, J.; Blyuss, O.; Saridogan, E.; Timms, J.F. Discovery of non-invasive biomarkers for the diagnosis of endometriosis. *Clin. Proteom.* **2019**, *16*, 14. [CrossRef] [PubMed]

11. Biomarkers Definitions Working Group. Biomarkers and surrogate endpoints: Preferred definitions and conceptual framework. *Clin. Pharmacol. Ther.* **2001**, *69*, 89–95. [CrossRef] [PubMed]

12. May, K.E.; Conduit-Hulbert, S.A.; Villar, J.; Kirtley, S.; Kennedy, S.H.; Becker, C.M. Peripheral biomarkers of endometriosis: A systematic review. *Hum. Reprod. Update* **2010**, *16*, 651–674. [CrossRef] [PubMed]

13. Halme, J.; Hammond, M.G.; Hulka, J.F.; Raj, S.G.; Talbert, L.M. Retrograde menstruation in healthy women and in patients with endometriosis. *Obstet. Gynecol.* **1984**, *64*, 151–154. [PubMed]

14. Lagana, A.S.; Vitale, S.G.; Salmeri, F.M.; Triolo, O.; Ban Frangez, H.; Vrtacnik-Bokal, E.; Stojanovska, L.; Apostolopoulos, V.; Granese, R.; Sofo, V. Unus pro omnibus, omnes pro uno: A novel, evidence-based, unifying theory for the pathogenesis of endometriosis. *Med. Hypotheses* **2017**, *103*, 10–20. [CrossRef] [PubMed]

15. Pluchino, N.; Taylor, H.S. Endometriosis and stem cell trafficking. *Reprod. Sci.* **2016**, *23*, 1616–1619. [CrossRef] [PubMed]

16. Lagana, A.S.; Salmeri, F.M.; Vitale, S.G.; Triolo, O.; Gotte, M. Stem cell trafficking during endometriosis: May epigenetics play a pivotal role? *Reprod. Sci.* **2017**, *25*, 978–979. [CrossRef]

17. Eggers, J.C.; Martino, V.; Reinbold, R.; Schafer, S.D.; Kiesel, L.; Starzinski-Powitz, A.; Schuring, A.N.; Kemper, B.; Greve, B.; Gotte, M. microRNA miR-200b affects proliferation, invasiveness and stemness of endometriotic cells by targeting ZEB1, ZEB2 and KLF4. *Reprod. Biomed. Online* **2016**, *32*, 434–445. [CrossRef]

18. Marki, G.; Bokor, A.; Rigo, J.; Rigo, A. Physical pain and emotion regulation as the main predictive factors of health-related quality of life in women living with endometriosis. *Hum. Reprod.* **2017**, *32*, 1432–1438. [CrossRef]

19. Lagana, A.S.; La Rosa, V.L.; Rapisarda, A.M.C. Anxiety and depression in patients with endometriosis: Impact and management challenges. *Int. J. Women Health.* **2017**, *9*, 323–330. [CrossRef]

20. Zheng, W.; Cao, L.; Zheng, X.; Yuanyuan, M.; Liang, X. Anti-Angiogenic Alternative and complementary medicines for the treatment of endometriosis: A review of potential molecular mechanisms. *Evid. Based Complement. Alternat. Med.* **2018**, *2018*, 4128984. [CrossRef]

21. Lousse, J.C.; Van Langendonckt, A.; Defrere, S.; Gonzalez Ramos, R.; Colette, S. Peritoneal endometriosis is an inflammatory disease. *Frontiers Biosci.* **2012**, *E4*, 23–40. [CrossRef]

22. Gazvani, R.; Templeton, A. Peritoneal environment, cytokines and angiogenesis in the pathophysiology of endometriosis. *Reprod.* **2002**, *123*, 217–226. [CrossRef] [PubMed]

23. Van Langendonckt, A.; Casanas-Roux, F.; Donnez, J. Oxidative stress and peritoneal endometriosis. *Fertil. Steril.* **2002**, *77*, 861–870. [CrossRef]

24. Oral, E.; Olive, D.L.; Arici, A. The peritoneal environment in endometriosis. *Hum. Reprod. Update* **1996**, 385–398. [CrossRef] [PubMed]

25. Wu, M.H.; Shoji, Y.; Chuang, P.; Tsai, S. Endometriosis: Disease pathophysiology and the role of prostaglandins. *Expert Rev Mol Med.* **2007**, *9*, 1–20. [CrossRef] [PubMed]

26. Sugino, N.; Karube-Harada, A.; Taketani, T.; Sakata, A.; Nakamura, Y. Withdrawal of ovarian steroids stimulates prostaglandin F2-alpha production through nuclear factor-kappaB activation via oxygen radicals in human endometrial stromal cells: Potential relevance to menstruation. *J. Reprod. Dev.* **2004**, *50*, 215–225. [CrossRef]

27. Banu, S.K.; Lee, J.; Speights, V.O.; Starzinski-Powitz, A.; Arosh, J.A. Cyclooxygenase-2 regulates survival, migration, and invasion of human endometriotic cells through multiple mechanisms. *Endocrinol* **2008**, *149*, 1180–1189. [CrossRef]

28. Wu, M.H.; Wang, C.A.; Lin, C.C.; Chen, L.-C.; Chang, W.-C.; Tsai, S.-J. Distinct regulation of cyclooxygenase-2 by interleukin-1 beta in normal and endometriotic stromal cells. *J. Clin. Endocrinol. Metab.* **2005**, *90*, 286–295. [CrossRef]

29. Lagana, A.S.; Garzon, S.; Gotte, M.; Vigano, P.; Franchi, M.; Ghezzi, F.; Martin, D.C. The pathogenesis of endometriosis: Molecular and cell biology insights. *Int. J. Mol. Sci.* **2019**, *20*, 5615. [CrossRef]

30. Laird, S.M.; Tuckerman, E.M.; Cork, B.A.; Li, T.C. Expression of nuclear factor kappa B in human endometrium; role in the control of interleukin 6 and leukaemia inhibitory factor production. *Mol. Hum. Reprod.* **2000**, *6*, 34–40. [CrossRef]

31. Page, M.; Tuckerman, E.M.; Li, T.C.; Laird, S.M. Expression of nuclear factor kappa-B components in human endometrium. *J. Reprod. Immunol.* **2002**, *54*, 1–13. [CrossRef]

32. King, A.E.; Critchley, H.; Kelly, R.W. The NF-kappaB pathway in human endometrium and first trimester decidua. *Mol. Hum. Reprod.* **2001**, *7*, 175–183. [CrossRef] [PubMed]

33. González Ramos, R.; Van Langendonckt, A.; Defrère, S.; Lousse, J.C.; Colette, S.; Devoto, L.; Donnez, J. Involvement of the nuclear factor-kappaB (NF-kappa B) pathway in the pathogenesis of endometriosis. *Fertil Steril* **2010**, *94*, 1985–1994. [CrossRef] [PubMed]

34. Lousse, J.C.; Van Langendonckt, A.; González Ramos, R.; Defrère, S.; Renkin, E.; Donnez, J. Increased activation of nuclear factor-kappa B (NF-kappa B) in isolated peritoneal macrophages of patients with endometriosis. *Fertil. Steril.* **2008**, *90*, 217–220. [CrossRef] [PubMed]

35. Agarwal, A.; Gupta, S.; Sikka, S. The role of oxidative stress in endometriosis. *Curr. Opin. Obstet. Gynecol.* **2006**, *18*, 325–332. [CrossRef] [PubMed]

36. Zeller, J.M.; Henig, I.; Radwanska, E.; Dmowski, W.P. Enhancement of human monocyte and peritoneal macrophage chemiluminescence activities in women with endometriosis. *Am. J. Reprod. Immunol. Microbiol.* **1987**, *13*, 78–82. [CrossRef]

37. Portz, D.M.; Elkins, T.E.; White, R.; Warren, J.; Adadevoh, S.; Randolph, J. Oxygen free radicals and pelvic adhesion formation: Blocking oxygen free radical toxicity to prevent adhesion formation in an endometriosis model. *Int. J. Fertil.* **1991**, *36*, 39–42. [CrossRef]

38. Wang, Y.; Sharma, R.K.; Falcone, T.; Goldberg, J.; Agarwal, A. Importance of reactive oxygen species in the peritoneal fluid of women with endometriosis or idiopathic infertility. *Fertil. Steril.* **1997**, *68*, 826–830. [CrossRef]

39. Polak, G.; Koziol-Montewka, M.; Gogacz, M.; Blaszkowska, I.; Kotarski, J. Total antioxidant status of the peritoneal fluid in infertile women. *Eur. J. Obstet. Gynecol. Reprod. Biol.* **2001**, *94*, 261–263. [CrossRef]

40. Wu, M.H.; Hsiao, K.Y.; Tsai, S.J. Endometriosis and possible inflammation markers. *Gynecol. Minim. Invasive Ther.* **2015**, *4*, 61–67. [CrossRef]

41. Lagana, A.S.; Salmeri, F.M.; Ban Frangez, H.; Ghezzi, F.; Vrtacnik-Bokal, E.; Granese, R. Evaluation of M1 and M2 macrophages in ovarian endometriomas from women affected by endometriosis at different stages of the disease. *Gynecol. Endocrinol.* **2019**, *30*, 1–4. [CrossRef]

42. Capobianco, A.; Monno, A.; Cottone, L.; Venneri, M.A.; Biziato, D.; Di Puppo, F.; Ferrari, S.; De Palma, M.; Manfredi, A.A.; Rovere-Querini, P. Proangiogenic Tie2(+) macrophages infiltrate human and murine endometriotic lesions and dictate their growth in a mouse model of the disease. *Am. J. Pathol.* **2011**, *179*, 2651–2659. [CrossRef] [PubMed]

43. Lagana, A.S.; Ghezzi, F.; Vetvicka, V. Endometriosis and risk of ovarian cancer: What do we know? *Arch. Gynecol. Obstet.* **2019**, *301*, 1–10. [CrossRef]

44. Wu, M.Y.; Yang, J.H.; Chao, K.H.; Hwang, J.L.; Yang, Y.S.; Ho, H.N. Increase in the expression of killer cell inhibitory receptors on peritoneal natural killer cells in women with endometriosis. *Fertil. Steril.* **2000**, *74*, 1187–1191. [CrossRef]

45. Lagana, A.S.; Triolo, O.; Salmeri, F.M.; Granese, R.; Palmara, V.I.; Ban Frangez, H.; Vrtcnik Bokal, E.; Sofo, V. Natural Killer T cell subsets in eutopic and ectopic endometrium: A fresh look to a busy corner. *Arch. Gynecol. Obstet.* **2016**, *293*, 941–949. [CrossRef] [PubMed]

46. Ho, H.N.; Wu, M.Y.; Chao, K.H.; Der Chen, C.; Chen, S.U.; Yang, Y.S. Peritoneal interleukin-10 increases with decrease in activated CD4+ T lymphocytes in women with endometriosis. *Hum. Reprod.* **1997**, *12*, 2528–2533. [CrossRef] [PubMed]

47. Nie, M.-F.; Xie, Q.; Wu, Y.-H.; He, H.; Zou, L.-J.; She, X.-L.; Wu, X.-Q. Serum and Ectopic Endometrium from Women with Endometriosis Modulate Macrophage M1/M2 Polarization via the Smad2/Smad3 Pathway. *J. Immun. Res.* **2018**, *2018*, 14. [CrossRef] [PubMed]

48. Kralickova, M.; Vetvicka, V. Immunological aspects of endometriosis: Review. *Ann. Transl. Med.* **2015**, *3*, 153. [CrossRef]

49. Osuga, Y.; Hirota, Y.; Hirata, T.; Takamura, M.; Urata, Y.; Harada, M.; Izumi, G.; Fujii, T.; Koga, K. Th2 Cells and Th17 cells in the development of endometriosis—Possible roles of interleukin-4 and interleukin-17A. *J. Endometr. Pelvic Pain Dis.* **2016**, *8*, 136–140. [CrossRef]

50. Asante, A.; Taylor, R.N. Endometriosis: The role of neuroangiogenesis. *Ann. Rev. Physiol.* **2011**, *73*, 163–182. [CrossRef]

51. Hanahan, D.; Folkman, J. Patterns and emerging mechanisms of the angiogenic switch during tumorigenesis. *Cell* **1996**, *86*, 353–364. [CrossRef]

52. Ahn, S.H.; Edwards, A.K.; Singh, S.S.; Young, S.L.; Lessey, B.A.; Tayade, C. Il-17A contributes to the pathogenesis of endometriosis bu triggering proinflammatory cytokines and angiogenic growth factors. *J. Immunol.* **2015**, *195*, 2591–2600. [CrossRef] [PubMed]

53. Gupta, M.K.; Qin, R.Y. Mechanism and its regulation of tumor-induced angiogenesis. *World J. Gastroenterol.* **2003**, *9*, 1144–1155. [CrossRef] [PubMed]

54. Strieter, R.M.; Polverini, P.J.; Kunkel, S.L.; Arenberg, D.A.; Burdick, M.D.; Kasper, J.; Dzuiba, J.; Van Damme, J.; Walz, A.; Marriott, D.; et al. The functional role of the ELR motif in CXC chemokine-mediated angiogenesis. *J. Biol. Chem.* **1995**, *270*, 27348–27357. [CrossRef] [PubMed]

55. Volpert, O.V.; Fong, T.; Koch, A.E.; Peterson, J.D.; Waltenbaugh, C.; Tepper, R.I.; Bouck, N.P. Inhibition of angiogenesis by interleukin 4. *J. Exp. Med.* **1998**, *188*, 1039–1046. [CrossRef]

56. Torisu, H.; Ono, M.; Kiryu, H.; Furue, M.; Ohmoto, Y.; Nakayama, J.; Nishioka, Y.; Sone, S.; Kuwano, M. Macrophage infiltration correlates with tumor stage and angiogenesis in human malignant melanoma: Possible involvement of TNFalpha and IL-1alpha. *Int. J. Cancer* **2000**, *85*, 182–188. [CrossRef]

57. Donnez, J.; Smoes, P.; Gillerot, S.; Casanas-Roux, F.; Nisolle, M. Vascular endothelial growth factor (VEGF) in endometriosis. *Hum. Reprod.* **1998**, *3*, 1686–1690. [CrossRef]

58. Machado, D.E.; Rodrigues-Baptista, K.C.; Perini, J.A. Soares de Moura, R. Euterpe oleracea extract (Açaí) is a promising novel pharmacological therapeutic treatment for experimental endometriosis. *PLoS ONE* **2016**, *11*, e0166059. [CrossRef]

59. Thambisetty, M.; Lovestone, S. Blood-based biomarkers of Alzheimers disease: Challenging but feasible. *Biomark. Med.* **2010**, *4*, 65–79. [CrossRef]

60. Mol, B.W.J.; Bayram, N.; Lijmer, J.G.; Wiegerinck, M.A.H.M.; Bongers, M.Y.; Van der Veen, F.; Bossuyt, P. The performance of CA-125 measurement in the detection of endometriosis: A meta-analysis. *Fertil. Steril.* **1998**, *70*, 1101–1108. [CrossRef]

61. Mihalyi, A.; Gevaert, O.; Kyama, C.M.; Simsa, P.; Pochet, N.; De Smet, F.; De Moor, B.; Meuleman, C.; Billen, J.; Blanckaert, N.; et al. Non-invasive diagnosis of endometriosis based on a combined analysis of six plasma biomarkers. *Hum. Reprod.* **2010**, *25*, 654–664. [CrossRef]

62. Agic, A.; Djalali, S.; Wolfler, M.M.; Halis, G.; Diedrich, K.; Hornung, D. Combination of CCR1 mRNA, MCP1, and CA125 measurements in peripheral blood as a diagnostic test for endometriosis. *Reprod. Sci.* **2008**, *15*, 906–911. [CrossRef] [PubMed]

63. Vodolazkaia, A.; El-Aalamat, Y.; Popovic, D. Evaluation of a panel of 28 biomarkers for the non-invasive diagnosis of endometriosis. *Hum. Reprod.* **2012**, *27*, 2698–2711. [CrossRef] [PubMed]

64. Ozhan, E.; Kokcu, A.; Yanik, K.; Gunaydin, M. Investigation of diagnostic potentials of nine different biomarkers in endometriosis. *Eur. J. Obstet. Gynecol.* **2014**, *178*, 128–133. [CrossRef] [PubMed]

65. Mosbah, A.; Nabiel, Y.; Khashaba, E. Interleukin-6, intracellular adhesion molecule-1, and glycodelin A levels in serum and peritoneal fluid as biomarkers for endometriosis. *Obstet. Gynecol.* **2016**, *134*, 247–251. [CrossRef] [PubMed]

66. Kocbek, V.; Vouk, K.; Bersinger, N.A.; Mueller, M.D.; Lanišnik Rižner, T. Panels of Cytokines and Other Secretory Proteins as Potential Biomarkers of Ovarian Endometriosis. *J. Mol. Diagn.* **2015**, *17*, 325–334. [CrossRef]

67. Pretice Crapper, E. Clinical Biomarkers for the Noninvasive Diagnosis of Endometriosis. 2016. Available online: http://hdl.handle.net/11375/20495 (accessed on 26 February 2020).

68. Reis, F.M.; Luisi, S.; Abrão, M.S.; Rocha, A.L.L.; Viganò, P.; Rezende, C.P.; Florio, P.; Petraglia, F. Diagnostic value of serum activin A and follistatin levels in women with peritoneal, ovarian and deep infiltrating endometriosis. *Hum. Reprod.* **2012**, *27*, 1445–1450. [CrossRef]

69. Vigano, P.; Infantino, M.; Lattuada, D.; Lauletta, R.; Ponti, E.; Somigliana, E.; Vignali, M.; DiBlasio, A.M. Intercellular adhesion molecule-1 (ICAM-1) gene polymorphisms in endometriosis. *Mol. Hum. Reprod.* **2003**, *9*, 47–52. [CrossRef]

70. Othman, E.E.R.; Hornung, D.; Salem, H.T.; Kalifa, E.A.; El-Metwally, T.H.; Al-Hendy, A. Serum cytokines as biomarkers for nonsurgical prediction of endometriosis. *Eur. J. Obstet. Gynecol. Repd. Biol.* **2008**, *137*, 240–246. [CrossRef]

71. Borrelli, G.M.; Abrão, M.S.; Mechsner, S. Can chemokines be used as biomarkers for endometriosis? A systematic review. *Hum. Reprod.* **2014**, *29*, 253–266. [CrossRef]

72. Martinez, S.; Garrido, N.; Coperias, J.L.; Pardo, F.; Desco, J.; Garcia-Velasco, J.A.; Simon, C.; Pellicer, A. Serum interleukin-6 levels are elevated in women with minimal-mild endometriosis. *Hum. Reprod.* **2007**, *22*, 836–842. [CrossRef]

73. Socolov, R.; Butureanu, S.; Angioni, S.; Sindilar, A.; Boiculese, V.L.; Cozma, L.; Socolov, D. The value of serological markers in the diagnosis and prognosis of endometriosis: A prospective case-control study. *Eur. J. Obstet. Gynecol. Reprod. Biol.* **2010**, *154*, 215–217. [CrossRef] [PubMed]

74. Kalu, E.; Sumar, N.; Giannopoulos, T.; Patel, P.; Croucher, C.; Sherriff, E.; Bansal, A. Cytokine profiles in serum and peritoneal fluid from infertile women with and without endometriosis. *J. Obstet. Gynaecol. Res.* **2007**, *33*, 490–495. [CrossRef] [PubMed]

75. Pizzo, A.; Salmeri, F.M.; Ardita, F.V.; Sofo, V.; Tripepi, M.; Marsico, S. Behaviour of cytokine levels in serum and peritoneal fluid of women with endometriosis. *Gynecol. Obstet. Investig.* **2002**, *54*, 82–87. [CrossRef] [PubMed]

76. Ohata, Y.; Harada, T.; Miyakoda, H.; Taniguchi, F.; Iwabe, T.; Terakawa, N. Serum interleukin-8 levels are elevated in patients with ovarian endometrioma. *Fertil. Steril.* **2008**, *90*, 994–999. [CrossRef]

77. Darai, E.; Detchev, R.; Hugol, D.; Quang, N.T. Serum and cyst fluid levels of interleukin (IL) -6, IL-8 and tumour necrosis factor-alpha in women with endometriomas and benign and malignant cystic ovarian tumours. *Hum. Reprod.* **2003**, *18*, 1681–1685. [CrossRef] [PubMed]

78. Xavier, P.; Belo, L.; Beires, J.; Rebelo, I.; Martinez-de-Oliveira, J.; Lunet, N.; Barros, H. Serum levels of VEGF and TNF-a and their association with C-reactive protein in patients with endometriosis. *Arch. Gynecol. Obstet.* **2006**, *273*, 227–231. [CrossRef]

79. Cho, S.H.; Oh, Y.J.; Nam, A.; Kim, H.Y.; Park, J.H.; Kim, J.H.; Cho, D.J.; Lee, B.S. Evaluation of Serum and Urinary Angiogenic Factors in Patients with Endometriosis. *Am. J. Reprod. Immunol.* **2007**, *58*, 497–504. [CrossRef]

80. Seeber, B.; Sammel, M.D.; Fan, X.; Gerton, G.L.; Shaunik, A.; Chittams, J.; Barnhart, K.T. Panel of markers can accurately predict endometriosis in a subset of patients. *Fertil. Steril.* **2008**, *89*, 1073–1081. [CrossRef]

81. Steff, A.M.; Gagné, D.; Pagé, M.; Rioux, A.; Hugo, P.; Gosselin, D. Insulin-like growth factor-1, soluble tumor necrosis factor receptor-1 and angiogenin in endometriosis patients. *Am. J. Reprod. Immunol.* **2004**, *51*, 166–173. [CrossRef]

82. Choi, Y.S.; Kim, S.; Oh, Y.S.; Cho, S.; Hoon Kim, S. Elevated serum interleukin-32 levels in patients with endometriosis: A cross-sectional study. *Am. J. Reprod. Immunol.* **2019**, *82*, e13149. [CrossRef]

83. Kikuchi, Y.; Ishikawa, N.; Hirata, J.; Imaizumi, E.; Sasa, H.; Nagata, I. Changes of peripheral blood lymphocyte subsets before and after operation of patients with endometriosis. *Acta Obstet. Gynecol. Scand.* **1993**, *72*, 157–161. [CrossRef] [PubMed]

84. Tuten, A.; Kucur, M.; Imamoglu, M.; Kaya, B.; Acikgoz, A.S.; Yilmaz, N.; Ozturk, Z.; Oncul, M. Copeptin is associated with the severity of endometriosis. *Arch. Gynecol. Obstet.* **2014**, *290*, 75–82. [CrossRef] [PubMed]

85. Carvalho, L.F.; Samadder, A.N.; Agarwal, A.; Fernandes, L.F.; Abrao, M.S. Oxidative stress biomarkers in patients with endometriosis: Systematic review. *Arch. Gynecol. Obstet.* **2012**, *286*, 1033–1040. [CrossRef] [PubMed]

86. Scutiero, G.; Iannone, P.; Bernardi, G.; Bonaccorsi, G.; Spadaro, S.; Volta, C.A.; Greco, P.; Nappi, L. Oxidative stress and endometriosis: A systematic review of the literature. *Oxidative Med. Cell Longev.* **2017**, *2017*, 7265238. [CrossRef] [PubMed]

87. Nasiri, N.; Moini, A.; Eftekhari-Yazdi, P.; Karimian, L.; Salman-Yazdi, R.; Arabipoor, A. Oxidative stress statues in serum and follicular fluid of women with endometriosis. *Cell. J.* **2017**, *18*, 582–587. [PubMed]

88. Verit, F.F.; Erel, O.; Celik, N. Serum paraoxonase-1 activity in women with endometriosis and its relationship with the stage of the disease. *Hum. Reprod.* **2008**, 100–104. [CrossRef]

89. Jackson, L.W.; Schisterman, E.F.; Dey-Rao, R.; Browne, R.; Armstrong, D. Oxidative stress and endometriosis. *Hum. Reprod.* **2005**, *20*, 2014–2020. [CrossRef]

90. Turkyilmaz, E.; Yildirim, M.; Cendek, B.D.; Baran, P.; Alisik, M.; Dalgaci, F.; Yavuz, A.F. Evaluation of oxidative stress markers and intra-extracellular antioxidant activities in patients with endometriosis. *Eur. J. Obstet. Gynecol. Reprod. Biol.* **2016**, *199*, 164–168. [CrossRef]

91. Prieto, L.; Quesada, J.F.; Cambero, O.; Pacheco, A.; Pellicer, A.; Codoceo, R.; Garcia-Velasco, J.A. Analysis of follicular fluid and serum markers of oxidative stress in women with infertility related to endometriosis. *Fertil. Steril.* **2012**, *98*, 126–130. [CrossRef]

92. Andrisani, A.; Dona, G.; Brunati, A.M.; Clari, G.; Armanini, D.; Ragazzi, E.; Ambrosini, G.; Bordin, L. Increased oxidation-related glutathionylation and carbonic anhydrase activity in endometriosis. *Reprod. Biomed. Online* **2014**, *28*, 773–779. [CrossRef]

93. Gurgan, T.; Bukulmez, O.; Yarali, H.; Tanir, M.; Akyildiz, S. Serum and peritoneal fluid levels of IGF I and II and insulin-like growth binding protein-3 in endometriosis. *J. Reprod. Med.* **1999**, *44*, 450–454. [CrossRef] [PubMed]

94. Steff, A.M.; Gagne, D.; Page, M.; Hugo, P.; Gosselin, D. Concentration of soluble intercellular adhesion molecule-1 in serum samples from patients with endometriosis collected during the luteal phase of the menstrual cycle. *Hum. Reprod.* **2004**, *19*, 172–178. [CrossRef] [PubMed]

95. Philippoussis, F.; Gagne, D.; Hugo, P.; Gosselin, D. Concentrations of alpha-fetoprotein, insulin-like growth factor binding protein-3, c-erbB-2, and epidermal growth factor in serum of patients with endometriosis. *J. Soc. Gynecol. Investig.* **2004**, *11*, 175–181. [CrossRef] [PubMed]

96. Garcia-Galiano, D.; Navarro, V.M.; Gaytan, F.; Tena-Sempere, M. Expanding roles of NUCB2/nesfatin-1 in neuroendocrine regulation. *J. Mol. Endocrinol.* **2010**, *45*, 281–290. [CrossRef]

97. Sengul, O.; Dilbaz, B.; Halici, Z.; Ferah, I.; Cadirci, E.; Yilmaz, F. Decreased serum nesfatin-1 levels in endometriosis. *Eur. J. Obstet. Gynecol. Reprod. Biol.* **2014**, *177*, 34–37. [CrossRef]

98. Tokmak, A.; Ugur, M.; Tonguc, E.; Var, T.; Moraloglu, O.; Ozaksit, G. The value of urocortin and CA-125 in the diagnosis of endometrioma. *Arch. Gynecol. Obstet.* **2011**, *283*, 1075–1079. [CrossRef]

99. Chmaj-Wierzchowska, K.; Kampioni, M.; Wilczak, M.; Sajdak, S.; Opala, T. Novel markers in the diagnostics of endometriomas: Urocortin, ghrelin and leptin or leukocytes, fibrinogen, and CA-125? *Taiwan. J. Obstet. Gynecol.* **2015**, *54*, 126–130. [CrossRef]

100. Florio, P.; Reis, F.M.; Torres, P.B.; Calonaci, F.; Toti, P.; Bocchi, C.; Linton, E.A.; Petraglia, F. Plasma urocortin levels in the diagnosis of ovarian endometriosis. *Obstet. Gynecol.* **2007**, *110*, 594–600. [CrossRef]

101. Mohamed, M.L.; El Behery, M.M.; Mansour, S.A.E.-A. Comparative study between VEGF-A and CA-125 in diagnosis and follow-up of advanced endometriosis after conservative laparoscopic surgery. *Arch. Gynecol. Obstet.* **2013**, *287*, 77–82. [CrossRef]

102. Bourlev, V.; Iljasova, N.; Adamyan, L.; Larsson, A.; Olovsson, M. Signs of reduced angiogenic activity after surgical removal of deeply infiltrating endometriosis. *Fertil. Steril.* **2010**, *94*, 52–57. [CrossRef]

103. Szubert, M.; Suzin, J.; Duechler, M.; Szuławska, A.; Czyz, M.; Kowalczyk-Amico, K. Evaluation of selected angiogenic and inflammatory markers in endometriosis before and after danazol treatment. *Reprod. Fertil. Dev.* **2014**, *26*, 414–420. [CrossRef] [PubMed]

104. Chen, L.; Fan, R.; Huang, X.; Xu, H.; Zhang, X. Reduced levels of serum pigment epithelium-derived factor in women with endometriosis. *Reprod. Sci.* **2012**, *19*, 64–69. [CrossRef]

105. Ozhan, E.; Kokcu, A.; Yanik, K.; Gunaydin, M. Investigation of diagnostic potentials of nine different biomarkers in endometriosis. *Eur. J. Obstet. Gynecol. Reprod. Biol.* **2014**, *178*, 128–133. [CrossRef] [PubMed]

106. Gajbhiye, R.; Sonawani, A.; Khan, S.; Suryawanshi, A.; Kadam, S.; Warty, N.; Raut, V.; Khole, V. Identification and validation of novel serum markers for early diagnosis of endometriosis. *Hum. Reprod.* **2012**, *27*, 408–417. [CrossRef] [PubMed]

107. Yi, Y.-C.; Wang, S.-C.; Chao, C.-C.; Su, C.-L.; Lee, Y.-L.; Chen, L.-Y. Evaluation of serum autoantibody levels in the diagnosis of ovarian endometrioma. *J. Clin. Lab Anal.* **2010**, *24*, 357–362. [CrossRef] [PubMed]

108. Nabeta, M.; Abe, Y.; Kagawa, L.; Haraguchi, R.; Kito, K.; Ueda, N.; Sugita, A.; Yokoyama, M.; Kusanagi, Y.; Ito, M. Identification of anti-α-enolase autoantibody as a novel serum marker for endometriosis. *Proteom. Clin. Appl.* **2009**, *3*, 1201–1210. [CrossRef]

109. Inagaki, J.; Matsuura, E.; Kaihara, K.; Kobayashi, K.; Yasuda, T.; Nomizu, M.; Sugiura-Ogasawara, M.; Katano, K.; Aoki, K. IgG antilaminin-1 autoantibody and recurrent miscarriages. *Am. J. Reprod. Immunol.* **2001**, *45*, 232–238. [CrossRef]

110. Inagaki, J.; Sugiura-Ogasawara, M.; Nomizu, M.; Nakatsuka, M.; Ikuta, K.; Suzuki, N.; Kaihara, K.; Kobayashi, K.; Yasuda, T.; Shoenfeld, Y.; et al. An association of IgG anti-laminin-1 autoantibodies with endometriosis in infertile patients. *Hum. Reprod.* **2003**, *18*, 544–549. [CrossRef]

111. Mathur, S.; Garza, D.E.; Smith, L.F. Endometrial autoantigens eliciting immunoglobulin (Ig) G, IgA, and IgM responses in endometriosis. *Fertil. Steril.* **1990**, *54*, 56–63. [CrossRef]

112. Odukoya, O.A.; Wheatcroft, N.; Weetman, A.P.; Cooke, I.D. The prevalence of endometrial immunoglobulin G antibodies in patients with endometriosis. *Hum. Reprod.* **1995**, *10*, 1214–1219. [CrossRef]

113. Long, X.; Jinag, P.; Zhou, L.; Zhang, W. Evaluation of novel serum biomarkers and the proteomic differences of endometriosis and adenomyosis using MALDI-TOF–MS. *Arch. Gynecol Obstet.* **2013**, *288*, 201–205. [CrossRef] [PubMed]

114. Wölfler, M.M.; Schwamborn, C.; Otten, D.; Hornung, D.; Liu, H.; Rath, W. Mass spectrometry and serum pattern profiling for analyzing the individual risk for endometriosis: Promising insights? *Fertil. Steril.* **2009**, *91*, 2331–2337. [CrossRef]

115. Zheng, N.; Pan, C.; Liu, W. New serum biomarkers for detection of endometriosis using matrix-assisted laser desorption/ionization time-of-flight mass spectrometry. *J. Int. Med. Res.* **2011**, *39*, 1184–1192. [CrossRef] [PubMed]

116. Wang, L.; Zheng, W.; Mu, L.; Zhang, S.-Z. Identifying biomarkers of endometriosis using serum protein fingerprinting and artificial neural networks. *Int. J. Gynaecol. Obstet.* **2008**, *101*, 253–258. [CrossRef]

117. Jing, J.; Qiao, Y.; Suginami, H.; Taniguchi, F.; Shi, H.; Wang, S. Two novel serum biomarkers for endometriosis screened by surface-enhanced laser desorption/ionization time-of-flight mass spectrometry and their change after laparoscopic removal of endometriosis. *Fertil. Steril.* **2008**, *92*, 1221–1227. [CrossRef]

118. Malin, E.; Bodil, R.; Gunnar, E.; Bodil, O. AXIN1 in Plasma or Serum Is a Potential New Biomarker for Endometriosis. *Int. J. Mol. Sci.* **2019**, *20*, 189. [CrossRef]

119. Signorile, P.G.; Baldi, A. Supporting evidences for potential biomarkers of endometriosis detected in peripheral blood. *Data Brief.* **2015**, *5*, 971–974. [CrossRef]

120. Signorile, P.G.; Baldi, A. Serum Biomarker of Endometriosis. *J. Cell Physiol.* **2014**, *229*, 1731–1735. [CrossRef]

121. Dutta, M.; Joshi, M.; Srivastava, S.; Lodh, I.; Chakravarty, B.; Chaudhury, K. A metabonomics approach as a means for identification of potential biomarkers for early diagnosis of endometriosis. *Mol. Biosyst.* **2012**, *8*, 3281–3287. [CrossRef]

122. Vouk, K.; Hevir, N.; Ribic-Pucelj, M.; Haarpaintner, G.; Scherb, H.; Osredkar, J.; Moller, G.; Prehn, C.; Lanisnik Rizner, T.; Adamski, J. Discovery of phosphatidylcholines and sphingomyelins as biomarkers for ovarian endometriosis. *Hum. Reprod.* **2012**, *27*, 2955–2965. [CrossRef]

123. Zachariah, R.; Schmid, S.; Radpour, R.; Buerki, N.; Fan, A.X.-C.; Hahn, S.; Holzgreve, W.; Zhong, X.Y. Circulating cell free DNA as a potential biomarker for minimal and mild endometriosis. *Reprod. Biomed. Online* **2009**, *18*, 407–411. [CrossRef]

124. Creed, J.; Maggrah, A.; Reguly, B.; Harbottle, A. Mitochondrial DNA deletions accurately detect endometriosis in symptomatic females of child-bearing age. *Biomark. Med.* **2019**, *13*, 291–306. [CrossRef] [PubMed]

125. Bartel, D.P. MicroRNAs: Genomics, biogenesis, mechanism, and function. *Cell* **2004**, *116*, 281–297. [CrossRef]

126. Weber, J.A.; Baxter, D.H.; Zhang, S.; Huang, D.Y.; Huang, K.H.; Lee, M.J.; Galas, D.J.; Wang, K. The microRNA spectrum in 12 body fluids. *Clin. Chem.* **2010**, *56*, 1733–1741. [CrossRef] [PubMed]

127. Ohlsson Teague, E.M.C.; Print, C.G.; Hull, M.L. The role of microRNAs in endometriosis and associated reproductive conditions. *Hum. Reprod. Update* **2009**, *16*, 142–165. [CrossRef] [PubMed]

128. Zhao, M.; Tang, Q.; Wu, W.; Xia, Y.; Chen, D.; Wang, X. miR-20a contributes to endometriosis by regulating NTN4 expression. *Mol. Biol. Rep.* **2014**, *41*, 5793–5797. [CrossRef]

129. Wang, W.T.; Zhao, Y.N.; Han, B.W.; Hong, S.J.; Chen, Y.Q. CirculatingMicroRNAsIdentifiedinaGenome-Wide Serum MicroRNA Expression Analysis as Noninvasive Biomarkers for Endometriosis. *J. Clin. Endocrinol. Metab.* **2013**, *98*, 281–289. [CrossRef]

130. Kozomara, A.; Birgaoanu, M.; Griffiths-Jones, S. miRBase: From microRNA sequences to function. *Nucleic Acids Res.* **2019**, *47*, D155–D162. [CrossRef]

131. Rekker, K.; Saare, M.; Roost, A.M.; Kaart, T.; Sõritsa, D.; Karro, H.; Sõritsa, A.; Simón, C.; Salumets, A.; Peters, M. Circulating miR-200-family micro-RNAs have altered plasma levels in patients with endometriosis and vary with blood collection time. *Fertil. Steril.* **2015**, *104*, 938–946. [CrossRef]

132. Nisenblat, V.; Sharkey, D.J.; Wang, Z.; Evans, S.F.; Healey, M.; Ohlsson Teague, E.M.C.; Print, C.G.; Robertson, S.A.; Hull, M.L. Plasma miRNAs display limited potential as diagnostic tools for endometriosis. *Clin. Endocrinol. Metab.* **2019**, *104*, 1999–2022. [CrossRef]

133. Vanhie, A.; Peterse, D.O.D.; Beckers, A.; Cuellar, A.; Fassbender, A.; Meuleman, C.; Mestdagh, P.; D'Hooghe, T. Plasma miRNAs as biomarkers for endometriosis. *Hum. Reprod.* **2019**, *34*, 1650–1660. [CrossRef]

134. Jia, S.Z.; Yang, Y.; Lang, J.; Sun, P.; Leng, J. Plasma miR-17–5p, miR-20a and miR-22 are down-regulated in women with endometriosis. *Hum. Reprod.* **2013**, *28*, 322–330. [CrossRef] [PubMed]

135. Suryawanshi, S.; Vlad, A.M.; Lin, H.M.; Mantia-Smaldone, G.; Laskey, R.; Lee, M.; Lin, Y.; Donnellan, N.; Klein-Patel, M.; Lee, T.; et al. Plasma MicroRNAs as novel biomarkers for endometriosis and endometriosis-associated ovarian cancer. *Clin. Cancer Res.* **2013**, *19*, 1213–1224. [CrossRef] [PubMed]

136. Cosar, E.; Mamillapalli, R.; Ersoy, G.S.; Cho, S.; Seifer, B.; Taylor, H.S. Serum microRNAs as diagnostic markers of endometriosis: A comprehensive array-based analysis. *Fertil. Steril.* **2016**, *106*, 402–409. [CrossRef] [PubMed]

137. Zhang, X.-Y.; Zheng, L.-W.; Li, C.-J.; Xu, Y.; Zhou, X.; Fu, L.-I.; Li, D.-D.; Sun, L.-T.; Zhang, D.; Cui, M.-H.; et al. Dysregulated Expression of Long Noncoding RNAs in Endometriosis. *Crit. Rev. Eukaryot. Expr.* **2019**, *29*, 113–121. [CrossRef]

138. Wang, W.-T.; Sun, Y.-M.; Huang, W.; He, B.; Zhao, Y.-N.; Chen, Y.-Q. Genome-wide long non-coding RNA Analysis identified circulating LncRNAs as novel non-invasive diagnostic biomarkers for gynecological disease. *Sci. Rep.* **2016**, *6*, 23343. [CrossRef]

139. Qiu, J.; Zhang, X.; Ding, Y.; Hua, K. 1856 circulating exosomal long noncoding RNA-TC0101441 as a non-invasive biomarker for the prediction of endometriosis severity and recurrence. *J. Minim. Invasive Gynecol.* **2019**, *26*, S170–S171. [CrossRef]

140. Gueye, N.A.; Stanhiser, J.; Valentine, L.; Kotlyar, A.; Goodman, L.; Falcone, T. Biomarkers for Endometriosis in saliva, urine, and peritoneal fluid. *Biomark. endometr.* **2017**, 141–163. [CrossRef]

141. Kuessel, C.; Jaeger-Lamsky, A.; Pateisky, P.; Rossberg, N.; Schulz, A.; Schmitz, A.A.P.; Staudigl, C.; Wenzl, R. Cytokeratin-19 as a biomarker in urine and in serum for the diagnosis of endometriosis—A prospective study. *Gynecol. Endocrinol.* **2014**, *30*, 38–41. [CrossRef]

142. Hawkins, S.M.; Creighton, C.J.; Han, D.Y.; Zariff, A.; Anderson, M.L.; Gunaratne, P.H.; Matzuk, M.M. Functional microRNA involved in endometriosis. *Molec Endocrinol.* **2011**, *25*, 821–832. [CrossRef]

143. Becker, C.M.; Louis, G.; Exarhopoulos, A.; Mechsner, S.; Ebert, A.D.; Zurakowski, D.; Moses, M.A. Matrix metalloproteinases are elevated in the urine of patients with endometriosis. *Fertil. Steril.* **2010**, *94*, 2343–2346. [CrossRef] [PubMed]

144. Tokushige, N.; Markham, R.; Crossett, B.; Ahn, S.B.; Nelaturi, V.L.; Khan, A.; Fraser, I.S. Discovery of a novel biomarker in the urine in women with endometriosis. *Fertil. Steril.* **2011**, *95*, 46–49. [CrossRef]

145. El-Kasti, M.M.; Wright, C.; Fye, H.K.S.; Roseman, F.; Kessler, B.M.; Becker, C.M. Urinary peptide profiling identifies a panel of putative biomarkers for diagnosing and staging endometriosis. *Fertil. Steril.* **2011**, *95*, 1261–1266. [CrossRef] [PubMed]

146. Cho, S.; Choi, Y.S.; Yim, S.Y.; Yang, H.I.; Jeon, Y.E.; Lee, K.E.; Kim, H.Y.; Seo, S.K.; Lee, B.S. Urinary vitamin D-binding protein is elevated in patients with endometriosis. *Hum. Reprod.* **2012**, *27*, 515–522. [CrossRef] [PubMed]

147. Potlog-Nahari, C.; Stratton, P.; Winkel, C.; Widra, E.; Sinaii, N.; Connors, S.; Nieman, L.K. Urine vascular endothelial growth factor-A is not a useful marker for endometriosis. *Fertil. Steril.* **2004**, *81*, 1507–1512. [CrossRef] [PubMed]

148. Chen, X.; Liu, H.; Sun, W.; Guo, Z.; Lang, J. Elevated urine histone 4 levels in women with ovarian endometriosis revealed by discovery and parallel reaction monitoring proteomics. *J. Proteom.* **2019**, *204*, 103398. [CrossRef]

149. Gmyrek, G.B.; Sozanski, R.; Jerzak, M.; Chrobak, A.; Wickiewicz, D.; Skupnik, A.; Sierazka, U.; Fortuna, W.; Gabrys, M.; Chelmonska-Syta, A. Evaluation of monocyte chemotactic protein-1 levels in peripheral blood of infertile women with endometriosis. *Eur. J. Obstet. Gynecol. Reprod. Biol.* **2005**, *122*, 199–205. [CrossRef]

150. Gungor, T.; Kanat-Pektas, M.; Karayalcin, R.; Mollamahmutoglu, L. Peritoneal fluid and serum leptin concentrations in women with primary infertility. *Arch. Gynecol. Obstet.* **2009**, *279*, 361–364. [CrossRef]

151. Huang, H.; Hong, H.; Tan, Y.; Sheng, J. Matrix metalloproteinase 2 is associated with changes in steroids hormones in the sera and peritoneal fluid of patients with endometriosis. *Fertil. Steril.* **2004**, *81*, 1235–1239. [CrossRef]

152. Morin, M.; Bellehumeur, C.; Therriault, M.J.; Metz, C.; Maheux, R.; Akoum, A. Elevated levels of macrophage migration inhibitory factor in the peripheral blood of women with endometriosis. *Fertil. Steril.* **2005**, *83*, 865–872. [CrossRef]

BIRC5/Survivin Expression as a Non-Invasive Biomarker of Endometriosis

Carolina Filipchiuk [1], Antonio Simone Laganà [2,*], Rubia Beteli [3], Tatiana Guida Ponce [4], Denise Maria Christofolini [3], Camila Martins Trevisan [4], Fernando Luiz Affonso Fonseca [5], Caio Parente Barbosa [3] and Bianca Bianco [1,3]

[1] Center of Natural and Human Sciences (CCNH), Universidade Federal do ABC, Santo André 09210-580, SP, Brazil; carol_f24@hotmail.com (C.F.); bianca.bianco@fmabc.br (B.B.)
[2] Department of Obstetrics and Gynecology, "Filippo Del Ponte" Hospital, University of Insubria, 2100 Varese, Italy
[3] Discipline of Sexual and Reproductive Health and Populational Genetics, Department of Collective Health, Faculdade de Medicina do ABC/Centro Universitário Saúde ABC, Santo André 09210-580, Brazil; rubs.fmabc@gmail.com (R.B.); denise.christofolini@fmabc.br (D.M.C.); caio.parente@fmabc.br (C.P.B.)
[4] Postgraduate Program in Health Sciences, Faculdade de Medicina do ABC/Centro Universitário Saúde ABC, Santo André 09210-580, Brazil; tatianaguidaponce@gmail.com (T.G.P.); camilatrevisan22@gmail.com (C.M.T.)
[5] Discipline of Clinical Analysis, Deparment of Patology, Faculdade de Medicina do ABC/Centro Universitário Saúde ABC, Santo André 09210-580, Brazil; profferfonseca@gmail.com
* Correspondence: antoniosimone.lagana@uninsubria.it

Abstract: The etiology of endometriosis is highly complex, and although it is a benign disease, it has several biological behaviors similar to malignant lesions, including cell invasion, neo-angiogenesis, and decreased apoptosis. Survivin is a protein encoded by the BIRC5 gene that plays a role in cell division by inhibiting apoptosis and regulating the process of mitosis in embryonic and cancer cells. Therefore, we aimed to evaluate the expression of BIRC5 in samples of peripheral blood of women with and without endometriosis. This study comprised of 40 women with endometriosis and 10 healthy women as controls. Peripheral blood samples were collected in the three phases of the menstrual cycle (follicular, ovulatory, and luteal). The expression of the BIRC5 gene was evaluated by RT-qPCR using the TaqMan methodology. The BIRC5 expression was significantly higher in all phases of the menstrual cycle in women with endometriosis, regardless of the disease stage. The accuracy of BIRC5 expression in the peripheral blood for the diagnosis endometriosis presented AUC of 0.887 ($p < 0.001$), with 97.2% of sensitivity and specificity of 65.5% considering the overall endometriosis group. Regarding the minimal/mild endometriosis group, the AUC presented a value of 0.925 ($p < 0.001$), with 100% of sensitivity and 79.3% of specificity, whereas in the moderate/severe endometriosis group the AUC was 0.868 ($p < 0.001$), with a sensitivity of 95.8% and specificity of 65.5%. These findings suggest that the expression of BIRC5 may be a potential noninvasive biomarker for the diagnosis of endometriosis.

Keywords: endometriosis; survivin; BIRC5; apoptosis; inhibitor of apoptosis protein

1. Introduction

Endometriosis is a common estrogen-dependent gynecological condition, which can affect women at a reproductive age [1]. It is defined as the presence of endometrial-like tissue outside of the uterus, often associated with chronic and inflammatory reaction [2]. The symptoms of endometriosis may vary from severe dysmenorrhea, dyspareunia, or chronic pelvic pain [1–3] to unexplained infertility, although the disease can be asymptomatic [4].

Cancer antigen 125 (CA125) plasma concentrations, a glycoprotein of epithelial origin, although largely used, are not reliable to diagnose endometriosis. Indeed, it may be elevated in several benign diseases and patients with non-ovarian malignancies, including cancers of the endometrium, lung, breast, pancreas, and colon [5], and it has no value in the diagnosis as a single test [3]. Indeed, according to guidelines of the European Society of Human Reproduction and Embryology (ESHRE), clinicians are recommended not to use immunological biomarkers, including CA125, in plasma, urine, or serum to diagnose endometriosis [6]. Despite considerable efforts towards searching for noninvasive diagnostic methods to detect endometriosis, the diagnosis can be suspected by ultrasound and/or other imaging methods [7] and confirmed only through laparoscopy with inspection of the abdominal cavity and histological confirmation of the lesion(s) [1,3]. As the surgery presents risks and also a high cost, a less invasive, but accurate test could lead to the diagnosis of the disease without the need for surgery, or at least it could help reduce the need for a surgical procedure for its confirmation [3].

The pathogenesis of endometriosis is still debated, although genetics, epigenetics, and immune elements may all play a pivotal role [8–10]. There are several theories to account for the origin of endometriosis and to explain how ectopic tissue can implant throughout the abdominal cavity [11]. However, there is no single theory that explains all of the different clinical presentations and pathological features in endometriosis [10]. A growing body of evidence has identified several comorbidities that are associated with endometriosis, including congenital uterine anomalies, autoimmune disease, allergy, cancers, and cardiovascular disease [12,13]. Melin et al. [14], based on 64,492 registers of the National Swedish Inpatient and Cancer Registrar data from 1969 to 2000, observed that women with endometriosis have an increased risk of some malignancies, particularly ovarian cancer. In addition, Wang et al. [15] in a recent meta-analysis comprising a total of 40,609 cases of epithelial ovarian cancer and 368,452 controls from 38 publications, also found that endometriosis was associated with an increased risk of epithelial ovarian cancer (OR = 1.42, 95% CI = 1.28–1.57). Endometriosis and cancer present similarities [16], such as cell invasion, unrestrained growth, neo-angiogenesis, and decreased apoptosis [17,18], although the first condition is clearly not neoplastic.

Inhibitors of apoptosis proteins (IAPs) have emerged as modulators in an evolutionarily conserved step in apoptosis, as negative regulatory proteins that prevent apoptotic cell death. Survivin, a member of the IAP family, is encoded by the *BIRC5* (baculoviral IAP repeat-containing 5) gene located at 17q25, and it plays a role in cell division by inhibiting apoptosis and regulating the process of mitosis in embryonic cells during embryogenesis and in cancer cells during tumorigenesis and tumor metastasis [19]. It also participates in chromosome division and segregation, proliferation, stress response, and angiogenesis [20]. In addition, survivin is considered a key element for the metastasis phenomenon [21–24] and, consequently, has received significant attention as a potential oncotherapeutic target [25].

Survivin expression in normal endometrium shows cyclic alterations dependent on the menstrual cycle [26–28]. In addition, survivin overexpression is shown to be present in hormone-dependent endometrial disorders, such as endometrial hyperplasia, carcinomas, and endometriosis [27–30]. Therefore, the aim of the present study was to evaluate the expression of *BIRC5* in samples of peripheral blood of women with and without endometriosis.

2. Materials and Methods

2.1. Participants

This case-control study was performed between February 2017 and December 2018 and comprised 50 women recruited at the Human Reproduction and Genetics Center of the Faculdade de Medicina do ABC, Santo Andre, Brazil. The design, analysis, interpretation of data, drafting, and revisions followed the Helsinki Declaration and the strengthening the reporting of observational studies in epidemiology (STROBE) statement, available through the enhancing the quality and transparency of health research (EQUATOR) network (www.equator-network.org). The study design was approved by the independent Research Ethics Committee of the "Faculdade de Medicina do ABC" (approve code

CAEE 64005816.8.0000.0082, approved on 1 February 2017). Each patient enrolled in this study signed an informed consent for all the procedures and to allow data and biological sample collection and analysis for research purposes. The study was non-advertised, and no remuneration was offered to encourage patients to give consent for the collection and analysis of their data. An independent data monitoring committee evaluated the interim and final data analysis of the study.

The endometriosis group comprised 40 women who had endometriosis diagnosed by laparoscopy and histological confirmation, classified according to the revised American Society for Reproductive Medicine (rASRM) score [31]. In this group, minimal/mild (stage I and II) endometriosis was found in 33.3% (12/36) of the cases, whereas moderate/severe (stage III and IV) endometriosis was found in 66.7% (24/36) of the cases. The surgical indication for all patients was infertility. The control group was carefully selected and comprised of 10 healthy and non-menopausal women who had no personal and/or familial history of endometriosis, autoimmune diseases, or cancer. All these women previously underwent tubal ligation for family planning reasons, and the absence of endometriosis was confirmed through inspection of the pelvic cavity.

2.2. Sample Collection

Fifteen milliliters of the peripheral blood samples were collected in a tube containing clot-separator gel and in a tube containing PAXgene Blood RNA (PreAnalytiX, BD Diagnostics®, Franklin Lakes, NJ, USA). After collection, the tubes for the biochemical dosages were centrifuged (1000 rpm for 10 min), the plasma was aliquoted into microtubes and frozen at −80 °C for further determination of follicle-stimulating hormone (FSH), luteinizing hormone (LH), progesterone, prolactin, and CA125 concentrations. The tube for RNA extraction was stored at −80 °C until extraction.

The samples for RNA extraction were collected in the three phases of the menstrual cycle (follicular, ovulatory, and luteal) for all women of the control group. Among the women of the endometriosis group, the samples were collected in 38.9% of women (14/36) in the follicular phase, 27.8% (10/36) in the ovulatory phase, and in 33.3% (12/36) in the luteal phase.

2.3. Hormonal Measurement

The hormonal profile was measured during the investigation into the cause of infertility. Progesterone and prolactin were measured at the luteal phase and FSH and LH at the follicular phase of the menstrual cycle. The hormones were measured by enzyme-linked fluorescent immunoassay (BioMerieux®, Hazelwood, MO, USA).

2.4. RT-qPCR

RNA extraction was carried out with Qiazol Lysis Reagent according to the manufacturer's instructions (Qiagen Inc., Valencia, CA, USA) and then total RNA was treated with DNase-I endonuclease (Thermo Fisher Scientific, Waltham, MA, USA). RNA sample concentrations were analyzed using a Nanodrop 2000 spectrophotometer (Thermo Fisher Scientific, Waltham, MA, USA) and the RNA integrity was analyzed via agarose gel electrophoresis to identify the 28S and 18S ribosomal rRNA. The cDNA synthesis was done with 1 µg of total RNA using a high capacity cDNA reverse transcription kit (Thermo Fisher Scientific, Waltham, MA, USA) following the manufacturer's guidelines.

The expression of BIRC5 (Hs04194392_s1) and glyceraldehyde3-phosphate dehydrogenase (GAPDH, Hs99999905_m1) genes was measured by RT-qPCR, based on the TaqMan methodology (ThermoFisher Scientific, Waltham, MA, USA) using the equipment StepOne Real-Time PCR System (Applied Biosystems, Foster City, CA, USA). PCR reactions were processed to a final volume of 20 mL containing 10 µL of 2× TaqMan Universal PCR Master Mix, 1.25 µL TaqMan assay (20×), 2 µL of sample cDNA, and 6.75 µL of RNAse-free water. Reactions were performed at 95 °C for 10 min, followed by 40 cycles of 95 °C for 15 s, and annealing/extension at 60 °C for 60 s. Each reaction was performed in triplicates. The gene expression results were obtained using the $2^{-\Delta Ct}$.

2.5. Statistical Analyses

Statistical analyses were performed using GraphPad Software (v.7, LLC, San Diego, CA, USA, https://www.graphpad.com). Data normality was verified with the Shapiro–Wilk test. Variables were presented by medians with 95% confidence intervals (CI). Differences between two groups were tested by Mann–Whitney or Kruskal–Wallis tests. A Spearman's correlation test was performed to analyze the correlation between hormonal levels and the *BIRC5* expression. To test for accuracy, receiver operator characteristic (ROC) analysis was used and specificity, sensibility, predictive values, and 95% confidence interval (95% CI) were calculated. Statistical significance was considered when $p < 0.05$.

3. Results

Table 1 shows the comparison of clinical and hormonal characteristics of women with and without endometriosis. Hormonal values were in accordance with the reference values for each phase of the menstrual cycle. CA125, FSH, and prolactin levels were significantly higher in women with endometriosis compared with the control group. Conversely, age, body mass index (BMI), LH, and progesterone levels were not significantly different between groups. Regarding the endometriosis stage, all the parameters were not significantly different between women with minimal/mild and moderate/severe disease.

Figure 1A shows the comparison of *BIRC5* expression among women with endometriosis and according to the disease stage and the control group. The *BIRC5* expression was also significantly higher in women with endometriosis, regardless of the endometriosis stage (minimal/mild and moderate/severe endometriosis). Figure 1B shows the comparison of *BIRC5* expression between women with and without endometriosis in different phases of the menstrual cycle. The *BIRC5* expression was significantly higher in all phases of the menstrual cycle in women with endometriosis.

The correlation between hormonal levels and *BIRC5* expression in peripheral blood of women with endometriosis is reported in Table 2. Spearman's correlation coefficient showed that the progesterone was correlated with *BIRC5* expression (rho = 0.382, $p = 0.045$).

Table 1. Comparison of clinical and hormonal characteristics of women with and without endometriosis.

Variable *	Endometriosis (*n* = 36)	Controls (*n* = 10)	*p* **
Age (years)	35 (33.0–38.0)	33 (32–34.5)	0.933
BMI (kg/m^2)	24.3 (23.1–25.4)	24.7 (23.8–25.7)	0.800
CA125 (mUI/mL)	49.8 (22.6–67.6)	18.9 (15.2–36.3)	<0.001
FSH (mUI/mL)	7.2 (6.8–8.2)	6.4 (6.1–6.9)	<0.001
LH (mUI/mL)	6.3 (4.3–8.3)	6.7 (5.0–8.3)	0.838
Progesterone (ng/mL)	8.9 (6.9–11.0)	5.9 (2.9–8.9)	0.061
Prolactin (ng/mL)	17.1 (11.9–22.6)	8.5 (6.5–15.1)	0.010

* Median and 95% confidence interval. BMI, body mass index; CA125, cancer antigen 125; FSH, follicle-stimulating hormone; LH, luteinizing hormone. ** Mann–Whitney test.

Table 2. Correlation between hormone levels and *BICR5* expression in peripheral blood of women with endometriosis.

	rho *	*p*
CA125	−0.191	0.265
FSH	0.276	0.115
LH	0.274	0.117
Progesterone	0.382	0.045
Prolactin	−0.030	0.873

* Spearman's correlation. CA125, cancer antigen 125; FSH, follicle-stimulating hormone; LH, luteinizing hormone.

Figure 1. (A) *BIRC5* expression in the peripheral blood samples of women with endometriosis according to the disease stage. (B) *BIRC5* expression in the peripheral blood samples of women with and without endometriosis in different phases of the menstrual cycle.

To estimate the accuracy of *BIRC5* expression in the peripheral blood to diagnostic endometriosis and also according to disease staging, the area under the ROC curve was analyzed (Figure 2).

Figure 2. The accuracy of *BIRC5* expression in the peripheral blood for the diagnosis of endometriosis. Red dotted line indicates line of no-discrimination.

Considering the overall endometriosis group, the area under the curve (AUC) was 0.887 (95% CI = 0.809–0.965; $p < 0.001$), with a cut-off value of $2^{-\Delta Ct} > 0.00030$, 97.2% of sensitivity and specificity of 65.5%; with a positive predictive value of 68.5% (95% CI 61.0–75.2) and a negative predictive value of 92.8% (95% CI 64.2–98.9). Regarding the minimal/mild endometriosis group, the AUC presented a value of 0.925 (95% CI = 0.848–1.0; $p < 0.001$), with a cut-off value of $2^{-\Delta Ct} > 0.0018$, sensitivity of 100% and specificity of 79.3%, positive predictive value 66.7% (95% CI 49.5–80.3), and negative predictive value 100%. For the moderate/severe endometriosis group, the AUC was 0.868 (95% CI = 0.775–0.962; $p < 0.001$), with a cut-off value of $2^{-\Delta Ct} > 0.00030$, sensitivity of 95.8% and specificity of 65.5%, with a positive predictive value of 69.7% (95% CI 58.0–79.3) and a negative predictive value of 95.0% (95% CI 73.3–99.2).

4. Discussion

In the current study, the expression pattern of *BIRC5* as a potential non-invasive biomarker was assessed in the peripheral blood samples taken during different phases of the menstrual cycle of women with and without endometriosis. Our results showed that *BIRC5* is differently expressed in women with endometriosis compared with healthy controls, regardless of the endometriosis stage.

Some findings have highlighted the main role of inflammation in endometriosis by acting on proliferation, apoptosis, and angiogenesis. Nevertheless, the mechanisms underlying this disease are still unclear [32]. Homeostasis maintenance of tissue is mainly regulated by cell death and some studies have shown that apoptosis increases during the menstrual cycle to retain cell homeostasis, removing aged cells from the functional layer of the endometrium [33]. The rate of apoptosis is decreased in endometrial cells of women with endometriosis, and therefore, it may contribute to the pathogenesis of the disease [34–38].

In apoptosis inhibition, survivin has a key role in both intrinsic and extrinsic pathways of apoptosis [39–44]. Considering the aspects of an immune response, survivin modulates the apoptotic threshold of neutrophils and its expression increases during inflammatory reactions in these cells. Survivin has also a contribution to T-cell development, maturation, activation, and homeostasis [20,42]. Its expression increases after the activation of naive T cells in lymphoid organs, showing the importance of survivin in the initiation of immune responses. The increased level of survivin has been documented in serum and lymphocytes of patients with different autoimmune diseases [20,42,43]. Numerous studies have shown that peritoneal leukocytes and their inflammatory mediators exert local effects, creating a microenvironment that may facilitate the development and progression of endometriotic lesions. Besides, some authors have suggested that endometriosis may have, at least in part, an autoimmune component [43,44].

Zwerts et al. [45] observed that the structures of the embryo show high expression of survivin, while the absence of its expression in endothelial cells contributes to the death of the embryo. Other studies also demonstrated that the presence of survivin is essential for normal development and organogenesis. Survivin's involvement in the regulation of endothelial cell survival and its influence in maintaining vascular integrity has paramount importance in neurogenesis, angiogenesis, and cardiogenesis. The survival of undifferentiated pluripotent stem cells is highly dependent on anti-apoptotic factors, such as survivin [46,47], and overexpression of survivin in embryonic stem cells, pluripotent cells and somatic stem cells [48,49], as well as the correlation between higher *BIRC5* expression and lower cell differentiation in cells derived from bone marrow [47] is probably due to the fact that bone marrow is a source of hematopoietic stem cells and mesenchymal stem cells [50,51].

All these findings corroborate different theories for the origin of endometriosis, such as the theory of endometrial stem cells [52] or the increase in transient progenitor cells in which circulating stem cells originating from bone marrow or the basal layer of the endometrium can differentiate into endometrial tissue in different anatomical locations; or the theory of genetic/epigenetic changes in which, regardless of the origin of the initial cell, genic variants or epigenetic changes associated with changes in the peritoneal environment, such as inflammatory, immunological and oxidative stress, could initiate diseases in their different forms (ovarian, peritoneal, deep, and lesions outside the pelvis) and thus explain its complexity [11,53], which may lead also to significant anatomical alterations and make the surgical approach difficult [54]. Recently, a systematic review that summarized the findings from 21 studies and 1263 women with endometriosis reported that survivin (gene and/or protein) expression is increased in endometriosis, regardless of the methodology used (real-time reverse transcription polymerase chain reaction (RT-PCR), quantitative PCR (RT-qPCR), immunohistochemistry, Western blot, or enzyme-linked immunosorbent assay (ELISA)), sample studied (endometrium or blood), the phenotype of the endometriosis (superficial, ovarian, and deep) or morphology of the endometriotic lesions (pigmented or non-pigmented) [43].

Zang et al. [28] observed that the presence of paracrine factors produced by normal endometrial stromal cells mediated the effect of progesterone on glandular endometriotic cells in vitro. The authors also found that endometriotic stromal cells have lost the ability to regulate apoptotic signaling in endometriotic gland cells that grow in ectopic sites, while these cells have not lost their ability to respond to paracrine factors produced by endometrial stromal cells. The observation of the cyclic expression of survivin in normal endometrial cells suggests that the expression of the BIRC5 gene is influenced by steroid hormones and deregulated by the increase in progesterone in the luteal phase. Progesterone is a potent antagonist of estrogen-induced endometrial proliferation and plays an important role in the pathogenesis of endometriosis [55]. The continuous use of progestogens, as well as the combined use of estrogens and progestogens in the treatment of endometriosis results in the inhibition of endometrial growth, with consequent atrophy of the lesions, in addition to being associated with anti-inflammatory action, suppression of metalloproteinases, and inhibition of angiogenesis [56]. In the present study, Spearman's correlation showed that progesterone level was correlated with BIRC5 expression (rho = 0.382, $p = 0.045$).

Acimovic et al. [57] studied survivin expression in 30 women with endometriosis and 10 women without the disease. The authors found a difference in the expression of survivin in peripheral blood between the groups ($p = 0.025$) and the results demonstrated that the accuracy of survivin as a diagnostic test for endometriosis was 70%, with a sensitivity of 66.7% and specificity of 80%. However, the study does not report the phase of the menstrual cycle during which the samples were collected. In our study, the expression of BIRC5 in the peripheral blood of women with endometriosis showed an accuracy of 88.7%, with a sensitivity of 97.2% and specificity of 65.5%. In minimum/mild endometriosis the accuracy was 92.5%, with 100% sensitivity and 79.3% specificity, whereas in moderate/severe disease the accuracy was 86.8% with 95.8% sensitivity and specificity of 65.5%. The data suggest that BIRC5 expression may be a potential minimally invasive biomarker in the diagnosis of endometriosis.

Some studies suggest that prolactin may also act as a probable prognostic biomarker to differentiate patients with endometriosis according to the stage of the disease and also as an indicator of endometriosis related-infertility since higher levels are observed in women with endometriosis when compared with infertile women without endometriosis; however, this relation is debatable [58]. Prolactin plays an important role in the immune system, participating in the inflammatory process, angiogenesis, and in the formation of thrombi and scarring [59]. In our study, we observed that women with endometriosis had higher levels of prolactin, despite being within the reference value, when compared to fertile women without the disease; in addition, we did not find a significant difference for prolactin values considering the stage of the disease (13.5 ng/mL (7.6–19.3) versus 15.2 ng/mL (10.5–20.2), respectively in minimal/mild and moderate/severe endometriosis; $p = 0.410$). Nonetheless, minimal/mild disease was found in only one-third of the women enrolled in this study. Indeed, 66.7% of the women in the endometriosis group were classified as advanced (III/IV) stages according to the rASRM, and this could be considered in line with the enrollment of women with endometriosis-associated infertility.

For the correct interpretation of our findings, some limitations of the present study should be taken into account. We studied infertile women with endometriosis and fertile women without the disease, and the mechanisms responsible for the association of infertility and endometriosis are still not fully elucidated. As women with endometriosis were undergoing assisted reproduction treatment and the strict inclusion and exclusion criteria of the study participants, we were unable to obtain samples from the same participant at different phases of the menstrual cycle.

5. Conclusions

In conclusion, increased expression of the BIRC5 gene in the peripheral blood of women with endometriosis may indicate their role in cell proliferation and anti-apoptotic activity in the development of the disease. The findings suggest that the expression of BIRC5 may be a potential noninvasive biomarker for the diagnosis of endometriosis.

Increased knowledge of the pathophysiologic mechanisms of endometriosis is crucial for an early and accurate diagnosis, which can reduce the costs associated with the management of the disease and help to avoid (or at least reduce) the negative impact on the physical and psychosocial health of the patients.

More studies however are needed to confirm the applicability of the proposed biomarker of endometriosis for clinical use.

Author Contributions: Conceptualization, F.L.A.F. and B.B.; Data curation, C.F., R.B., T.G.P., and C.M.T.; Formal analysis, C.F., C.M.T., and F.L.A.F.; Investigation, C.F., R.B., and F.L.A.F.; Project administration, B.B.; Validation, B.B.; Writing—original draft, C.F.; Writing—review & editing, A.S.L., R.B., T.G.P., D.M.C., C.M.T., F.L.A.F., C.P.B., and B.B. All authors have read and agreed to the published version of the manuscript.

Acknowledgments: The authors thank CAPES for granting Carolina Filipchiuk a PhD scholarship. The authors are also grateful to the FAPESP (#2017/10045-2) for granting Rubia Beteli a scientific Initiation scholarship.

References

1. Chapron, C.; Marcellin, L.; Borghese, B.; Santulli, P. Rethinking mechanisms, diagnosis and management of endometriosis. *Nat. Rev. Endocrinol.* **2019**, *15*, 666–682. [CrossRef]

2. Zondervan, K.T.; Becker, C.M.; Koga, K.; Missmer, S.A.; Taylor, R.N.; Viganò, P. Endometriosis. *Nat. Rev. Dis. Primers* **2018**, *4*, 9. [CrossRef]

3. Kiesel, L.; Sourouni, M. Diagnosis of endometriosis in the 21st century. *Climacteric* **2019**, *22*, 296–302. [CrossRef] [PubMed]

4. Barbosa, C.P.; Souza, A.M.; Bianco, B.; Christofolini, D.; Bach, F.A.; Lima, G.R. Frequency of endometriotic lesions in peritoneum samples from asymptomatic fertile women and correlation with CA125 values. *Sao Paulo Med. J.* **2009**, *127*, 342–345. [CrossRef]

5. Bast, R.C., Jr.; Badgwell, D.; Lu, Z.; Marquez, R.; Rosen, D.; Liu, J.; Baggerly, K.A.; Atkinson, E.N.; Skates, S.; Zhang, Z.; et al. New tumor markers: CA125 and beyond. *Int. J. Gynecol. Cancer* **2005**, *15* (Suppl. 3), 274–281. [CrossRef]

6. Dunselman, G.A.; Vermeulen, N.; Becker, C.; Calhaz-Jorge, C.; D'Hooghe, T.; De Bie, B.; Heikinheimo, O.; Horne, A.W.; Kiesel, L.; Nap, A.; et al. European Society of Human Reproduction and Embryology. ESHRE guideline: Management of women with endometriosis. *Hum. Reprod.* **2014**, *29*, 400–412. [CrossRef]

7. Barra, F.; Biscaldi, E.; Scala, C.; Laganà, A.S.; Vellone, V.G.; Stabilini, C.; Ghezzi, F.; Ferrero, S. A Prospective Study Comparing Three-Dimensional Rectal Water Contrast Transvaginal Ultrasonography and Computed Tomographic Colonography in the Diagnosis of Rectosigmoid Endometriosis. *Diagnostics* **2020**, *10*, 252. [CrossRef]

8. Laganà, A.S.; Garzon, S.; Götte, M.; Viganò, P.; Franchi, M.; Ghezzi, F.; Martin, D.C. The Pathogenesis of Endometriosis: Molecular and Cell Biology Insights. *Int. J. Mol. Sci.* **2019**, *20*, 5615. [CrossRef]

9. Sofo, V.; Götte, M.; Laganà, A.S.; Salmeri, F.M.; Triolo, O.; Sturlese, E.; Retto, G.; Alfa, M.; Granese, R.; Abrão, M.S. Correlation between dioxin and endometriosis: An epigenetic route to unravel the pathogenesis of the disease. *Arch. Gynecol. Obstet.* **2015**, *292*, 973–986. [CrossRef] [PubMed]

10. Wang, Y.; Nicholes, K.; Shih, I.M. The Origin and Pathogenesis of Endometriosis. *Annu. Rev. Pathol.* **2020**, *15*, 71–95. [CrossRef]

11. Alkatout, İ.; Meinhold-Heerlein, I.; Keckstein, J.; Mettler, L. Endometriosis: A concise practical guide to current diagnosis and treatment. *J. Turk. Ger. Gynecol. Assoc.* **2018**, *19*, 173–175. [CrossRef] [PubMed]

12. Alderman, M.H.; Yoder, N.; Taylor, H.S. The Systemic Effects of Endometriosis. *Semin. Reprod. Med.* **2017**, *35*, 263–270. [CrossRef]

13. Freytag, D.; Mettler, L.; Maass, N.; Günther, V.; Alkatout, I. Uterine anomalies and endometriosis. *Minerva Med.* **2020**, *111*, 33–49. [CrossRef]

14. Melin, A.; Sparén, P.; Persson, I.; Bergqvist, A. Endometriosis and the risk of cancer with special emphasis on ovarian cancer. *Hum. Reprod.* **2006**, *21*, 1237–1242. [CrossRef]

15. Wang, C.; Liang, Z.; Liu, X.; Zhang, Q.; Li, S. The Association between Endometriosis, Tubal Ligation, Hysterectomy and Epithelial Ovarian Cancer: Meta-Analyses. *Int. J. Environ. Res. Public Health* **2016**, *13*, 1138. [CrossRef]

16. Králíčková, M.; Laganà, A.S.; Ghezzi, F.; Vetvicka, V. Endometriosis and risk of ovarian cancer: What do we know? *Arch. Gynecol. Obstet.* **2020**, *301*, 1–10. [CrossRef]

17. Moga, M.A.; Bălan, A.; Dimienescu, O.G.; Burtea, V.; Dragomir, R.M.; Anastasiu, C.V. Circulating miRNAs as Biomarkers for Endometriosis and Endometriosis-Related Ovarian Cancer-An Overview. *J. Clin. Med.* **2019**, *8*, 735. [CrossRef]

18. Karnezis, A.N.; Leung, S.; Magrill, J.; McConechy, M.K.; Yang, W.; Chow, C.; Kobel, M.; Lee, C.H.; Huntsman, D.G.; Talhouk, A.; et al. Evaluation of endometrial carcinoma prognostic immunohistochemistry markers in the context of molecular classification. *J. Pathol. Clin. Res.* **2017**, *3*, 279–293. [CrossRef]

19. Wheatley, S.P.; McNeish, I.A. Survivin: A protein with dual roles in mitosis and apoptosis. *Int. Rev. Cytol.* **2005**, *247*, 35–88. [CrossRef]

20. Zafari, P.; Rafiei, A.; Esmaeili, S.A.; Moonesi, M.; Taghadosi, M. Survivin a pivotal antiapoptotic protein in rheumatoid arthritis. *J. Cell. Physiol.* **2019**, *234*, 21575–21587. [CrossRef]

21. Marsicano, S.R.; Kuniyoshi, R.K.; Gehrke, F.S.; Alves, B.C.; Azzalis, L.A.; Fonseca, F.L. Survinin expression in patients with breast cancer during chemotherapy. *Tumour Biol.* **2015**, *36*, 3441–3445. [CrossRef] [PubMed]

22. Rivadeneira, D.B.; Caino, M.C.; Seo, J.H.; Angelin, A.; Wallace, D.C.; Languino, L.R.; Altieri, D.C. Survivin promotes oxidative phosphorylation, subcellular mitochondrial repositioning, and tumor cell invasion. *Sci. Signal.* **2015**, *8*, ra80. [CrossRef]

23. Ausserlechner, M.J.; Hagenbuchner, J. Mitochondrial survivin–an Achilles' heel in cancer chemoresistance. *Mol. Cell Oncol.* **2015**, *3*, e1076589. [CrossRef]

24. Galbo, P.M., Jr.; Ciesielski, M.J.; Figel, S.; Maguire, O.; Qiu, J.; Wiltsie, L.; Minderman, H.; Fenstermaker, R.A. Circulating CD9+/GFAP+/survivin+ exosomes in malignant glioma patients following survivin vaccination. *Oncotarget* **2017**, *8*, 114722–114735. [CrossRef]

25. Wheatley, S.P.; Altieri, D.C. Survivin at a glance. *J. Cell Sci.* **2019**, *132*, jcs223826. [CrossRef]

26. Konno, R.; Yamakawa, H.; Utsunomiya, H.; Ito, K.; Sato, S.; Yajima, A. Expression of survivin and Bcl-2 in the normal human endometrium. *Mol. Hum. Reprod.* **2000**, *6*, 529–534. [CrossRef]

27. Lehner, R.; Enomoto, T.; McGregor, J.A.; Shroyer, L.; Haugen, B.R.; Pugazhenthi, U.; Shroyer, K.R. Correlation of survivin mRNA detection with histologic diagnosis in normal endometrium and endometrial carcinoma. *Acta Obstet. Gynecol. Scand.* **2002**, *81*, 162–167. [CrossRef]

28. Zhang, H.; Li, M.; Zheng, X.; Sun, Y.; Wen, Z.; Zhao, X. Endometriotic stromal cells lose the ability to regulate cell-survival signaling in endometrial epithelial cells in vitro. *Mol. Hum. Reprod.* **2009**, *15*, 653–663. [CrossRef]

29. Takai, N.; Miyazaki, T.; Nishida, M.; Nasu, K.; Miyakawa, I. Survivin expression correlates with clinical stage, histological grade, invasive behavior and survival rate in endometrial carcinoma. *Cancer Lett.* **2002**, *184*, 105–116. [CrossRef]

30. Pallares, J.; Martínez-Guitarte, J.L.; Dolcet, X.; Llobet, D.; Rue, M.; Palacios, J.; Prat, J.; Matias-Guiu, X. Survivin expression in endometrial carcinoma: A tissue microarray study with correlation with PTEN and STAT-3. *Int. J. Gynecol. Pathol.* **2005**, *24*, 247–253. [CrossRef]

31. Canis, M.; Donnez, J.G.; Guzick, D.S.; Halme, J.K.; Rock, J.A.; Schenken, R.S.; Vernon, M.W. Revised American Society for Reproductive Medicine classification of endometriosis: 1996. *Fertil. Steril.* **1997**, *67*, 817–821. [CrossRef]

32. Burney, R.O.; Giudice, L.C. Pathogenesis and pathophysiology of endometriosis. *Fertil. Steril.* **2012**, *98*, 511–519. [CrossRef] [PubMed]

33. Vetvicka, V.; Laganà, A.S.; Salmeri, F.M.; Triolo, O.; Palmara, V.I.; Vitale, S.G.; Sofo, V.; Králíčková, M. Regulation of apoptotic pathways during endometriosis: From the molecular basis to the future perspectives. *Arch. Gynecol. Obstet.* **2016**, *294*, 897–904. [CrossRef]

34. Kokawa, K.; Shikone, T.; Nakano, R. Apoptosis in the human uterine endometrium during the menstrual cycle. *J. Clin. Endocrinol. Metab.* **1996**, *81*, 4144–4147.

35. Gebel, H.M.; Braun, D.P.; Tambur, A.; Frame, D.; Rana, N.; Dmowski, W.P. Spontaneous apoptosis of endometrial tissue is impaired in women with endometriosis. *Fertil. Steril.* **1998**, *69*, 1042–1047. [CrossRef]

36. Vaskivuo, T.E.; Stenbäck, F.; Karhumaa, P.; Risteli, J.; Dunkel, L.; Tapanainen, J.S. Apoptosis and apoptosis-related proteins in human endometrium. *Mol. Cell. Endocrinol.* **2000**, *165*, 75–83. [CrossRef]

37. Uegaki, T.; Taniguchi, F.; Nakamura, K.; Osaki, M.; Okada, F.; Yamamoto, O.; Harada, T. Inhibitor of apoptosis proteins (IAPs) may be effective therapeutic targets for treating endometriosis. *Hum. Reprod.* **2015**, *30*, 149–158. [CrossRef]

38. Vallée, A.; Lecarpentier, Y. Curcumin and Endometriosis. *Int. J. Mol. Sci.* **2020**, *21*, 2440. [CrossRef]

39. Riedl, S.J.; Shi, Y. Molecular mechanisms of caspase regulation during apoptosis. *Nat. Rev. Mol. Cell Biol.* **2004**, *5*, 897–907. [CrossRef]

40. Okada, H.; Mak, T.W. Pathways of apoptotic and non-apoptotic death in tumour cells. *Nat. Rev. Cancer* **2004**, *4*, 592–603. [CrossRef]

41. Altieri, D.C. Survivin, versatile modulation of cell division and apoptosis in cancer. *Oncogene* **2003**, *22*, 8581–8589. [CrossRef] [PubMed]

42. Altznauer, F.; Martinelli, S.; Yousefi, S.; Thürig, C.; Schmid, I.; Conway, E.M.; Schöni, M.H.; Vogt, P.; Mueller, C.; Fey, M.F.; et al. Inflammation-associated cell cycle-independent block of apoptosis by survivin in terminally differentiated neutrophils. *J. Exp. Med.* **2004**, *199*, 1343–1354. [CrossRef] [PubMed]

43. Bianco, B.; Filipchiuk, C.; Christofolini, D.M.; Barbosa, C.P.; Montagna, E. The role of survivin in the pathogenesis of endometriosis. *Minerva Med.* **2020**, *111*, 21–32. [CrossRef]

44. Matarese, G.; De Placido, G.; Nikas, Y.; Alviggi, C. Pathogenesis of endometriosis: Natural immunity dysfunction or autoimmune disease? *Trends Mol. Med.* **2003**, *9*, 223–228. [CrossRef]

45. Zwerts, F.; Lupu, F.; De Vriese, A.; Pollefeyt, S.; Moons, L.; Altura, R.A.; Jiang, Y.; Maxwell, P.H.; Hill, P.; Oh, H.; et al. Lack of endothelial cell survivin causes embryonic defects in angiogenesis, cardiogenesis, and neural tube closure. *Blood* **2007**, *109*, 4742–4752. [CrossRef]

46. Lee, M.O.; Moon, S.H.; Jeong, H.C.; Yi, J.-Y.; Lee, T.-H.; Shim, S.H.; Rhee, Y.-H.; Lee, S.-H.; Oh, S.-J.; Lee, M.-Y.; et al. Inhibition of pluripotent stem cell-derived teratoma formation by small molecules. *Proc. Natl. Acad. Sci. USA* **2013**, *110*, E3281–E3290. [CrossRef]

47. Gil-Kulik, P.; Krzyżanowski, A.; Dudzińska, E.; Karwat, J.; Chomik, P.; Świstowska, M.; Kondracka, A.; Kwaśniewska, A.; Cioch, M.; Jojczuk, M.; et al. Potential Involvement of *BIRC5* in Maintaining Pluripotency and Cell Differentiation of Human Stem Cells. *Oxid. Med. Cell. Longev.* **2019**, *2019*, 8727925. [CrossRef]

48. Mull, A.N.; Klar, A.; Navara, C.S. Differential localization and high expression of SURVIVIN splice variants in human embryonic stem cells but not in differentiated cells implicate a role for SURVIVIN in pluripotency. *Stem Cell Res.* **2014**, *12*, 539–549. [CrossRef]

49. Altieri, D.C. Survivin–The inconvenient IAP. *Semin. Cell Dev. Biol* **2015**, *39*, 91–96. [CrossRef]

50. Maijenburg, M.W.; Kleijer, M.; Vermeul, K.; Mul, E.P.J.; van Alphen, F.P.J.; van der Schoot, C.E.; Voermans, C. The composition of the mesenchymal stromal cell compartment in human bone marrow changes during development and aging. *Haematologica* **2012**, *97*, 179–183. [CrossRef]

51. Reagan, M.R.; Rosen, C.J. Navigating the bone marrow niche: Translational insights and cancer-driven dysfunction. *Nat. Rev. Rheumatol.* **2016**, *12*, 154–168. [CrossRef] [PubMed]

52. Laganà, A.S.; Salmeri, F.M.; Vitale, S.G.; Triolo, O.; Götte, M. Stem Cell Trafficking During Endometriosis: May Epigenetics Play a Pivotal Role? *Reprod. Sci.* **2018**, *25*, 978–979. [CrossRef] [PubMed]

53. Koninckx, P.R.; Ussia, A.; Adamyan, L.; Wattiez, A.; Gomel, V.; Martin, D.C. Pathogenesis of endometriosis: The genetic/epigenetic theory. *Fertil. Steril.* **2019**, *111*, 327–340. [CrossRef] [PubMed]

54. Alkatout, I. Laparoscopic hysterectomy: Total or subtotal?–Functional and didactic aspects. *Minim. Invasive Ther. Allied Technol.* **2020**. [CrossRef]

55. García-Gómez, E.; Vázquez-Martínez, E.R.; Reyes-Mayoral, C.; Cruz-Orozco, O.P.; Camacho-Arroyo, I.; Cerbón, M. Regulation of Inflammation Pathways and Inflammasome by Sex Steroid Hormones in Endometriosis. *Front. Endocrinol.* **2020**, *10*, 935. [CrossRef]

56. Laschke, M.W.; Menger, M.D. Anti-angiogenic treatment strategies for the therapy of endometriosis. *Hum. Reprod. Update* **2012**, *18*, 682–702. [CrossRef]

57. Acimovic, M.; Vidakovic, S.; Milic, N.; Jeremic, K.; Markovic, M.; Milosevic-Djeric, A.; Lazovic-Radonjic, G. Survivin and VEGF as Novel Biomarkers in Diagnosis of Endometriosis. *J. Med. Biochem.* **2016**, *35*, 63–68.

58. Mirabi, P.; Alamolhoda, S.H.; Golsorkhtabaramiri, M.; Namdari, M.; Esmaeilzadeh, S. Prolactin concentration in various stages of endometriosis in infertile women. *JBRA Assist. Reprod.* **2019**, *23*, 225–229. [CrossRef]

59. Marschalek, J.; Ott, J.; Husslein, H.; Kuessel, L.; Elhenicky, M.; Mayerhofer, K.; Franz, M.B. The impact of GnRH agonists in patients with endometriosis on prolactin and sex hormone levels: A pilot study. *Eur. J. Obstet. Gynecol. Reprod. Biol.* **2015**, *195*, 156–159. [CrossRef]

Genetic Characterization of Endometriosis Patients: Review of the Literature and a Prospective Cohort Study on a Mediterranean Population

Stefano Angioni [1,*], Maurizio Nicola D'Alterio [1,*], Alessandra Coiana [2], Franco Anni [3], Stefano Gessa [4] and Danilo Deiana [1]

[1] Department of Surgical Science, University of Cagliari, Cittadella Universitaria Blocco I, Asse Didattico Medicna P2, Monserrato, 09042 Cagliari, Italy; danideiana82@gmail.com

[2] Department of Medical Science and Public Health, University of Cagliari, Laboratory of Genetics and Genomics, Pediatric Hospital Microcitemico "A. Cao", Via Edward Jenner, 09121 Cagliari, Italy; acoiana@unica.it

[3] Department of Medical Science and Public Health, University of Cagliari, Cittadella Universitaria di Monserrato, Asse Didattico E, Monserrato, 09042 Cagliari, Italy; francoanni@gmail.com

[4] Laboratory of Molecular Genetics, Service of Forensic Medicine, AOU Cagliari, Via Ospedale 54, 09124 Cagliari, Italy; stefagessa@libero.it

[*] Correspondence: sangioni@yahoo.it (S.A.); mauridalte84@gmail.com (M.N.D.)

Abstract: The pathogenesis of endometriosis is unknown, but some evidence supports a genetic predisposition. The purpose of this study was to evaluate the recent literature on the genetic characterization of women affected by endometriosis and to evaluate the influence of polymorphisms of the wingless-type mammalian mouse tumour virus integration site family member 4 (WNT4), vezatin (VEZT), and follicle stimulating hormone beta polypeptide (FSHB) genes, already known to be involved in molecular mechanisms associated with the proliferation and development of endometriotic lesions in the Sardinian population. **Materials and Methods:** In order to provide a comprehensive and systematic tool for those approaching the genetics of endometriosis, the most cited review, observational, cohort and case-control studies that have evaluated the genetics of endometriosis in the last 20 years were collected. Moreover, 72 women were recruited for a molecular biology analysis of whole-blood samples—41 patients affected by symptomatic endometriosis and 31 controls. The molecular typing of three single nucleotide polymorphisms (SNPs) was evaluated in patients and controls: rs7521902, rs10859871 and rs11031006, mapped respectively in the WNT4, VEZT and FSHB genes. In this work, the frequency of alleles, genotypes and haplotypes of these SNPs in Sardinian women is described. **Results:** From the initial search, a total of 73 articles were chosen. An analysis of the literature showed that in endometriosis pathogenesis, the contribution of genetics has been well supported by many studies. The frequency of genotypes observed in the groups of the study population of 72 women was globally coherent with the law of the Hardy–Weinberg equilibrium. For the SNP rs11031006 (FSHB), the endometriosis group did not show an increase in genotypic or allelic frequency due to this polymorphism compared to the control group ($p = 0.9999$, odds ratio (OR) = 0.000, 95% confidence interval (CI), 0.000–15.000 and $p = 0.731$, OR = 1639, 95% CI, 0.39–683, respectively, for the heterozygous genotype and the polymorphic minor allele). For the SNP rs10859871 (VEZT), we found a significant difference in the frequency of the homozygous genotype in the control group compared to the affected women ($p = 0.0111$, OR = 0.0602, 95% CI, 0.005–0.501). For the SNP rs7521902 (WNT4), no increase in genotypic or allelic frequency between the two groups was shown ($p = 0.3088$, OR = 0.4133, 95% CI, 0.10–1.8 and $p = 0.3297$, OR = 2257, 95% CI, 0.55–914, respectively, for the heterozygous genotype and the polymorphic minor allele). **Conclusion:** An analysis of recent publications on the genetics of endometriosis showed a discrepancy in the results obtained in different populations. In the Sardinian population, the results obtained do not show a significant association between the investigated variants of the genes and a greater risk of developing endometriosis, although several other studies in the literature have shown the opposite. Anyway, the data underline the importance of evaluating genetic variants in different populations. In fact, in different ethnic groups, it is possible that specific risk alleles could act differently in the pathogenesis of the disease.

Keywords: endometriosis; genetic polymorphisms; SNPs; pathogenesis; aetiology; Mediterranean population; Sardinian population

1. Introduction

Endometriosis is a chronic disease of the reproductive age with a prevalence of 5%, reaching its peak between 25 and 35 years of age [1]. The scientific community agrees in recognizing a multifactorial aetiology of endometriosis, with possible genetic, hormonal, immunological and environmental factors as causes. Studies on family aggregation and twins have emphasized the genetic component, demonstrating how predisposition generated by certain susceptibility genes plays an important role in the development, maintenance and recurrence of the disease [2–5]. Nonetheless, studies on the genetics of endometriosis are complicated by various factors: the phenotypic heterogeneity of the disease; the still unknown prevalence in the population, burdened by the absence of registries and diagnostic underestimation; the invasiveness of diagnostic methods; and various co-morbidities that can generate bias [3]. In the field of research on the genetic basis of endometriosis, Simpson is considered a pioneer. In 1980, he verified in a sample of 123 women with histological diagnosis of endometriosis that 6.9% of first-degree relatives (mother and sisters) were affected, while the disease prevalence in controls (first-degree female relatives of the corresponding "husbands") was less than 1% [6]. In 1999, Treloar's work on an Australian population demonstrated a concordance ratio of 2:1 between monozygotic and dizygotic twins and a correspondent genetic risk of 2.34 to affect a sister. The study results show that 51% of genetic influence is responsible for developing endometriosis [7]. There is therefore enough evidence on how endometriosis is clearly heritable, although in what manner is not yet clear. The increased genetic risk in first-degree relatives (5–8%) suggests polygenic and multifactorial inheritance rather than monogenic. However, this recurrence risk is higher than the expected risk for a polygenic pathology (2–5%). The other, more likely, hypothesis is that phenotypic heterogeneity reflects genetic heterogeneity and that therefore not all forms of endometriosis are the same disease; in fact, some forms of endometriosis, due to their characteristics, behave almost like Mendelian pathologies [2]. The aim of this study was to evaluate the recent literature on the genetic characterization of women affected by endometriosis and to evaluate the influence of polymorphisms of the WNT4, VEZT and FSHB genes, known to be involved in molecular mechanisms associated with proliferation and development of endometriotic lesions in a particular Mediterranean population, the Sardinian population. The people of the Mediterranean island of Sardinia are particularly well suited for genetic studies, as is evident from a number of successes in complex trait and disease mapping [8].

The wingless-type mammalian mouse tumour virus integration site family member 4 (WNT4) gene is positioned on chromosome 1p36.23-p35 and codifies a protein which is essential in developing the female reproductive system [9–14]. It critically regulates the appropriate postnatal uterine maturation, as well as ovarian antral follicle growth [10]. The WNT class is an extensive group of secreted glycoproteins, codified through 19 different genes implicated in the WNT signalling pathway [9]. WNT-mediated signal transduction pathways address the specific mobilization of groups of genes which are responsible for managing several cellular responses, including cell growth, differentiation, movement, migration, polarity, cell survival and immune response [9]. A study published by Jordan et al. [15] demonstrated that WNT4 is the first signalling molecule causing the chain of events which ends with sex determination, through local secernment of growth factors. Imperfections in WNT4 activity play a role in the development of three important organs deriving from the primordial urogenital ridge—the kidneys, adrenal glands and gonads [9]. This may demonstrate the significant position of WNT4 at an early embryological stage of development. The loss of WNT4 in knockout mice determines the total absence of the Mullerian duct and its derivatives [11]. Apart from being crucial for epithelial–stromal cell communication in the endometrium, WNT signalling is likely important for endometrial maturation and differentiation and embryonic implantation [16]. An association between endometriosis and markers located in or near WNT4 has been highlighted in a number of extensive studies on gene mapping [17,18]. The expression of WNT4 has also been detected at the level of the peritoneum, leading to the consideration of a possible metaplastic hypothesis in promoting the transformation of peritoneal cells into endometriosic cells, through pathways with a role in the development of the female genital tract [12]. Pagliardini et al. demonstrated that a single nucleotide polymorphism (SNP), rs7521902, located 21 kb up/downstream of the WNT4 region, has a susceptibility locus for endometriosis. The functional significance of this SNP in endometriosis remains to be explained [10]. While the SNP rs7521902 was connected to endometriosis susceptibility in British, Australian, Italian and Japanese women [10,18,19], in Belgian [13] and Brazilian women this association was not found [9]. The different genetic backgrounds of the cohorts may be identified as the reason for the lack of association between this polymorphism and endometriosis.

The vezatin (VEZT) gene is located on chromosome 12 locus 12q22; it codifies vezatin, a significant element of the cadherin–catenin complex, which plays a crucial role in the formation and sustenance of adherent joints [20–24]. According to Kussel-Andermann et al., vezatin was found to be a plasma membrane component with a short extracellular domain, a transmembrane domain and an extended intracellular domain. Its intracellular domain connects to myosin VIIA as part of the adherens junctional complex in epithelial cells [21]. Furthermore, several studies on co-immunoprecipitation showed that the system between vezatin and myosin VIIA is able to interact with the system between E-cadherin and catenin, although the specificity of this interaction remains to be determined [21,22]. Also, VEZT is fundamental for implantation; embryos from mice with silenced VEZT cannot develop after the blastocyst stage, because of a loss of adhesion between cells [25]. It has been highlighted that VEZT protein is extensively expressed in human endometrium and myometrium. During the secretory phase of the menstrual cycle, VEZT expression increases in the glandular epithelium in a significant way. The mRNA expression of adherens junction members (E-cadherin and A- and B-catenin) is also enhanced in the secretory phase with respect to the proliferative phase. This indicates that progesterone could be responsible for activating cell-to-cell adhesion [20]. The VEZT promoter does not contain a reaction point for the progesterone receptor (PR), but it contains a nuclear factor kappa B (NF-kB) binding site. As a pro-inflammatory transcription factor, NF-kB is involved in the pathogenesis of endometriosis, showing cycle control in the endometrium and reciprocal management with PR [26]. Therefore, variations in VEZT levels in endometrial glandular cells are likely to occur in response to the dynamic oscillation in progesterone and associated NF-kB changes [20]. Considering the studied physiological roles of VEZT, its potential for a functional role in endometriosis is a likely option, since VEZT has been demonstrated to be upregulated in ectopic endometrium with respect to eutopic endometrium in patients suffering from endometriosis [20,23,24].

The follicle-stimulating hormone beta polypeptide (FSHB) gene, positioned on chromosome 11 locus 11p14.1, codifies subunit b of the hormone-specific follicle-stimulating hormone (FSH), with a crucial role in the growth of ovarian follicles and production of oestrogens [27–29]. Recently, some evidence for an association between endometriosis and SNPs of FSHB was reported in independent targets from the UK Biobank, firmly supporting this result [28]. FSH and luteinizing hormone (LH) are related gonadotropin hormones sharing the same alpha subunit. A connection between these SNPs on chromosome 11 with concentrations of both hormones indicates a common mechanism of regulation, with both being key elements in managing follicle development in the ovary, influencing oestradiol release during the proliferative phase of the cycle and contributing to a role for oestradiol in endometriosis risk [27]. Data from the ENCODE project [30] show that the SNP rs11031006 modifies the sequence of 11 protein-binding motifs, including that of oestrogen receptor α, with a possible effect on hormonal feedback inhibition. Recently, allele G of this SNP has been proven to be significantly associated with higher levels of serum FSH [29].

1.1. Review of the Literature

This review aims to provide a comprehensive and systematic tool for those approaching the genetics of endometriosis. Computerized literature searches were conducted using the Medline/PubMed database and a manual search of relevant and frequently cited publications in the English language from 1999 to 2019. Additional articles were identified by manually searching references from the retrieved eligible articles. Keywords included: endometriosis combined with genes, genetics, SNPs, genome-wide association study (GWAS), WNT4, VEZT, FSHB, next-generation sequencing (NGS) and epigenetics. Review, observational, cohort and case-control studies that evaluated the genetics of endometriosis are herein described.

1.2. Cohort Study

The study was carried out through molecular typing of the following single nucleotide polymorphisms (SNPs): rs7521902, rs10859871 and rs11031006, mapped, respectively, in the WNT4, VEZT and FSHB genes. In this work, we set out to describe the frequency of alleles and genotypes of these SNPs among Sardinian women, and to evaluate their impact on the susceptibility to develop endometriosis. The choice of which polymorphisms were to be analysed fell to WNT4, VEZT and FSHB genes because of their hypothetical correlation with endometriosis, according to recent findings in the literature. Several GWAS meta-analyses have reported a possible pathogenetic role [16,27]. In particular, an association study published in 2017 analysed these SNPs in a Greek population, highlighting a significant connection with the disease [29]. The molecular biological examinations of single-substitution polymorphisms in our study were carried out from whole blood drawn exclusively from Sardinian patients, upon their informed consent. We chose to limit the study to only patients of Sardinian origin, considering the peculiarity of this island, which can be seen as a genetic macro-isolate. The choice of limiting the selection of the target population to patients of Sardinian origin for at least three generations was not intended to exclude the possible influence of genetic features from non-Sardinian distant ancestors. It was, rather, an attempt to make the target more homogeneous.

The genetic analysis of complex traits is simplified in isolated populations such as this one, in which inbreeding and the "founder effect" reduce the genetic diversity of complex and polygenic diseases such as endometriosis. The goal was to identify a genetic characterization of the disease in the Sardinian population, to shed light on the etiopathogenetic mechanisms of endometriosis, and to provide predictive markers for a non-invasive diagnosis of the disease.

Patients and Study Design

The present clinical study represents the initial application, on a small scale, of a study protocol conducted at the Department of Obstetrics and Gynaecology of the Hospital "Duilio Casula" of Monserrato, University of Cagliari, in collaboration with the Laboratory of Genetics and Genomics of the Pediatric Hospital Microcitemico "A. Cao" of Cagliari. Written consent was obtained from the local ethics committee (EndoSNPs, Prot. PG/2019/13157). In line with the Declaration of Helsinki 1975, revised in Hong Kong in 1989, the clinical trial was registered (ClinicalTrials.gov ID: NCT02388854). This study involved a total of 72 women who underwent surgery, 41 representing the cases with clinical and histological diagnosis of endometriosis, and 31 representing the corresponding controls—women without a diagnosis of endometriosis who underwent surgery for benign indications different from endometriosis and chronic pelvic pain. For each patient, a data collection folder was prepared in a database elaborated for the purpose. Apart from personal records, data on geographic origin and anthropometric measurements (weight, height, body mass index (BMI)), the data collection form contained data on habits such as cigarette smoking and alcohol intake, and clinical data on possible co-morbidities or previous surgical interventions. In patients with a diagnosis of endometriosis, data on this pathology were obviously included (familiarity, staging, location of lesions, transvaginal ultrasound data, gynaecological examination, symptomatology, number and type of surgical operations, histological data), type and duration of drug therapy (nonsteroidal anti-inflammatory drugs (NSAIDs), hormone therapy and antibiotics). The diagnosis of endometriosis was clinical, related to ultrasound and histology reports. The staging used was the revised classification proposed by the American Fertility Society/American Society for Reproductive Medicine (AFS/ASRM) [30], which is still the most widespread and widely used, in clinical and academic fields, to describe the severity of endometriosis in a standardized format. Localizations of deep infiltrating endometriosis (DIE) infiltrating the bladder or bowel were classified as severe. For each main symptom (dysmenorrhea, chronic pelvic pain, dyspareunia, intestinal symptoms, urinary symptoms), a score was assigned based on the intensity perceived by the patient (visual analogue scale (VAS) 0–3: mild; 4–7: moderate; 8–10: severe). For the controls, women who had never had a diagnosis or a suspicion of endometriosis were selected. The close and remote pathological medical history of these patients was also negative for dysmenorrhea, dyspareunia, chronic pelvic pain and infertility/sub-fertility, as one of the inclusion criteria was to have given birth to at least 2 children. A common criterion to be included in the study was geographic origin. All participants had an exclusively Sardinian origin for at least 3 generations (maternal and paternal grandparents from Sardinia).

2. Results

2.1. Review of the Literature

2.1.1. Gene Polymorphisms

Single nucleotide polymorphisms are present in the population with an allelic frequency >1%, and represent the most common type of genetic variation in humans (90% of polymorphisms). They are present with alternative allelic variants and follow a Mendelian inheritance. Their wide dissemination in the genetic makeup (one in every 100–300 base pairs) makes them interesting in studies on allelic association and usable as molecular markers. Single nucleotide polymorphisms (SNPs) can generate synonymous or non-synonymous mutations if present in coding regions of genes, or lead to alterations of the gene product if present in intronic or intergenic regions [2]. Variations in the genome may determine different individual susceptibilities to a disease, or different pharmacological responses. SNPs are therefore useful to identify "disease genes" through association studies based on population screening [2]. Technological advances in the field of molecular biology, especially through polymerase chain reaction (PCR) techniques, have stimulated interest in identifying certain gene polymorphisms and their influence on susceptibility in developing endometriosis. The choice of candidate genes falls to those genes whose polymorphic variants are hypothesized to be involved in the pathophysiological molecular mechanisms underlying the disease: genes involved in steroidogenesis and in receptorial activity of sex hormones, genes involved in inflammatory and immune response processes, genes regulating metabolism, genes affecting the processes of tissue remodelling and neoangiogenesis, and DNA repair genes [31,32].

2.1.2. Genes Involved in Stereidogenesis and Receptorial Activity of Sex Hormones

Endometriosic and endometrial tissues are responsive to the effect of sexual steroid hormones, especially oestrogens. It is no coincidence that the risk factors of this disease include early menarche and late-onset menopause, conditions that notoriously involve extended exposure to endogenous oestrogens throughout life. Therefore, among the most common pathogenetic hypotheses is that there is possible dysregulation of the ligand-receptorial signalling involving the main sex hormones, oestrogens and progesterone [33,34]. The choice of candidate genes for various association studies is based on this mechanism. The two estrogenic receptor (ER) isoforms (ER-beta and ER-alpha) are codified by two genes (ESR2 and ESR1) with tissue-specific distributions, and have different capacities in connecting ligands (oestrogen and antioestrogen) and starting the transcription of target genes. The influence of ESR1 gene polymorphisms was studied in women affected by endometriosis in different populations, both European and Asian, but with inconsistent results. For the ESR2 gene, the studied polymorphism is localized in region 3'UTR of the gene, on nucleotide 1730 (1730 adenine (A) → guanine (G)), and it is recognized by the restriction enzyme AluI. This polymorphism has been related to a risk of severe stage IV endometriosis in women of Japanese origin [35], but no significant association with the development of the disease in Italian and Korean women was seen [36]. The pathogenetic hypothesis that there is involvement of the corresponding receptors and their malfunctioning in determining those phenomena involved in the development of endometriosis is based on the dysregulation of tissue sensitivity influenced by progesterone. In particular, as an object of numerous studies on their role in the onset and development of ovarian carcinoma, the polymorphism of progesterone receptor (PR) gene, called PROGINS, seems to compromise the perfect receptor–ligand functionality in target tissues, making them less sensitive to progesterone and altering the hormonal balance in favour of oestrogenic activity. The PROGINS polymorphism was found more frequently in women suffering from endometriosis. A statistically significant association was found in affected women from Italy [37], Austria [38] and Brazil [39], while similar studies on women from India [40], Australia [41] and Germany [42] came to exactly opposite conclusions. Other more or less recent studies focused their research on gene polymorphisms of the androgen receptor (AR). Androgens play an important role, although not sufficiently clarified, in endometrial physiology and physiopathology, counteracting the effect of oestrogen on cell proliferation [43–46]. The AR gene is localized on the Xq11.2-q12 chromosome; the corresponding protein has eight domains with transactivation function, all distributed in exon 1. Here, we find a polymorphic microsatellite consisting of a cytosine–adenine–guanine (CAG) sequence, variously repeated in individuals, on which the length of glutamine residues in the amino-terminal end of the AR protein depends, with repercussions on its functionality [47,48]. In this case, the results are very different regarding the ethnic group used as a sample. Shaik's work on a female Indian population concluded that the presence of 19–21 CAG repeats of the AR gene could be considered a susceptibility marker for endometriosis and uterine leiomyoma [49], confirming the results obtained from a previous work on Taiwanese women [50], but in stark contrast to Lattuada's results on Italian women [51].

2.1.3. Genes Involved in Inflammation and Immune Response

The development of the inflammatory process is an integral part of the pathophysiology of endometriosis. Polymorphisms of numerous cytokines have become the objects of many studies, but with conflicting results. In their work on a female Taiwanese population, Hsieh et al. demonstrated an association between susceptibility to endometriosis and the presence of gene polymorphisms: −509C/T in the region promoter of the transforming growth factor-β1 (TGF-β1) gene, −627A/C in the region promoter of the interleukin 10 (IL-10) gene, and 881T/C in the IL2 beta receptor gene [52]. A 2017 study focused on TGF-β1, in particular on how it affects the development and progression of the disease with regard to hypoxia. The results support the hypothesis that TGF-β1 is involved in the pathogenesis of endometriosis through the regulation of vascular endothelial growth factor (VEGF) expression. TGF-β not only increased its levels, but also had an additive effect at the transcriptional level on hypoxia itself, increasing the expression of VEGF up to 87% [53]. The polymorphisms of the gene coding for cytokine TNF-α, with regard to its key role in the development of the acute phase of inflammatory processes and regulation of the immune response, have also been at the centre of several works: variations in promoter regions do not appear to be associated with an increased risk of endometriosis in Korean, Taiwanese and Caucasian women [54]. Several lines of evidence prove that endometriosis is characterized by specific modifications of the immune system, in particular endowing endometriosic cells with the ability to elude the mechanisms of immunosurveillance and thus guarantee easier implantation and development in ectopic sites. Among these mechanisms, we can hypothesize changes in the expression of human leukocyte antigens (HLAs), important for immunological recognition, secretion of circulating antigens competing with surface antigens, critical for self/non-self-recognition, and production of immunosuppressive or proapoptotic factors against T cell effector [55]. The HLA system or major histocompatibility complex (MHC) is the gene complex which boasts the largest number of polymorphisms in the human genome. Wang's study of 2001 on Chinese women reported the influence of polymorphisms of the HLA-B gene, but not the HLA-A gene, on the susceptibility to the development of endometriosis [56], whereas Ishi in 2003 reported a significant association with HLA-DRB1*1403 and HLA-DQB1*03031 alleles in Japanese women, but not with HLADPB1 [57]. In this case, too, we detect conflicting results. PTPN22 is a coding gene for a protein involved in the responsiveness of B and T lymphocyte receptors, whose mutations may be responsible for the onset of autoimmune diseases. The associations observed between PTPN22 (C1858T) and the risk of endometriosis suggest that this polymorphism could be a useful marker of susceptibility to the disease [58].

2.1.4. Genes Involved in the Processes of Tissue Remodeling and Neoangiogenesis

Vascular endothelial growth factor (VEGF) and endothelial growth factor receptor (EGFR) are molecular factors known to be involved in the regulation of neoangiogenesis, tissue remodelling and proliferation, phenomena also necessary for the growth of ectopic foci of endometrial tissue. Specifically, VEGF induces the proliferation, migration and differentiation of endothelial cells and capillary formation. Several studies have shown high levels of VEGF in peritoneal fluid and serum, and increased expression of mRNA and proteins in patients with endometriosis [59]. Furthermore, VEGF causes an increase in vascular permeability and a release of proteases such as metalloproteases (MMPs), enzymes able to "cut" the proteins of matrix and basement membrane, important for cellular invasion and tissue remodelling. It can also prevent apoptosis of different cell types. Perini's group study in 2014 on Brazilian women indicated a risk association with −1154G> polymorphism A of the VEGF gene [59]. EGFR is a transmembrane glycoprotein which plays an important role in the control of growth, differentiation and cell motility. The EGFR +2073A/T polymorphism, a candidate as a susceptibility gene, was studied by Hsieh et al. in 122 Taiwanese women and 139 controls, showing an association with a high risk of disease. These results were subsequently denied when reported to the Japanese population [60].

2.1.5. Genes Regulating Metabolism

Glutathione S-transferase mu M1 (GSTM1), glutathione S-transferase P1 (GSTP1), glutathione S-transferase theta T1 (GSTT1), N-acetyltransferase 1 (NAT1) and N-acetyltransferase 2 (NAT2) genes all encode phase II enzymes involved in the metabolism of xenobiotics, including toxic compounds such as dioxin and polycyclic aromatic hydrocarbons. In particular, a 2015 meta-analysis by Guo on the association between variants of GST, GSTM1 and GSTT1 genes, which encode for glutathione S transferase, and the development of endometriosis showed a significant increase in risk. Women with GSTM1-null genotype compared to other genotypes recorded a summary OR of 1.96, demonstrating an approximately double risk of endometriosis. Women with GSTT1-null genotype compared to other genotypes recorded a summary OR of 1.77, showing an 80% risk of endometriosis. Nevertheless, the existence of bias in this meta-analysis indicates that the magnitude of risk could be smaller or even non-existent [61]. Many gene polymorphisms corresponding to phase I enzymes involved in, among other things, oestrogen metabolism were investigated as variants associated with a greater susceptibility to disease, for example CYP1A1 6235T/C, CYP17A1 −34T/C and CYP19A1 microsatellite TTTA repeat [62,63].

2.1.6. Genes Related to the Process of DNA Repair

Many studies have proposed oxidative stress as a factor involved in the pathophysiology of endometriosis [64]. An excess of reactive oxygen species causes DNA damage, base modifications and chromosomal aberrations, which would justify the metaplastic features of the disease. The DNA repair system from oxidative stress involves the intervention of enzymes encoded by genes including X-ray repair cross-complementing 1 and 3 (XRCC1 and XRCC3) and XPD (also known as excision repair cross-complementing (ERCC)), whose defective functioning decisively contributes to develop endometriosic lesions. Attar et al. in 2010 reported no significant differences between the frequency of genotypes and polymorphic alleles of APE1, XRCC1, XPD, XPG and HOGG1 genes in patients with and without endometriosis, whilst a significant increase in disease frequency would appear to be associated with the XRCC3 Thr/Thr genotype [65].

2.1.7. Genome-Wide Association Study (GWAS) and Next-Generation Sequencing (NGS)

So far, we have discussed works adopting an investigative approach based on the a priori selection of polymorphisms of candidate genes known to have hypothetical biological roles in the pathogenesis of endometriosis, and their subsequent research on DNA samples. A radical change in perspective was applied in the so-called hypothesis-free methods, such as the analysis of family linkage, association studies on the genomic scale, or genome-wide studies (GWASs), up to the most recent new generation sequencing technique, next-generation sequencing (NGS), which targets the entire genome, without pre-selecting a particular gene or gene region, therefore with no initial pathogenetic hypothesis. Among its main advantages, this type of approach can detect alterations of unexpected molecular pathways perhaps shared by apparently very different pathologies. Analyses of family linkage and genome-wide association studies are different though complementary approaches to the identification of genetic risk variants across the whole spectrum of allele frequencies. A linkage analysis aims to identify those genetic variants which are rare in the general population, but are responsible for the family aggregation of a given pathology, while a GWAS aims to identify genetic common variants in the general population associated with the risk of the disease [66]. Studies of family linkage have analysed the association between a known marker and the unknown gene/disease, assuming their proximity to the chromosome and the consequent co-segregation in affected families. In 2005, an impressive linkage study was carried out by Treloar's group on 1176 English and Australian families, each with at least two members, mainly sister pairs, with a surgical diagnosis of endometriosis, for a total of 4985 genotyped individuals, 2709 of them women with endometriosis. This study found a strongly significant linkage on chromosome 10q26 and another region suggestive of linkage on chromosome 20p13 [67]. The fine-mapping of the 10q26 region using 11,984 SNPs in 1144 affected families and 1190 controls was described in a study by Painter's group in 2011, which identified three signs of significant association with endometriosis [68]. Among them, the only one to be replicated in an independent cohort was rs11592737, located in the CYP2C19 gene, an important candidate gene involved in oestrogenic metabolism, particularly in the conversion of oestradiol to oestrone [69]. However, despite the valuable contribution of this method to the study of monogenic pathologies, this technique was shown to be less accurate when applied to multifactorial diseases such as endometriosis, able to identify extensive chromosome regions containing hundreds of genes with too large and inaccurate linkage peaks. This fact, together with the lack of sensitivity and the difficulty of independently replicating the positive results related to the need for a large number of affected families with more generations available to test, has made this method obsolete, opening the way to the more promising GWAS. A GWAS is a survey on all, or almost all, genes of an individual of a particular species to determine the gene variations between them. Later, attempts are made to associate the observed differences with some specific traits, such as a disease. In these cases, samples from hundreds or thousands of individuals are evaluated, usually looking for single nucleotide polymorphisms (SNPs). Instead of reading whole gene sequences, these systems usually identify SNP markers of groups of gene variations (haplotypes). If some gene variations are significantly more frequent in sick individuals, then the variations are said to be associated with the disease. These variations are then considered indicative of the region where the disease-causing mutation is likely to be found. The first GWAS on endometriosis was carried out on a Japanese population in 2010, on a sample of 1432 cases and 1318 controls. The study identified a significant association ($p = 5.6 \times 10^{-12}$; OR 1.44 (1.30–1.59)) with the SNP rs10965235 located on the CDKN2B-AS1 gene on chromosome 9 and with the SNP rs16826658 ($p = 1.7 \times 10^{-6}$ OR 1.2 (1.11–1.29)) located on the WNT4 gene on chromosome 1 [18]. The first gene regulates some onco-suppressors such as CDKN2B, CDKN2A and ARF; its inactivation has been correlated with the development of endometriosic foci and endometrial carcinoma [70]. The second one is a very important gene involved in the development of the female genital apparatus, indispensable for the formation of Müllerian ducts [12]. It has a sequence that regulates ESR1 and ESR2 genes, and it is still among the main candidate genes for endometriosis and ovarian cancer. A subsequent GWAS of 2016 also focused on this gene. Using a sample of 7090 individuals (2594 cases and 4496 controls), the study found the marker in the region of the WNT4 gene, with the strongest association with the risk of endometriosis: the SNP rs3820282 [71]. In 2011, a subsequent GWAS was conducted through the International Endogene Consortium (IEC) by Painter's group on British and Australian women, analysing 3194 cases of surgically diagnosed endometriosis and 7060 controls [19]. The study divided the sample of affected individuals into two categories based on the severity of the pathology (stage I–II and stage III–IV), and detected a strongly significant linkage, in particular in the "severe" subgroup, with two SNPs: rs1250248 ($p = 3.2 \times 10^{-8}$; OR 1.30 (1.19–1.43)), located on the FN1 gene on chromosome 2, involved in cell adhesion and migration, and rs12700667, ($p = 1.5 \times 10^{-9}$; OR 1.38 (1.24–1.53)), located on an intergenic region of chromosome 7p15 containing regulatory elements, located upstream of three candidate genes: miRNA148a (88kb), the closest, encoding a microRNA implicated in the important Wnt β-catenin signalling pathway for the homeostasis of sex hormones; NFE2L3 (331 kb), encoding a transcription factor involved in the processes of phlogosis, differentiation and carcinogenesis, highly expressed in the placenta; and the HOXA 10-11 genes, coding for homeobox A transcription factors, considered important in the spatial and temporal regulation of uterine development about 1.35 Mb downstream. Thanks to the data of this GWAS, it was also possible to refute the conclusions of later works, such as the study of Grechukhina in 2012, which reported a high frequency (31% vs. 5% case-control) of SNP rs61764370 in the 3'UTR region of the Kirsten rat sarcoma viral oncogene homolog (KRAS) gene in women with endometriosis [72]. The KRAS gene was considered a strong candidate gene; in fact, KRAS activation determined the development of peritoneal endometriosis in 47% of mice and endometriosis-like ovarian lesions in 100%. SNP rs61764370 interrupts the link between the LCS6 complementary site and let-7 miRNA, altering the expression of the KRAS gene and favouring the development of the disease. The analysis conducted in 2012 by Hien Luong and Painter denied this risk association [73]. A meta-analysis of the GWASs of the IEC and the Japanese group, carried out in 2012, confirmed the associations previously reported in the respective studies and identified further significant new loci of association localized on GREB1 genes, involved in estrogenic regulation; VEZT, involved in cell growth, migration and adhesion; and ID4, an ovarian tumour suppressor [17]. Another interesting GWAS of 2017 was a meta-analysis of 11 case-control datasets, for a total of 17,045 cases of endometriosis and 191,596 controls. Five additional new loci significantly associated with the risk of endometriosis ($p < 5 \times 10^{-8}$) of genes involved in sexual steroid hormone pathways (FN1, CCDC170, ESR1, SYNE1 and FSHB) were identified, for a total of 16 genomic regions associated with endometriosis risk in one or more populations [27]. At present, 19 independent single nucleotide polymorphisms (SNPs) have been validly associated with endometriosis, explaining 5.19% of disease variance [27]. In particular, a recent study investigated in a Greek population three of these SNPs: rs7521902, rs10859871 and rs11031006, mapped respectively on WNT4, VEZT and FSHB genes, highlighting a significant association with endometriosis [29]. In recent years, thanks above all to the reduction in cost and time of examination, an innovative DNA reading technique has come forward forcefully: next-generation sequencing (NGS). Through NGS, it is possible to analyse a large number of DNA fragments in parallel, until the sequences of many genes are obtained simultaneously, even the entire coding region (exome sequencing) or the whole genome (whole genome sequencing) of an individual. Instead of screening several variants, the most common ones, scattered throughout the genome as in the genome arrays of GWASs, with an NGS reading it is possible to search for the rarest variants in a population. A study of families affected by endometriosis using NGS was conducted in 2014 by Chettier et al.; out of 13 pairs of affected sisters, five shared genomic regions (in chromosomes 2, 5, 9 and 11) where rare gene variants associated with endometriosis are located [74]. In February 2016, Er's research group focused on the molecular characterization of endometriosis associated with ovarian cancer through targeted NGS of 409 cancer-related genes by identifying gene variants on the PIK3CA and ARID1A genes, related to endometriosis with a high risk of malignant transformation [75]. Most GWA variants associated with the risk of endometriosis are not codified and the genes responsible for association signals have not been identified. A direct approach to identifying target genes could be identifying variants encoding common proteins associated with the risk of endometriosis. Large international exon sequencing projects have identified exome variants modifying the coding of corresponding proteins (nonsynonymous codification, alternative splicing sites or stopping codon gain or loss), classifying them according to their frequency. The role of protein-coding variants associated with endometriosis risk was therefore directly tested by genotyping through a specific Illumina array (Illumina exome chip) designed to allow the simultaneous capture of rare, low-frequency and common frequency exonerated variants. In all, 7164 patients with endometriosis and 210,005 controls were analysed. The initial association between disease and variations in encoding the CUBN, CIITA and PARP4 genes was not confirmed when replicating the study [76]. There is therefore no clear evidence of the existence of codifying variants of common or low-frequency proteins which can influence the risk of endometriosis. Variants capable of directly modifying the sequence and function of protein amino acids would have provided immediate gene targets. The causal SNPs are probably located in non-codifying sequences, but are involved in functions regulating gene expression and are able to influence the development and progression of disease [77]. If GWASs have identified various susceptibility loci, the biggest challenge of the post-GWAS era is therefore to understand the functional consequences of these loci. Studying the association between genetic variations and gene expression offers a way to link risk variants with the corresponding target genes. Gene expression varies in different individuals, and the level of expression of certain genes is under the control of particular regulatory variants indicated as expression quantitative traits loci (eQTLs), which can influence the abundance of specific transcripts [78]. Various study groups have identified three eQTLs capable of altering the transcription of potential target genes: LINC0039 and CDC42 on chromosome 1, CDKN2A-AS1 on chromosome 9 and VEZT on chromosome 12. Further functional studies are needed to confirm the role of causal genes in different susceptibility loci [79].

2.1.8. Epigenetics

During the past five years, evidence has emerged that endometriosis may be an epigenetic disease. Epigenetics proves to be the common denominator of a pathology in which both genetic and environmental components play pathogenetic roles. Many large-scale profiling studies on gene expression have unequivocally demonstrated that many genes are deregulated in endometriosis [80]. Several aspects related to possible post-transcriptional interference that may result in changes in endometriosic tissues, compared to healthy ones, have been investigated. These modifications are expressed at different levels (transcriptional, post-transcriptional, post-translational) and through different mechanisms (methylation, histone modification, activators, repressors, miRNAs). In particular, changes in terms of hypermethylation and silencing of genes which are normally expressed during the proliferative phase of the cycle and regulate the modalities of cell adhesion have been studied, such as HOXA-10, E-cadherin, the GATA family of transcription factors and the group of nuclear receptors for steroids (SR), which includes the progesterone receptors in two isoforms, PR-A and PR-B. The opposite transcriptional activity of the two isoforms has been demonstrated to be due to binding of the Hic-5 differential co-regulator. This type of change affects the resistance of endometriosis to treatment with progesterone [81]. Expression by endometrial tissue of the two receptors for progesterone, PR-A and PR-B, and their relationship influences the reaction of tissue to exposure to progestins. A prevalence of PR-A results in resistance to therapy and loss of cell adhesion. In vitro studies have shown that deacetylase inhibitors show promise as therapies for the treatment of endometriosis. In particular, trichostatin A has been shown to reactivate the expression of E-cadherin, an intercellular adhesion protein, which is hypermethylated and therefore silenced in endometriotic cell lines, with a concomitant reduction in invasiveness [80]. MiRNAs are a class of endogenous NcRNAs of about 22 nucleotides, which play a key role in regulating gene expression. As well as DNA methylation and histone modification, they implement this regulation without any change in DNA sequence, but inhibit or induce miRNA degradation. A profiling study of miRNA expression identified 48 out of 287 miRNAs differentially expressed in healthy women and women with endometriosis. The target genes of these miRNAs include many genes involved in endometriosis (Erα, ERβ, PR, TGFβ), suggesting that miRNA deregulation may play a pathogenetic role [80]. Acetylation, methylation and phosphorylation are the most well-known and studied post-translational histone modifications. These changes alter the interaction of histone with DNA and nuclear proteins. In general, histone acetylation is associated with transcriptional activation and deacetylation with transcriptional repression [82,83]. Studies on animals seemed to suggest that HDAC2 is expressed aberrantly in ectopic endometrium. Furthermore, Sun et al. (2003) reported that treatment of endometriotic stromal cells with prostaglandin E2 (PGE2) resulted in increased acetylation of histone H3 bound to StAR promoter, with concomitant induction of co-activator CBP/p300, binding of CREB protein, and possible involvement in the pathogenesis of endometriosis [84]. So far, studies on epigenetics have barely scratched the surface of this area, and further research will allow us to shed light on the pathophysiology of endometriosis, and on the complex mechanisms regulating the activation or silencing of different genetic targets. Such knowledge will provide a basis for the identification of new drugs and diagnostic biomarkers.

2.2. Cohort Study

The patients' average age was 35 years (median 33 years in the group of cases, 36 years in the group of controls). The median values of body mass index (BMI) in the two groups were uniform (21 for cases vs. 22 for controls). Among the affected women, we found comorbidities in nine: two cases of haemorrhoidal disease, one of serous cystadenoma, borderline mucinous cystadenoma associated with breast cancer, mitral valve prolapse, umbilical hernia, anxiety disorder, hyperinsulinemia, and irritable colon. Among the controls, nine women had a pathological medical history: HashimotO's thyroiditis (5), type 2 diabetes mellitus, hypercholesterolaemia, uterine prolapse (1), renal ptosis (1), gastro-oesophageal reflux disease (1), breast fibroadenoma (1) (Table 1).

Table 1. Clinical and personal data of the study population. BMI, body mass index.

Clinical and Personal Data of the Study Population			
Patients	**Total (n = 72)**	**Endometriosis (n = 41)**	**No Endometriosis (n = 31)**
Age (median, interval)	35 (20–68)	33 (20–45)	36 (26–68)
BMI (median, interval)	21 (15–30)	21 (17–30)	22 (15–30)
Comorbidity	18	9	9
Parity		0.25	2.3

In the sample of women diagnosed with endometriosis, six were at stage I (minimum disease), with superficial lesions; five were at stage II (mild disease), with extended foci (up to 4 cm) in different locations; 14 were at stage III (moderate disease), mostly cases of ovarian endometrioma; and 16 were at stage IV (severe disease), in which we included cases of deep endometriosis with extended nodular formations (5–6 cm) and infiltrating contiguous structures such as the rectum, pararectal spaces, ureters and retroperitoneum. Table 2 shows, for each stage, the data related to age and BMI at the time of diagnosis, which was almost uniform among the subgroups; number of term pregnancies; surgical interventions for the treatment of the disease, performed laparoscopically in all cases, two completed with intestinal resection; and extent and severity of symptoms (the percentage of symptoms perceived as severe (score 3) was higher in stage IV (94%) than in stage I (40%)). In stages II and III, the degree of symptom severity perceived by women showed similar scores (60% vs. 64%), proving that symptomatology is not always connected linearly to the surgical stage of the disease. None of the women in the group of affected patients reported a family medical history positive for endometriosis.

Table 2. Distribution of clinical anamnestic data of the group of affected women.

Stage	I	II	III	IV
Number of patients	6	5	14	16
Age (median)	35	22	37	31
Parity (number of patients with at least one pregnancy)	0	1	5	2
BMI (median)	21	20	20	20
Number of patients with previous surgical intervention for endometriosis	0	2	10	14
Dysmenorrhea				
Mild	2	0	0	1
Moderate	1	2	6	1
Severe	2	3	7	14
Chronic pelvic pain				
Mild	0	1	2	0
Moderate	2	2	3	6
Severe	0	0	3	6
Dyspareunia				
Mild	2	1	4	2
Moderate	1	2	2	6
Severe	0	1	3	6
Intestinal symptoms	2	0	7	10
Urinary symptoms	2	0	3	3
Severe symptomatology percentage *	40%	60%	64%	94%

* Percentage of women who attributed a maximum severity score (visual analogue scale (VAS) 7–10) to at least one symptom (dysmenorrhea, chronic pelvic pain, dyspareunia, intestinal or urinary symptoms); mild (0–3); moderate (4–7); severe (8–10).

The frequency of genotypes observed in the groups of the reference population, 72 individuals, was globally consistent with the Hardy–Weinberg equilibrium law (Table 3).

Table 3. Expected and observed frequencies and Hardy–Weinberg equilibrium (HWE) p-values for SNPs investigated in total population.

SNP	TEST	A1 Minor Allele	A2 Major Allele	GENO	Observed (HET)	Expected (HET)	P
SNP1(FSHB)G>A	ALL	A	G	1/7/62	0.1	0.1203	0.2396
SNP2(VEZT)A>C	ALL	C	A	8/27/32	0.403	0.4358	0.5766
SNP3(WNT4)C>A	ALL	A	C	0/10/55	0.1538	0.142	1

Applying the HWE test to all components of the study population (cases + controls), there are no consistent differences between expected and observed genotypic frequencies, as shown by the p-values calculated for each investigated SNP. The p-values obtained are equal to 0.2396 for rs11031006 (FSHB), 0.5766 for rs10859871 (VEZT) and 1 for rs7521902 (WNT4); they allow us to accept the starting hypothesis, according to which there is no difference among the examined groups concerning the considered parameters. For each SNP, checking the expected and observed genotypic/allelic frequencies in single groups of affected cases and healthy controls, a modest significance in deviation from the Hardy–Weinberg equilibrium is highlighted, regarding the group of positive controls for genotypes containing allele C of the polymorphism rs10859871 (VEZT) (HWE p-value = 0.0435.) This violation of the proportions of the Hardy–Weinberg equilibrium could constitute a bias selection (Table 4).

Table 4. Expected and observed frequencies and HWE *p*-values for SNPs investigated in groups of affected cases and healthy controls.

SNP	TEST	A1 Minor Allele	A2 Major Allele	GENO	Observed (HET)	Expected (HET)	P
SNP1(FSHB)G>A	AFF	A	G	1/4/34	0.1026	0.142	0.187
SNP1(FSHB)G>A	UNAFF	A	G	0/3/28	0.09677	0.09209	1
SNP2(VEZT)A>C	AFF	C	A	1/19/18	0.5	0.3999	0.2255
SNP2(VEZT)A>C	UNAFF	C	A	7/8/14	0.2759	0.4709	0.0435
SNP3(WNT4)C>A	AFF	A	C	0/7/27	0.2059	0.1847	1
SNP3(WNT4)C>A	UNAFF	A	C	0/3/28	0.09677	0.09209	1

The following data are related to the study on genetic association between the considered SNPs and endometriosis.

rs11031006 (FSHB): Patients with endometriosis did not have an increase in genotypic or allelic frequency for this polymorphism compared to the control group ($p = 0.9999$, OR = 0.000, 95% CI, 0.000–15.000 and $p = 0.731$, OR = 1639, 95% CI, 0.393–683, respectively, for heterozygous genotype GA and polymorphic minor allele A) (Table 5, Figure 1). We also verified whether, by stratifying the sample of cases based on the severity of the situation (considering only women with stage III and IV endometriosis), a possible association with the investigated polymorphism would emerge; however, no correlation was found.

Table 5. Genotypic and allelic frequencies of rs11031006 (FSHB).

Genotipic Test		Controls		Cases				
		N°	%	N°	%	P Value	Odds Ratio	95% CI
	A A	0	0.000%	1	2.56%			1.00 Reference
SNP1 (FSHB)	G A	3	9.68%	4	10.26%	>0.9999	0.000	0.000 to 15.000
	G G	28	90.32%	34	87.18%	>0.9999	0.91	0.215 to 3.631
	Total	31	100.00%	39	100.00%			

Allelic Test		Controls		Cases				
		N°	%	N°	%	P Value	Odds Ratio	95% CI
	A	3	4.84%	6	7.69%			
SNP1 (FSHB)	G	59	95.16%	72	92.30%	0.7311	1639	0.393 to 683
	Total	62	100.00%	78	100.00%			

rs10859871 (VEZT): In the case of the polymorphism of the VEZT gene, we found a significant difference in frequency of homozygous genotype CC in the healthy control group compared to the affected women ($p = 0.0111$, OR = 0.0602, 95% CI, 0.005–0.501) (Table 6).

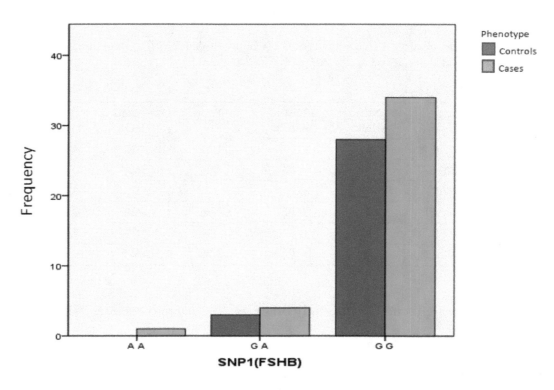

Figure 1. Distribution of AA, GA and GG genotypes obtained for the rs11031006 polymorphism (FSHB).

Table 6. Genotypic and allelic frequencies of rs10859871 (VEZT).

Genotipic Test		Controls		Cases				
		N°	%	N°	%	P Value	Odds Ratio	95% CI
SNP2 (VEZT)	A A	14	48.28%	18	47.37%			1.00 Reference
	A C	8	27.59%	19	50.00%	0.2931	1847.000	0.662 to 5.08
	C C	7	24.14%	1	2.63%	0.0111	0.06015	0.005 to 0.501
	Total	29	100.00%	38	100.00%			

Allelic Test		Controls		Cases				
		N°	%	N°	%	P Value	Odds Ratio	95% CI
SNP2 (VEZT)	C	22	37.93%	21	27.63%	0.2627	0.6248	0.300 to 129
	A	36	62.07%	55	72.36%			
	Total	58	100.00%	76	100.00%			

The same result was replicated by applying the analysis to the sub-group of affected women with moderate to severe endometriosis (stage III–IV) versus healthy controls, confirming a protective role for the homozygosity of the allelic variant ($p = 0.02703$). No significant differences between the groups concerning the allelic frequency of the minor allele C ($p = 0.2627$, OR = 0.6248, 95% CI, 0.300–129) were reported (Figure 2).

rs7521902 (WNT4): Patients with endometriosis did not have an increase in genotypic or allelic frequency of this polymorphism compared to the control group ($p = 0.3088$, OR = 0.4133, 95% CI, 0.10–1.8 and $p = 0.3297$, OR = 2257, 95% CI, 0.55–914, respectively, for heterozygous genotype CA and polymorphic minor allele A) (Table 7, Figure 3). No association was found between this SNP and the disease, even when limiting the analysis to the sample of severe surgical cases (stage III and IV).

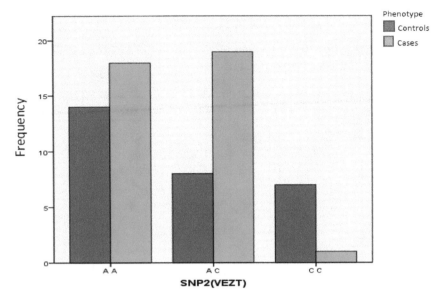

Figure 2. Distribution of AA, AC and CC genotypes obtained for polymorphism rs10859871 (VEZT).

Table 7. Genotypic and allelic frequencies of rs7521902 (WNT4).

Genotipic Test		Controls		Cases		P Value	Odds Ratio	95% CI
		N°	%	N°	%			
	C A	3	9.68%	7	20.59%			1.00 Reference
SNP3 (WNT4)	C C	28	90.32%	27	79.41%	0.3088	0.4133	0.108 to 1.811
	Total	31	100.00%	34	100.00%			

Allelic Test		Controls		Cases		P Value	Odds Ratio	95% CI
		N°	%	N°	%			
	A	3	4.84%	7	10.29%	0.3297	2257	0.557 to 914
SNP3 (WNT4)	C	59	95.16%	61	89.71%			
	Total	62	100.00%	68	100.00%			

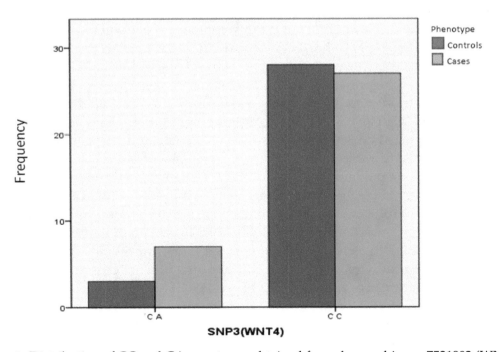

Figure 3. Distribution of CC and CA genotypes obtained for polymorphism rs7521902 (WNT4).

3. Discussion

Our analysis of the recent literature shows evidence of many genes possibly implicated in different pathogenetic mechanisms of endometriosis (Figure 4).

Figure 4. Pathogenetic targets of the most important genes related to endometriosis.

Nevertheless, it is clear that there are differences in genetic associations in endometriosis between different populations around the world. Therefore, it is important to study the genetic basis of this condition in several populations and to replicate the previous results, in order to define the role of significant variants of the risk of endometriosis. In this study, we specifically wanted to test the association between rs11031006 (FSHB), rs10859871 (VEZT) and rs7521902 (gene polymorphisms) and greater susceptibility to the development of endometriosis in a native Sardinian population. SNP rs7521902 WNT4 has been repeatedly associated in the literature with greater susceptibility to endometriosis in women of different ethnicities, including British, Australian, Italian and Japanese [10,16,17]. In the present study, no association between the risk C allele of this SNP and increased risk of endometriosis was detected. These data are consistent with those previously reported by Sundqvist et al. and Mafra et al. [9,13] in a Belgian population. Similarly, no association was detected in a study conducted on 800 Brazilian women (400 with and 400 without endometriosis) [9], or in another conducted on Chinese women (646 with and 766 without endometriosis) [14]. The SNP rs11031006 (FSHB) is another polymorphism candidate for a pathogenetic role, under its possible effect on the inhibition of hormonal feedback; although a significant association in a Greek population was reported, our results in a Sardinian population do not appear to be in line with the literature. The SNP rs10859871 is located in chromosomal region 12q22, 17 kb upstream of the VEZT 187 gene. VEZT is a transmembrane protein with a short extracellular and long intracellular domain, which clips on myosin VIIA as part of the adherent junctional complex in epithelial cells [21,22]. In the blood and endometrium, the C allele at risk of endometriosis of rs10859871 SNP in previous works was associated with increased expression of VEZT, and a pathogenetic role had been hypothetically attributed to this over-expression of VEZT [20]. In the case of gene polymorphism rs10859871 (VEZT), in our study, we instead show a significant and unexpected protective role in the pathology, in sharp contrast to the results obtained in other association studies conducted on populations with different ethnicities. We believe that this is the result of bias due to the small sample. As proof, the preliminary calculation of the Hardy–Weinberg equilibrium indeed signalled a significant deviation precisely in the group of positive controls for this polymorphism, compromising the validity of the results. Therefore, the obtained results did not highlight a significant association between the studied gene variants and a greater risk of developing the disease, although several other studies in the literature show the opposite. This is not surprising, if we consider that the obtained results refer to a Sardinian population known for its unique characteristics. The Sardinian population has always aroused considerable interest in human genetics, both for the peculiar distribution of different genetic variants and for the numerous genetically based diseases particularly frequent on the island. The Sardinian population, even if placed within European variability, shows singular characteristics: some frequent variants in Sardinia are rare or even absent in other populations, and vice versa. For example, the lack of significance of the SNP rs7521902 WNT4 as an endometriosis risk variant in the population of our study is largely due to a minimum allelic frequency (MAF), very low in the Sardinian population (0.0971). In other words, if a gene variant in a given ethnic population is quite rare, a large sample of individuals will be needed to test its frequency in terms relevant to the study. Similarly, the results in our study related to the SNP rs10859871 (VEZT), curiously not in line with what is highlighted in the literature, may have experienced interference because of the reduced size of the sample. It is equally true that most of the SNPs analysed in association studies or detected in GWASs do not fall within regions codifying the gene, and functional studies on them are insufficient. It is easy to hypothesize that the regulatory effect of these polymorphic variants on the expression of certain genes is in turn influenced by the modulation of other factors and co-factors expressed on other regions of the genome whose location and function we do not know. There is also more and more evidence for the role of epigenetic influences, which, through environmental, food-related and/or misunderstood factors and through methylation mechanisms of sequences and histone acetylation, can induce modifications in DNA gene expression without changing its sequence, but simply by turning on or off certain target genes. Since the pathogenesis of endometriosis is extremely complex, involving both genetic background and environmental conditions, studies with conflicting results in several cases have made it difficult to interpret these data. The lack of confirmation of the previous results is therefore largely attributed to an insufficient sample, to population differences and the interaction with genetic and/or non-genetic factors. For this reason, it appears mandatory to extend the case histories of the study in order to reveal or confirm the influence of these gene variants on the Sardinian population.

4. Materials and Methods

4.1. Sampling and Genotyping

After collecting their informed consent, we took a sample of whole blood from each patient (9mL EDTA tube) for genetic analysis. On each sample, a label indicating the date of acquisition and an alphanumeric code (single coding) was affixed, through which only authorized personnel could trace the patient's identity through a special data collection file. The samples were stored in a freezer at a temperature of $-30\,°C$, locked and accessible only by authorized personnel. Genomic DNA was extracted from whole blood with a Qiagen Extraction Kit (QIAmp $^®$ DNA Mini Kit (QIAGEN GmbH, Hilden, Germany), according to the protocol illustrated in the kit manual. Subsequently, genomic DNA extracted from whole blood was read in a NanoDrop photometer 3300^{Tm} ThermoFisher Scientific (www.termofisher.com) at wavelengths of 260, 280 and 260nm/280nm, to assess its quality and quantity. The extracted nuclear DNA was subsequently aliquoted for the next phases of PCR. The analysis of rs7521902, rs10859871 and rs11031006 SNPs examined in the study was carried out by sequencing with the Sanger method. For each selected SNP, the minimum allelic frequency (MAF) in the Sardinian population was preliminarily verified, using the online PheWeb dataset (http://sardinia-pheweb.sph.umich.edu) (Table 8).

Table 8. Minimum allelic frequency (MAF) in Sardinian population of single nucleotide polymorphisms (SNPs) under investigation. WNT4, wingless-typemammalian mouse tumour virus integration site family member 4; VEZT, vezatin; FSHB, follicle stimulating hormone beta polypeptide.

Gene	SNP	MAF Sardinia
WNT4	rs7521902	0.0971
VEZT	rs10859871	0.407
FSHB	rs11031006	0.106

Each DNA sample was amplified with PCR (final volume 25 µL) according to the following protocol: to 75 ng of genomic DNA, 2.5 µL of the specific Taq Polymerase ThermoFisher Scientific (www.termofisher.com) 10× buffer and 1.5 µL of $MgCl_2$ solution (25 mM) was added 0.2 µL of a 2.5 mM dNTP solution, 0.125 µL of Taq Polymerase (5 U/µL), and the forward and reverse primers (25 pmol/µLeach) specific to each analysed region. For each fragment, the same amplification file was used in which initial denaturation was foreseen at 95 °C for 10 min, 30 amplification cycles at 95 °C for 30 min, 60 °C for 30 min, 72 °C for 40 min and a final extension at 72 °C for 10 min. The PCR products were then sequenced using a BigDye Terminator v3.1 Cycle Sequencing Kit ThermoFisher Scientific (www.termofisher.com), according to the manufacturer's instructions. The primers used for sequencing were the same ones used for the amplification of the fragments. Sequence reactions were subsequently subjected to electrophoresis with an ABI3130XL genetic analyser instrument (Applied Biosystems–ThermoFisher) and analysed with SeqScapev3.0 software (ThermoFisher).

4.2. Statistical Analysis

Data were tabulated in a specific database and analysed through specific software. For statistical analysis, Plink v.1.7, SPSS Statistics for Windows v.18 (IBM Corp., Armonk, NY, USA) and GraphPad Prism v.8 (GraphPad Software, La Jolla, CA, USA) software were used, applying addictive, allelic, dominant and recessive models. To examine the differences in frequency of genotypes and alleles among the groups of cases and controls, and to consider a possible association among the SNPs and the pathology under study, Fisher's exact test was used. All of the examined SNPs had a >98% callrate. We considered a 2-tailed p-value < 0.05 to be statistically significant. The odds ratio (OR) and 95% confidence interval (CI) were calculated. The studied genetic variants were evaluated in advance for deviation from the Hardy–Weinberg equilibrium (HWE), comparing the observed and expected genotype frequencies in the groups of the reference sample, through Fisher's exact test.

5. Conclusions

Our data underline the importance of evaluating genetic variants in different populations, in an attempt to define the genetic architecture of endometriosis and the extent of the effects of specific risk alleles in different ethnic groups. An important advantage of the analysis of genetic associations for different ethnic populations is that it can also shed light on the decomposition of the different disequilibrium linkage of populations. At the genomic level, this "trans-ethnic fine mapping" is an important method to restrict the signal to a causal variant [29]. To test this aspect further, exploration of the loci is needed, analysing the surrounding variants, for example through GWASs. GWASs allow the examination of a high number of SNPs and rare variants (up to 4.5 million) in a very large population, to find possible associations with a disease. Recent GWAS meta-analyses, identifying some genetic loci associated with endometriosis, have marked a starting point to define the molecular basis at the origin of the disease, representing the proverbial tip of the iceberg. Studies in very large populations are needed to identify new polymorphisms and to understand their molecular mechanisms. At the moment, the identified gene polymorphisms cannot be used in clinical practice to predict the risk of developing endometriosis or as diagnostic/prognostic markers, but this constitutes a concrete goal for the near future. In fact, defining the genetic alterations predisposing the onset of endometriosis has several potential benefits. First, it could allow us to identify patients at risk of developing endometriosic pathology during the pre-pubescent phase, and contribute to a non-invasive diagnosis in adulthood. Moreover, it could help to better define the molecular mechanisms responsible for its onset and, consequently, represent a rational basis for determining specific therapeutic molecules for this disease.

Author Contributions: Conceptualization, D.D. and S.A.; methodology, S.A..; software, F.A.; validation, S.A.; formal analysis, S.G. and A.C.; investigation, D.D.; data curation, F.A.; writing—original draft preparation, S.A., M.N.D. and D.D.; writing—review and editing, M.N.D., S.A. and D.D.; visualization, M.N.D.; supervision, S.A.; project administration, S.A.; funding acquisition, D.D. All authors have read and agreed to the published version of the manuscript.

Acknowledgments: This publication was created as part of a research project financed with the resources of P.O.R. SARDEGNA F.S.E. 2014-2020-Asse III "Istruzione e Formazione, Obiettivo Tematico: 10, Obiettivo Specifico: 10.5, Azione dell'accordo fi Partenariato:10.5.12 "Avviso di chiamata per il finanziamento di Progetti di ricerca–Anno 2017.

Abbreviations

SNP	Single nucleotide polymorphism
PCR	Polymerase chain reaction
UTR	Untranslated region
AR	Androgen receptor
ER	Estrogenic receptor
PR	Progesterone receptor
A	Adenine
T	Thymine
C	Cytosine
G	Guanine
TGF-β	Transforming growth factor β
IL	Interleukin
VEGF	Vascular endothelial growth factor
TNF	Tumour necrosis factor
HLA	Human leukocyte antigen
MHC	Major histocompatibility complex
EGFR	Endothelial growth factor receptor
mRNA	Messenger ribonucleic acid
MMP	Matrix metalloproteinase
GSTM1	Glutathione S-transferase mu, M1
GSTP1	Glutathione S-transferase P1
GSTT1	Glutathione S-transferase theta, T1
NAT	N-acetyltransferase
CYP	Cytochrome P450
XRCC	X-ray repair cross-complementing
ERCC	Excision repair cross-complementing
GWAS	Genome-wide association study
NGS	Next-generation sequencing
KRAS	Kirsten rat sarcoma viral oncogene homolog
eQTLs	Expression quantitative traits loci
MiRNA	Micro RNA
NcRNA	Non-coding RNA

References

1. Alio, L.; Angioni, S.; Arena, S.; Bartiromo, L.; Bergamini, N.; Berlanda, N.; Bonanni, V.; Bonin, C.; Buggio, L.; Candiani, M.; et al. Endometriosis: Seeking optimal management in women approaching menopause. *Climacteric* **2019**, *22*, 329–338. [CrossRef] [PubMed]

2.   Deiana, D.; Gessa, S.; Anardu, M.; Danilidis, A.; Nappi, L.; D'Alterio, M.N.; Pontis, A.; Angioni, S. Genetic of endometriosis: A comprehensive review. *Gynecol. Endocrinol.* **2019**, *35*, 553–558. [CrossRef] [PubMed]

3.   Melis, I.; Agus, M.; Pluchino, N.; Sardo, A.D.S.; Litta, P.; Melis, G.B.; Angioni, S. Alexithymia in women with deep endometriosis? *A pilot. Study. J. Endometr. Pelvic. Pain Dis.* **2014**, *6*, 26–33.

4.   Angioni, S. New insights on endometriosis. *Minerva Ginecol.* **2017**, *69*, 438–439. [PubMed]

5.   Locci, R.; Nisolle, M.; Angioni, S.; Foidart, J.M.; Munat, C. Expression of the gamma 2 chain of laminin-332 in eutopic and ectopic endometrium of patients with endometriosis. *Rep. Biol. Endocrinol.* **2013**, *11*, 94. [CrossRef] [PubMed]

6.   Simpson, J.L.; Elias, S.; Malinak, L.R.; Buttram, V.C., Jr. Heritable aspects of endometriosis. Genetic studies. *Am. J. Obstet. Gynecol.* **1980**, *137*, 327–331. [CrossRef]

7.   Treloar, S.A.; O'Connor, D.T.; O'Connor, V.M.; Martin, N.G. Genetic influences on endometriosis in an Australian twin sample. *Fertil. Steril.* **1999**, *71*, 701–710. [CrossRef]

8.   Lettre, G.; Hirschhorn, J.N. Small island, big genetic discoveries. *Nat. Genet.* **2015**, *47*, 1224–1225. [CrossRef]

9.   Mafra, F.; Catto, M.; Bianco, B.; Barbosa, C.P.; Christofolini, D. Association of WNT4 polymorphisms with endometriosis in infertile patients. *J. Assist. Reprod. Genet.* **2015**, *32*, 1359–1364. [CrossRef]

10. Pagliardini, L.; Gentilini, D.; Vigano', P.; Panina-Bordignon, P.; Busacca, M.; Candiani, M.; Di Blasio, A.M. An Italian association study and meta-analysis with previous GWAS confirm WNT4, CDKN2BAS and FN1 as the first identified susceptibility loci for endometriosis. *J. Med. Genet.* **2013**, *50*, 43–46. [CrossRef]

11. Vainio, S.; Heikkilä, M.; Kispert, A.; Chin, N.; McMahon, A.P. Female development in mammals is regulated by Wnt-4 signalling. *Nature* **1999**, *397*, 405–409. [CrossRef] [PubMed]

12. Gaetje, R.; Holtrich, U.; Engels, K.; Kissler, S.; Rody, A.; Karn, T.; Kaufmann, M. Endometriosis may be generated by mimicking the ontogenetic development of the female genital tract. *Fertil. Steril.* **2007**, *87*, 651–656. [CrossRef] [PubMed]

13. Sundqvist, J.; Xu, H.; Vodolazkaia, A.; Fassbender, A.; Kyama, C.; Bokor, A.; Gemzell-Danielsson, K.; D'Hooghe, T.M.; Falconer, H. Replication of endometriosis-associated single-nucleotide polymorphisms from genome-wide association studies in a Caucasian population. *Hum. Reprod.* **2013**, *28*, 835–839. [CrossRef] [PubMed]

14. Wu, Z.; Yuan, M.; Li, Y.; Fu, F.; Ma, W.; Li, H.; Wang, W.; Wang, S. Analysis of WNT4 polymorphism in Chinese Han women with endometriosis. *Reprod. Biomed. Online* **2015**, *30*, 415–420. [CrossRef] [PubMed]

15. Jordan, B.K.; Mohammed, M.; Ching, S.T.; Délot, E.; Chen, X.N.; Dewing, P.; Swain, A.; Rao, P.N.; Elejalde, B.R.; Vilain, E. Up-regulation ofWNT-4 signaling and dosage-sensitive sex reversal in humans. *Am. J. Hum. Genet.* **2001**, *68*, 1102–1109. [CrossRef]

16. Rahmioglu, N.; Nyholt, D.R.; Morris, A.P.; Missmer, S.A.; Montgomery, G.W.; Zondervan, K.T. Genetic variants underlying risk of endometriosis: Insights from meta-analysis of eight genome-wide association and replication datasets. *Hum. Reprod. Update* **2014**, *20*, 702–716. [CrossRef]

17. Nyholt, D.R.; Low, S.K.; Anderson, C.A.; Painter, J.N.; Uno, S.; Morris, A.P.; MacGregor, S.; Gordon, S.D.; Henders, A.K.; Martin, N.G.; et al. Genome-wide association meta-analysis identified new endometriosis risk loci. *Nat. Genet.* **2012**, *44*, 1355–1359. [CrossRef]

18. Uno, S.; Zembutsu, H.; Hirasawa, A.; Takahashi, A.; Kubo, M.; Akahane, T.; Aoki, D.; Kamatani, N.; Hirata, K.; Nakamura, Y. A genome-wide association study identifies genetic variants in the CDKN2BAS locus associated with endometriosis in Japanese. *Nat. Genet.* **2010**, *42*, 707–710. [CrossRef]

19. Painter, J.N.; Anderson, C.A.; Nyholt, D.R.; Macgregor, S.; Lin, J.; Lee, S.H.; Lambert, A.; Zhao, Z.Z.; Roseman, F.; Guo, Q.; et al. Genome-wide association study identifies a locus at 7p15.2 associated with the development of endometriosis. *Nat. Genet.* **2011**, *43*, 51–54. [CrossRef]

20. Haldsworth-Carson, S.J.; Fung, J.N.; Luong, H.T.; Sapkota, Y.; Bowdler, L.M.; Wallace, L.; Teh, W.T.; Powell, J.E.; Girling, J.E.; Healey, M.; et al. Endometrial vezatin and it association with endometriosis risk. *Hum. Reprod.* **2016**, *31*, 999–1013. [CrossRef]

21. Küssel-Andermann, P.; El-Amraoui, A.; Safieddine, S.; Nouaille, S.; Perfettini, I.; Lecuit, M.; Cossart, P.; Wolfrum, U.; Petit, C. Vezatin, a novel transmembrane protein, bridges myosin VIIA to the cadherin-catenins complex. *Embo J.* **2000**, *19*, 6020–6029. [CrossRef] [PubMed]

22. Blaschuk, O.W.; Rowlands, T.M. Plasma membrane components of adherens junctions. *Mol. Membr. Biol.* **2002**, *19*, 75–80. [CrossRef] [PubMed]

23. Luong, H.T.T.; Painter, J.N.; Sapkota, Y.; Niholt, D.R.; Rogers, P.A.; Montgomery, G.W. Identifying the functional role of VEZT Gene for endometriosis risk. *Ann. Transl. Med.* **2015**, *3*, AB028.

24. Pagliardini, L.; Gentilini, D.; Sanchez, A.M.; Candiani, M.; Viganò, P.; Di Blasio, A.M. Replication and meta-analysis of previous genome-wide association studies confirm vezatin as the locus with the strongest evidence for association with endometriosis. *Hum. Reprod.* **2015**, *30*, 987–993. [CrossRef] [PubMed]

25. Meola, J.; Rosa, E.; Silva, J.C.; Dentillo, D.B.; Da Silva, W.A., Jr.; Veiga-Castelli, L.C.; Bernardes, L.A.; Ferriani, R.A.; De Paz, C.C.; Giuliatti, S.; et al. Differentially expressed genes in eutopic and ectopic endometrium of women with endometriosis. *Fertil. Steril.* **2010**, *93*, 1750–1773. [CrossRef]

26. Guo, S.-W. Nuclear factor-kappab (NF-κB): An unsuspected major culprit in the pathogenesis of endometriosis that is still at large? *Gynecol. Obstet. Investig.* **2007**, *63*, 71–97. [CrossRef]

27. Sapkota, Y.; Steinthorsdottir, V.; Morris, A.P.; Fassbender, A.; Rahmioglu, N.; De Vivo, I.; Buring, J.E.; Zhang, F.; Edwards, T.L.; Jones, S.; et al. Meta-analysis identifies five novel loci associated with endometriosis highlighting key genes involved in hormone metabolism. *Nat. Commun.* **2017**, *8*, 15539. [CrossRef]

28. Ruth, K.S.; Beaumont, R.N.; Tyrrell, J.; Jones, S.E.; Tuke, M.A.; Yaghootkar, H.; Wood, A.R.; Freathy, R.M.; Weedon, M.N.; Frayling, T.M.; et al. Genetic evidence that lower circulating FSH levels lengthen menstrual cycle, increase age at menopause and impact female reproductive health. *Hum. Reprod.* **2016**, *31*, 473–481. [CrossRef]

29. Matalliotakis, M.; Zervou, M.I.; Matalliotaki, C.; Ramhioglu, N.; Koumantakis, G.; Kalogiannidis, I.; Prapas, I.; Zondervan, K.; Spandidos, D.A.; Matalliotakis, I.; et al. The role of gene polymorphisms in endometriosis. *Molec. Med. Rep.* **2017**, *16*, 5881–5886. [CrossRef]

30. Revised American Society for Reproductive Medicine classification of endometriosis: 1996. *Fertil. Steril.* **1997**, *67*, 817–821. [CrossRef]

31. Vercellini, P.; Viganò, P.; Somigliana, E.; Fedele, L. Endometriosis: Pathogenesis and treatment. *Nat. Rev. Endocrinol.* **2014**, *10*, 261–275. [CrossRef] [PubMed]

32. Laganà, A.S.; Garzon, S.; Gotte, M.; Viganò, P.; Franchi, M.; Ghezzi, F.; Martin, D.C. Pathogenesis of Endometriosis: Molecular and Cell Biology Insights. *Int. J. Mol. Sci.* **2019**, *20*, 5615. [CrossRef] [PubMed]

33. Angioni, S.; Cofelice, V.; Pontis, A.; Tinelli, R.; Socolov, R. New trends of progestins treatment of endometriosis. *Gynecol. Endocrinol.* **2014**, *30*, 769–773. [CrossRef] [PubMed]

34. Angioni, S.; Cofelice, V.; Sedda, F.; Stochino Loi, E.; Multinu, F.; Pontis, A.; Melis, G.B. Progestins for symptomatic endometriosis: Results of clinical studies. *Curr. Drug. Ther.* **2015**, *10*, 91–104. [CrossRef]

35. Wang, Z.; Yoshida, S.; Negoro, K.; Kennedy, S.; Barlow, D.; Maruo, T. Polymorphisms in the estrogen receptor beta gene but not estrogen receptor alpha gene affect the risk of developing endometriosis in a Japanese population. *Fertil. Steril.* **2004**, *81*, 1650–1656. [CrossRef]

36. Lee, G.H.; Kim, S.H.; Choi, Y.M.; Suh, C.S.; Kim, J.G.; Moon, S.Y. Estrogen receptor beta gene +1730 G/A polymorphism in women with endometriosis. *Fertil. Steril.* **2007**, *88*, 785–788. [CrossRef]

37. Lattuada, D.; Somigliana, E.; Vigano, P.; Candiani, M.; Pardi, G.; Di Blasio, A.M. Genetics of endometriosis: A role for the progesterone receptor gene polymorphism PROGINS? *Clin. Endocrinol.* **2004**, *61*, 190–194. [CrossRef]

38. Wieser, F.; Schneeberger, C.; Tong, D.; Tempfer, C.; Huber, J.C.; Wenzl, R. PROGINS receptor gene polymorphism is associated with endometriosis. *Fertil. Steril.* **2002**, *77*, 309–312. [CrossRef]

39. De Carvalho, C.V.; Nogueira-De-Souza, N.C.; Costa, A.M.; Baracat, E.C.; Girao, M.J.; D'Amora, P.; Schor, E.; da Silva, I.D. Genetic polymorphisms of cytochrome P450cl7alpha (CYP17) and progesterone receptor gene (PROGINS) in the assessment of endometriosis risk. *Gynecol. Endocrinol.* **2007**, *23*, 29–33. [CrossRef]

40. Govindan, S.; Ahmad, S.N.; Vedicherla, B.; Kodati, V.; Jahan, P.; Rao, K.P.; Ahuja, Y.R.; Hasan, Q. Association of progesterone receptor gene (PROGINS) with endometriosis, uterine fibroids and breast cancer. *Cancer Biomark.* **2007**, *3*, 73–77. [CrossRef]

41. Treloar, S.A.; Zhao, Z.Z.; Armitage, T.; Duffy, D.L.; Wicks, J.; O'Connor, D.T.; Martin, N.G.; Montgomery, G.W. Association between polymorphisms in the progesterone receptor gene and endometriosis. *Mol. Hum. Reprod.* **2005**, *11*, 641–647. [CrossRef] [PubMed]

42. Van Kaam, K.J.; Romano, A.; Schouten, J.P.; Dunselman, G.A.; Groothuis, P.G. Progesterone receptor polymorphism +331G/A is associated with a decreased risk of deep infiltrating endometriosis. *Hum. Reprod.* **2007**, *22*, 129–135. [CrossRef] [PubMed]

43. Slayden, O.D.; Nayak, N.R.; Burton, K.A.; Chwalisz, K.; Cameron, S.T.; Critchley, H.O.; Baird, D.T.; Brenner, R.M. Progesterone antagonist increase androgen receptor expression in the rhesus macaque and human endometrium. *J. Clin. Endocrinol. Metab.* **2001**, *86*, 2668–2679. [CrossRef] [PubMed]

44. Mertens, H.J.; Heinemann, M.J.; Theunissen, P.H.; de Jong, F.H.; Evers, J.L. Androgen, estrogen and progesterone receptor expression in the human uterus during the mestrual cycle. *Eur. J. Obstet. Gynecol. Reprod. Biol.* **2001**, *98*, 58–65. [CrossRef]

45. Tuckermann, E.M.; Okon, M.A.; Li, T.; Laird, S.M. Do androgens have a direct effect on endometrial function? An in vitro study. *Fertil. Steril.* **2000**, *74*, 771–779. [CrossRef]

46. Carneiro, M.M.; Morsch, D.M.; Camargos, A.F.; Reis, F.M.; Spritzer, P.M. Androgen receptor and 5α-reductase are expressed in pelvic endometriosis. *Int. J. Obstet. Gynaecol.* **2008**, *115*, 113–117. [CrossRef]

47. Gelmann, P.E. Molecular Biology of the AR. *J. Clin. Oncol.* **2002**, *20*, 3001–3015. [CrossRef]

48. Rajender, S.; Singh, L.; Thangaraj, K. Phenotypic heterogeneity of mutations in androgen receptor gene. *Asian J. Androl.* **2007**, *9*, 147–179.

49. Shaik, N.A.; Govindan, S.; Kodati, V.; Rao, K.P.; Hasan, Q. Polymorphic (CAG) repeats in the androgen receptor gene: A risk marker for endometriosis and uterine leiomyomas. *Hematol. Oncol. Stem Cel. Ther.* **2009**, *2*, 289–293. [CrossRef]

50. Hsieh, Y.Y.; Chang, C.C.; Tsai, F.J.; Wu, J.Y.; Tsai, C.H.; Tsai, H.D. Androgen receptor trinucleotide polymorphism in endometriosis. *Fertil. Steril.* **2001**, *76*, 412–413. [CrossRef]

51. Lattuada, D.; Viganò, P.; Somigliana, E.; Odorizzi, M.P.; Vignali, M.; Di Biasio, A.M. Androgen receptor gene cytosine, adenine, and guanine trinucleotide repeats in patients with endometriosis. *J. Soc. Gynecol. Investig.* **2004**, *11*, 237–240. [CrossRef] [PubMed]

52. Hsieh, Y.Y.; Chang, C.C.; Tsai, F.J.; Hsu, Y.; Tsai, H.D.; Tsai, C.H. Polymorphisms for interleukin-4 (IL-4)—590 promoter, IL-4 intron3, and tumor necrosis factor alpha -308 promoter: Non-association with endometriosis. *J. Clin. Lab. Anal.* **2002**, *16*, 121–126. [CrossRef] [PubMed]

53. Yu, Y.X.; Xiu, Y.L.; Chen, X.; Li, Y.L. Transforming Growth Factor-beta 1 involved in the pathogenesis of endometriosis through regulating expression of vascular endothelial growth factor under hypoxia. *Chin. Med. J.* **2017**, *130*, 950–956. [CrossRef] [PubMed]

54. Wieser, F.; Fabjani, G.; Tempfer, C.; Schneeberger, C.; Zeillinger, R.; Huber, J.C.; Wenzl, R. Tumor necrosis factor–alpha promoter polymorphisms and endometriosis. *J. Soc. Gynecol. Investig.* **2002**, *9*, 313–318. [CrossRef]

55. Somigliana, E.; Viganò, P.; Vignali, M. Endometriosis and unexplained recurrent spontaneous abortion: Pathological states resulting from aberrant modulation of natural killer cell function? *Hum. Reprod. Update* **1999**, *5*, 41–52. [CrossRef] [PubMed]

56. Wang, X.; Lin, Q.; Guo, S. Study on polymorphism of human leukocyte antigen I in patients with endometriosis. *Zhanghua Fu Chan Ke Za Zhi* **2001**, *36*, 150–152.

57. Ishii, K.; Takakuwa, K.; Kashima, K.; Tamura, M.; Tanaka, K. Associations between patients with endometriosis and HLA class II; the analysis of HLA-DQB1 and HLA- DPB1 genotypes. *Hum. Reprod.* **2003**, *18*, 985–989. [CrossRef]

58. Pabalan, N.; Jarjanazi, H.; Christofolini, D.M.; Bianco, B.; Barbosa, C.P. Association of the protein tyrosine phosphatase non receptor 22 polymorphism (PNTN22) with endometriosis: A meta-analysis. *Rev. Artic. Einstein* **2017**, *15*, 105–111. [CrossRef]

59. Perini, J.A.; Cardoso, J.V.; Berardo, P.T.; Vianna-Jorge, R.; Nasciutti, L.E.; Bellodi-Privato, M.; Machado, D.E.; Abrao, M.S. Role of vascular endothelial growth factor polymorphisms (−2578C > A, −460T > C, −1154G > A, +405G > C and + 936C > T) in endometriosis: A case-control study with Brazilians. *BMC Womens Health* **2014**, *14*, 117. [CrossRef]

60. Hsieh, Y.Y.; Chang, C.C.; Tsai, F.J.; Lin, C.C.; Tsai, C.H. T homozygote and allele of epidermal growth factor receptor 2073 gene polymorphism are associated with higher susceptibility to endometriosis and leiomyomas. *Fertil. Steril.* **2005**, *83*, 796–799. [CrossRef]

61. Guo, S.W. Glutathione S-transferases M1/T1 gene polymorphism and endometriosis: A meta-analysis of genetic association studies. *Mol. Hum. Reprod.* **2005**, *11*, 729–743. [CrossRef] [PubMed]

62. Arvanitis, D.A.; Koumantakis, G.E.; Gouemenou, A.G.; Metalliokatis, E.E.; Spandidos, D.A. CYP1A1, CYP19, and GSTM1 polymorphisms increase the risk of endometriosis. *Fertil. Steril.* **2003**, *79*, 707–709. [CrossRef]

63. Hsieh, Y.Y.; Chang, C.C.; Tsai, F.J.; Lin, C.C.; Tsai, C.H. Cytochrome P450c17alpha 5'- untranslated region *T/C polymorphism in endometriosis. *J. Genet.* **2004**, *83*, 189–192. [CrossRef] [PubMed]

64. Lambrinoudaki, I.V.; Augoulea, A.; Christodoulakos, G.E.; Economou, E.V.; Kaparos, G.; Kontoravdis, A.; Papadias, C.; Creatsas, G. Measurable serum markers of oxidative stress response in women with endometriosis. *Fertil. Steril.* **2009**, *91*, 46–50. [CrossRef]

65. Attar, R.; Cacina, C.; Sozen, S.; Attar, E.; Agachan, B. DNA repair genes in endometriosis. *Gen. Mol. Res.* **2010**, *9*, 629–636. [CrossRef]

66. Rahmioglu, N.; Montgomery, G.W.; Zondervan, K.T. Genetics of endometriosis. *Womens Health* **2015**, *11*, 577–586. [CrossRef]

67. Treloar, S.A.; Wicks, J.; Nyholt, D.R.; Montgomery, G.W.; Bahlo, M.; Smith, V.; Dawson, G.; Mackay, I.J.; Weeks, D.E.; Bennett, S.T.; et al. Genome-wide Linkage Study in 1,176 affected sister pair families identifies a significant susceptibility locus for endometriosis on chromosome 10q26. *Am. J. Hum. Genet.* **2005**, *77*, 365–376. [CrossRef]

68. Painter, J.N.; Nyholt, D.R.; Morris, A.; Zhao, Z.Z.; Henders, A.K.; Lambert, A.; Wallace, L.; Martin, N.G.; Kennedy, S.H.; Treloar, S.A.; et al. High-density fine-mapping of a chromosome 10q26 linkage peak suggests association between endometriosis and variants close to CYP2C19. *Fertil. Steril.* **2011**, *95*, 2236–2240. [CrossRef]

69. Cribb, A.E.; Knight, M.J.; Dryer, D.; Guernsey, J.; Hender, K.; Tesch, M.; Saleh, T.M. Role of a polymorphic human CYP450 enzymes in estrone oxidation. *Cancer Epidemiol. Biomark. Prev.* **2006**, *15*, 551–558. [CrossRef]

70. Martini, M.; Ciccarone, M.; Garganese, G.; Maggiore, C.; Evangelista, A.; Rahimi, S.; Zannoni, G.; Vittori, G.; Larocca, L.M. Possible involvement of hMLH1, p16INK4a and PTEN in the malignant transformation of endometriosis. *Int. J. Cancer* **2002**, *102*, 398–406. [CrossRef]

71. Powell, J.E.; Fung, J.N.; Shakhbazov, K.; Sapkota, Y.; Cloonan, N.; Hemani, G.; Hillman, K.M.; Kaufmann, S.; Luong, H.T.; Bowdler, L.; et al. Endometriosis risk alleles at 1p36.12 act through inverse regulation of CDC42 and LINC00339. *Hum. Mol. Genet.* **2016**, *25*, 5046–5058. [PubMed]

72. Grechukhina, O.; Petracco, R.; Popkhadze, S.; Massasa, E.; Paranjape, T.; Chan, E.; Flores, I.; Weidhaas, J.B.; Taylor, H.S. A polymorphism in a let-7 microRNA binding site of KRAS in women with endometriosis. *EMBO Mol. Med.* **2012**, *4*, 202–217. [CrossRef] [PubMed]

73. Luong, H.T.; Nyholt, D.R.; Painter, J.N.; Chapman, B.; Kennedy, S.; Treloar, S.A.; Zondervan, K.T.; Montgomery, G.W. No evidence for genetic association with the let-7 microRNA-binding site or the common KRAS variants in risk of endometriosis. *Hum. Reprod.* **2012**, *12*, 3616–3621. [CrossRef] [PubMed]

74. Chettier, R.; Albertsen, H.M.; Ward, K. Next Generation Sequencing of families with endometriosis identifies new genomic regions likely to contribute to heritability. *Fertil. Steril.* **2014**, *102*, 76–77. [CrossRef]

75. Er, T.K.; Su, Y.F.; Wu, C.C.; Chen, C.C.; Wang, J.; Hsieh, T.H.; Herreros-Villanueva, M.; Chen, W.T.; Chen, Y.T.; Liu, T.C.; et al. Targeted next-generation sequencing for molecular diagnosis of endometriosis-associated ovarian cancer. *J. Mol. Med.* **2016**, *94*, 835–847. [CrossRef]

76. Sapkota, Y.; Vivo, I.; Steinthorsdottir, V.; Fassbender, A.; Bowdler, L.; Buring, J.E.; Edwards, T.L.; Jones, S.; Dorien, O.; Peterse, D.; et al. Analysis of potential protein-modifying variants in 9000 endometriosis patients and 150000 controls of European ancestry. *Sci. Rep.* **2017**, *7*, 11380. [CrossRef]

77. Fung, J.N.; Montgomery, G.W. Genetics of endometriosis: State of art on genetic risk factors for endometriosis. *Best. Pract. Res. Clin. Obstetr. Gynecol.* **2018**, *50*, 61–71. [CrossRef]

78. Freedman, M.L.; Monteiro, A.N.; Gayther, S.A.; Coetzee, G.A.; Risch, A.; Plass, C.; Casey, G.; De Biasi, M.; Carlson, C.; Duggan, D.; et al. Principles for the post- GWAS functional characterization of cancer risk. *Nat. Genet.* **2011**, *43*, 513–518. [CrossRef]

79. Westra, H.J.; Peters, M.J.; Esko, T.; Yaghootkar, H.; Schurmann, C.; Kettunen, J.; Christiansen, M.W.; Fairfax, B.P.; Schramm, K.; Powell, J.E.; et al. Systematic identification of trans eQTLs as putative drivers of known disease associations. *Nat. Genet.* **2013**, *45*, 1238–1243. [CrossRef]

80. Guo, S.W. Epigenetics of endometriosis. *Mol. Hum. Reprod.* **2009**, *15*, 587–607. [CrossRef]

81. Wu, Y.; Starzinski-Powitz, A.; Guo, S.W. Trichostatin A, a histone deacetylase inhibitor, attenuates invasiveness and reactivates E-cadherin expression in immortalized endometriotic cells. *Reprod. Sci.* **2007**, *14*, 374–382. [CrossRef] [PubMed]

82. Jenuwein, T.; Allis, C.D. Translating the histone code. *Science* **2001**, *293*, 1074–1080. [CrossRef] [PubMed]

Differential Diagnosis of Endometriosis by Ultrasound: A Rising Challenge

Marco Scioscia [1]⬤, **Bruna A. Virgilio** [1], **Antonio Simone Laganà** [2,*]⬤, **Tommaso Bernardini** [1], **Nicola Fattizzi** [1], **Manuela Neri** [3,4] and **Stefano Guerriero** [3,4]⬤

[1] Department of Obstetrics and Gynecology, Policlinico Hospital, 35031 Abano Terme, PD, Italy; marcoscioscia@gmail.com (M.S.); bruna81@tiscali.it (B.A.V.); tbernardini@casacura.it (T.B.); nfattizzi@casacura.it (N.F.)

[2] Department of Obstetrics and Gynecology, "Filippo Del Ponte" Hospital, University of Insubria, 21100 Varese, VA, Italy

[3] Obstetrics and Gynecology, University of Cagliari, 09124 Cagliari, CA, Italy; manu.neri11@hotmail.it (M.N.); gineca.sguerriero@tiscali.it (S.G.)

[4] Department of Obstetrics and Gynecology, Azienda Ospedaliero Universitaria, Policlinico Universitario Duilio Casula, 09045 Monserrato, CA, Italy

*   Correspondence: antoniosimone.lagana@uninsubria.it

Abstract: Ultrasound is an effective tool to detect and characterize endometriosis lesions. Variances in endometriosis lesions' appearance and distorted anatomy secondary to adhesions and fibrosis present as major difficulties during the complete sonographic evaluation of pelvic endometriosis. Currently, differential diagnosis of endometriosis to distinguish it from other diseases represents the hardest challenge and affects subsequent treatment. Several gynecological and non-gynecological conditions can mimic deep-infiltrating endometriosis. For example, abdominopelvic endometriosis may present as atypical lesions by ultrasound. Here, we present an overview of benign and malignant diseases that may resemble endometriosis of the internal genitalia, bowels, bladder, ureter, peritoneum, retroperitoneum, as well as less common locations. An accurate diagnosis of endometriosis has significant clinical impact and is important for appropriate treatment.

Keywords: endometriosis; adenomyosis; bowel; rectum; ovary; bladder; ureter; abdominal wall; vagina

1. Introduction

Endometriosis is a common, chronic, and debilitating gynecological condition that affects between 5–15% of women within their reproductive ages [1,2]. It is characterized by the growth of tissue that mimics endometrial tissue and exhibits the same responses to hormonal changes [1]. However, this abnormal tissue growth occurs outside the uterus, usually on other organs inside the pelvis and abdominal cavity, thus creating endometriosis implants. These endometriosis implants lead to local inflammatory reactions that promote fibrosis and adhesion formation, which create resistance between organs and may result in an altered pelvic anatomy [3]. This cascade of events often causes menstrual and/or chronic pelvic pain, infertility, or malfunction of the affected abdominopelvic organs [1].

In the past decades, ultrasound has become a valuable tool to accompany pelvic bimanual examinations. Currently, both methods are used for the first-line examination and diagnosis of endometriosis [4]. When a patient presents with persistent symptoms of suspected endometriosis, a comprehensive and detailed evaluation of the pelvis by ultrasound is usually prescribed. However, the accuracy of the ultrasound in detecting deep-infiltrating endometriosis depends on the experience of the sonographer. Variances in endometriosis lesion appearance and distorted anatomy secondary to adhesions and fibrosis present as major difficulties during the complete sonographic evaluation of pelvic endometriosis [5].

Therefore, a trained ultrasound operator is needed to detect most of the endometriosis lesions, and is required to make sound judgments and to plan the appropriate treatment [5,6]. It is also important for expert evaluations to include a differential diagnosis (DD) of endometriosis to exclude all other abdominopelvic diseases. Although misdiagnoses represent a small number of cases with unknown prevalence (Figure 1), the clinical impact of a DD is great because the appropriate treatment largely varies based on the diagnosis.

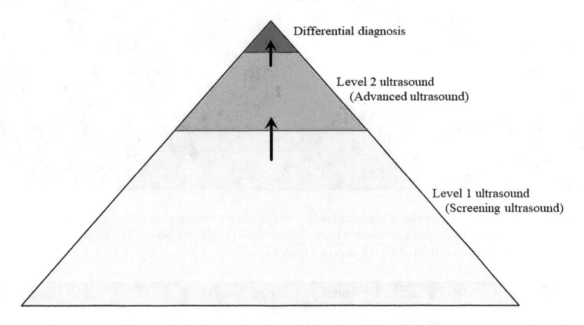

Figure 1. A pyramid chart that represents the distribution of ultrasound scans for endometriosis according to complexity. Although differential diagnosis must be considered in each exam, the number of cases where it makes a difference is relatively small, although it is fundamental.

2. What a Comprehensive Ultrasound for Endometriosis Should Investigate

Traditionally, a routine pelvic ultrasound only evaluates uterine and ovarian lesions, which leads to the detection of elementary lesions, such as endometriomas [7]. However, the evaluation should include the anterior and posterior pelvic compartments to assess the mobility of pelvic organs [7–10] and to improve the assessment of endometriosis, as suggested by the International Deep Endometriosis Analysis (IDEA) consensus [11]. The use of a systematic ultrasound approach can enhance the detection of different endometriosis locations within the pelvis [12–14], with a detection rate that is similar to that of magnetic resonance [15,16].

Endometriosis can extend to organs other than internal genitalia, such as the bowels, bladder [1,16], and retroperitoneal structures (e.g., ureters, parametria, nerves) [17], which significantly complicates the ultrasound evaluation [18]. Although all these locations appear similar on an ultrasound (nodular, sometimes flat, hypoechoic lesions with the absence of colored Doppler spots), and they present specific features according to the organ or tissue involved. In fact, deep-infiltrating endometriosis (DIE) of hollow organs induces a retraction of margins with a subsequent irregular profile of both external and internal surfaces (i.e., bladder, bowels, and vagina), whereas DIE of dense organs (i.e., peritoneal and retroperitoneal organs) maintains a nodular hypoechoic structure [11]. Less frequently, some lesions may display vascularity with small cysts (i.e., bladder; Figure 2). Cystic endometriosis of retroperitoneal organs is a rare event that mainly occurs in patients with a history of pelvic surgery (Figure 3).

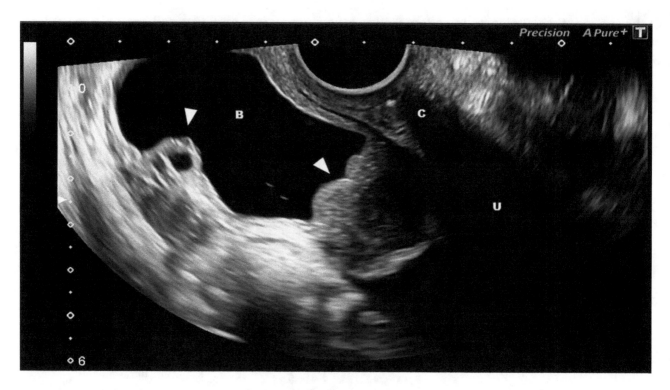

Figure 2. Bifocal endometriosis of the bladder (arrow). The two lesions present different characteristics as the one on the right-hand side presents a typical solid aspect while the left one is a cystic endometriosis location. Abbreviations: B, bladder; C, cervix; U, uterus.

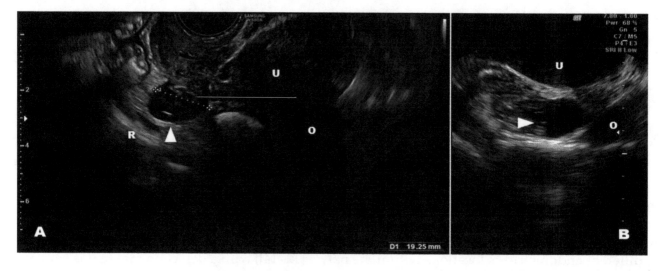

Figure 3. Cystic endometriosis (arrow) of the retroperitoneum in two patients on medical therapy with previous pelvic surgery for endometriosis. (**A**) shows an endometriosis cyst of the rectovaginal septum and (**B**) shows a cyst of the mesometrium. Abbreviations: U, uterus; R, rectum; O, Ovary.

3. Sonographic Differential Diagnosis

During a comprehensive evaluation, the sonographer should be able to correctly identify all significant endometriosis lesions, the presence of other benign diseases (i.e., fibroids, uterine malformations, etc.), and any suspected malignancies. It is also important that the DD includes examination for adenomyosis [12,19–21] and endometrioma [22,23]. It is far more difficult for gynecologists to identify and characterize diseases of organs other than the internal genitalia. However, the ultrasound operator must be competent in identifying not only normal and altered pelvic anatomy due to endometriosis and other gynecological diseases, but also other diseases that are typically identified by other specialists (e.g., radiologist, gastroenterologist, urologist). Furthermore, gynecologists also have to consider that the presence of endometriosis does not exclude other clinical conditions that may require further evaluation by another specialist.

Several gynecological and non-gynecological conditions can mimic DIE, which are summarized in Table 1. In some cases, clinical signs can help differentiate diseases even when a pelvic bimanual examination is suggestive of endometriosis. Several studies have demonstrated the possibility of a DD of endometriosis lesions with benign (e.g., adenomyoma vs. myoma or endometrioma vs. other cysts) [19,22,24–26] and malignant genital diseases (e.g., ovarian cancer) [26,27].

Table 1. Endometriosis possible anatomic locations, anatomical features, and differential diagnosis.

Anatomic Locations	Anatomical Aspect	Possible Differential Diagnosis
Internal genitalia		
Ovary	Cystic	Hemorrhagic corpus luteum Hemorrhagic cyst Dermoid cyst Tubovarian abscess Mucinous cystoadenoma Ovarian cystic adenomyoma Malignancy
Tube	Cystic	Tubovarian abscess
Uterus (adenomyosis)	Focal, solid (buds)	Endometrial malignancy
	Solid adenomyoma	Non-encapsulated myomas
	Cystic adenomyoma	Myomas with cystic degeneration/necrosis Suspected sarcoma/STUMP
Vagina	Solid nodulus	Cervical malignancy Vaginal malignancy
	Cystic	Benign vaginal cyst
Peritoneum		
Broad anterior/posterior ligament	Solid	Peritoneal carcinomatosis
Douglas pouch	Solid	Peritoneal carcinomatosis Advanced cervical malignancy
Prevesical peritoneum	Solid	Post-cesarean adhesions Peritoneal carcinomatosis Advanced cervical malignancy
Uterosacral ligaments	Solid	Peritoneal carcinomatosis Advanced cervical malignancy
Round ligaments	Solid	Peritoneal carcinomatosis Advanced endometrial malignancy
Retroperitoneal tissues		
Paracervix/parametrium	Solid	Advanced cervical malignancy
Mesometrium	Solid	Pedunculated infraligamentary fibroid Ovarian malignancy
	Cystic	Varicocele

Table 1. *Cont.*

Anatomic Locations	Anatomical Aspect	Possible Differential Diagnosis
Mesorectum	Solid	Colonic malignancy Downward dislocated appendix
	Cystic	Retrorectal dermoid cyst
Presacral space	Cystic	Tarlov cyst Ganglioneuroma
Vesicovaginal septum	Solid	Bladder malignancy
Bowel		
Rectosigmoid	Solid	Colonic polyp Diverticulosis Colonic malignancy
Caecum and appendix	Solid	Appendicitis Appendiceal tumors
Ileum	Solid	Malignancy
Urinary tract		
Bladder	Solid	Bladder malignancy Cervical malignancy Uterine leiomyomas/adenomyomas Hypertrophic traumatic bladder
	Cystic	Bladder malignancy Intravesical ureterocele Small bowel attached to the prevesical peritoneum
Ureter	Solid	Ureteric stone
External genitalia		
Perineum	Solid	Postpatum scar Chron disease
Mons pubis	Solid	Abscess Hematoma Muscular strain
Abdominal wall		
Umbilicus	Solid	Omphalitis Umbilical granuloma
Abdominal muscle	Solid	Strain Benign tumor (desmoid)
	Cystic	Hematoma
Inguinal canal	Solid	Complete small hernia

3.1. Internal Genitalia

The ovary is the most common site of endometriosis (Table 1). Additionally, the "typical" endometrioma in premenopausal women is the easiest to identify by ultrasound due to its specific characteristics (e.g., unilocular cysts with ground-glass echogenicity of the fluid content, polar clot/debris, and poor vascularization on color Doppler evaluation) [28,29]. This should be differentiated by hemorrhagic corpora lutea especially when fine strands of fibrin are seen in the fluid content of the cyst, through the evidence of rich peripheral vascularization and its transient nature. Sometimes a correct diagnosis is not easy, especially in the presence of multiple cysts, because it can be very difficult to distinguish an endometrioma from other adnexal masses, such as some dermoid cysts, hemorrhagic cysts, tubovarian abscesses, mucinous cystadenomas, or ovarian cystic adenomyomas [24–26]. The presence of intracystic vascularization certainly poses doubts about malignancy (e.g., borderline tumor, endometrioid cancer) [23] also because 1% of the masses presumed to be endometriomas are malignant [30]. Furthermore, the ultrasound characteristics of pre- and postmenopausal endometriomas differ. Postmenopausal endometriomas are less frequently unilocular and are less likely to have ground-glass content; however, those with typical ground-glass content have a high risk of malignancy [28].

Superficial endometriosis of the fallopian tubes is undetectable, but it can be suspected by the presence of a tubovarian complex with tube dilatation at the location of the endometriomas. Sonographic diagnosis of tubovarian abscesses is not easy in such cases, but the clinical presentations of tube wall edema and positive color/power Doppler intensities are suggestive [31], regardless of the presence of an endometrioma (abscess superimposed to the endometriosis tubovarian complex). Solid localizations of the fallopian tubes are certainly difficult to detect but they do not require a DD in the presence of other pelvic endometriosis lesions.

Adenomyosis is characterized by an altered junctional zone with an area that is isoechoic to the endometrial tissue (for the deepening of ectopic endometrial glands and stroma), and its ultrasound classification has been well described [19,32]. It can often present as an irregularity of the junctional zone (e.g., echogenic subendometrial lines and buds, an interrupted junctional zone) with or without myometrial cystic lesions, which appear either as focal or diffuse lesions or as adenomyomas. Solid lesions, which are referred to as buds, that originate from the endometrium must be differentiated from non-endophytic endometrial cancers, such as uterine clear-cell carcinoma and uterine papillary serous carcinoma. Buds do not develop from endometrial hyperplasia, but instead they arise from an atrophic endometrium [33]. The age of onset, which largely overlaps [34], clinical presentation [35], and endometrial thickness (women with symptomatic adenomyosis or perimenopausal menstrual alterations are often on hormonal therapy) may not help in the DD; however, the myometrial vascularization may provide some clues. In adenomyosis cases, the vessel distribution (i.e., arcuate, radial, and basal arteries) within the myometrium and the lesion is not altered [19,32], whereas the neoangiogenesis that occurs in tumoral lesions is detected by color/power Doppler and the identification of aberrant vessels, even in cases of endometrial cancer in which the endometrium does not appear particularly irregular [36].

Adenomyomas are defined as benign tumors that include components derived from endometrial glands, stroma, muscular cells, and fibrosis [20]. These lesions are mostly found within the myometrium, and their sonographic characteristics resemble those of myomas. Nevertheless, in some cases they can be differentiated from myomas [21]. The correct preoperative diagnosis between myomas and adenomyomas is of key importance for surgeons because the surgical removal of adenomyomas is very difficult, if not impossible. The ultrasound characteristics of adenomyomas have been reported [12,19], and their DD mainly consists of the absence of both the pseudocapsule and vascularization compared with that of myomas. In fact, non-encapsulated myomas that lack the typical refraction at the mass border maintain the typical circumferential vascularization of fibroids, whereas adenomyomas exhibit an anatomical myometrial pattern of vessels (i.e., arcuate, radial, and basal arteries). Lacunas are not necessarily a sign of adenomyomas because uterine fibroids may exhibit cystic degeneration secondary to a limited blood supply. In fact, the thick hyperechoic wall of the cystic glands of adenomyomas is poorly represented during hormonal therapy, thus a clear DD may not be possible. Clinical symptoms may support the findings of the sonographic examination because uterine myomas with cystic degeneration are poorly symptomatic, unless they are submucosal. However, adenomyomas may present with abnormal uterine bleeding and periodic pain during ovulation and menstruations. In cases of uterine masses with strong vascularity, usually hypervascular myomas, a DD that includes adenomyosis, occult degeneration (leiomyosarcoma or smooth uterine muscle of uncertain malignant potential [STUMP]), or a benign fibroid is not possible [21].

Endometriosis of the vagina occurs in approximately 12% of women with revised American Society for Reproductive Medicine (rASRM) stage IV endometriosis [17]. It presents as a nodular thickening of the vaginal wall that causes pain under a gentle pressure with the probe [37] and that does not modify with probe compression [22]. It infiltrates the recto-vaginal septum, usually in the posterior or lateral-posterior upper third of the vagina, and it presents as a hypoechoic lesion with a negative/minimal color Doppler signaling. Its DD must include advanced cervical cancer with vaginal infiltration. The normal appearance of the uterine cervix with different vascularization as well as symptoms after intercourse (endometriosis is associated to dyspareunia, whereas cervical cancer is associated with postcoital bleeding) can lead to a correct diagnosis. A DD that includes rare tumors, such as those of primary vaginal cancer, is mainly clinical because of its clinical appearance and the age of diagnosis (more frequent in postmenopausal women).

Endometriosis of the vagina rarely presents as cystic and is usually a part of a larger solid nodulus. Vaginal cysts have been reported to occur in approximately 1% of all women, and they are located in the anterolateral vaginal wall [38]. These cysts are asymptomatic remnants of the Wolffian duct and present as regular hypo- or anechoic cysts. Less frequently, they can be located on the posterolateral vaginal wall within vaginal scars (i.e., episiotomy and birth lacerations). The key aspects for a DD are the location (endometriosis is always on the posterior vaginal wall) and the absence of tenderness.

3.2. Peritoneal and Retroperitoneal Endometriosis Lesions

The pelvic peritoneum is almost always involved in advanced-stage endometriosis [3,17]. The typical appearance is a nodular thickening of the peritoneum, which is sometimes nodular or flat, like a plaque (this is very often found beneath the ovary on the ovarian fossa), and hypoechoic with negative color Doppler signaling. These lesions may grow inward into tissues from a superficial site of origin, deepening further into the mesometrium (endophytic growth) and reaching subperitoneal structures, such as ligaments (e.g., uterosacral and round), ureters, and superficial nerves (e.g., hypogastric nerve). The DD includes peritoneal carcinomatosis that presents as nodular or sheet-like, exophytic, hypoechoic, vascularized structures and is almost always associated with ascites [39].

The peritoneum over the uterus and bladder can be clearly evaluated by a transvaginal scan with an unemptied bladder, and any lesions with enough thickness (nodule) can be identified [40]. Although superficial, plain lesions cannot be detected, alterations in the peritoneal profile due to retractive fibrosis and adhesions have sometimes been reported [22]. The presence of adhesions in prevesical peritoneum due to a cesarean section with the absence of the uterine sliding sign are often misleading and impossible to differentiate from endometriosis. The two clinical conditions (adhesions and endometriosis) can coexist, and it is important to evaluate if a peritoneal lesion of endometriosis deepens into the vesicovaginal septum to the bladder.

Retroperitoneal endometriosis near the uterus (i.e., paracervical and parametrial) is common [17,41], and ultrasound is a valid tool to identify these lesions [11,42–45]. A DD that includes the spread of cervical cancer warrants attention [46]. Endometriosis of the broad posterior ligaments may infiltrate deeply into the mesometrium and paracervical tissues, reaching organs, such as the ureter [47], and appearing as a solid nodule in most cases. Retroperitoneal cystic endometriosis is not very common (Figure 3B), and it typically occurs in women who previously had pelvic surgery for endometriosis. However, it should be differentiated from a pelvic varicocele. A misplaced appendix may be easily confused with endometriosis of the mesorectum, which is usually superficial and presents as a peritoneal implant of endometriosis (Figure 4) [48]. Cystic endometriosis beneath the rectum is very rare [49] compared with benign cysts of sacral nerve roots.

3.3. The Bowels

Colonic endometriosis is not a rare condition. It affects 37% of women with severe endometriosis [13], and its correct diagnosis is essential for the proper planning of treatment [15,48,50,51]. Recently, the ultrasound detection rate of endometriosis foci of the bowels has increased, exhibiting both high sensitivity and specificity [46,52]. Additionally, its accuracy is as high as other imaging techniques, such as magnetic resonance, rectal endoscopy sonography, and double contrast barium enema [11,12,15,53]. Bowel lesions can present as different shapes; however, they exhibit an anechoic appearance without posterior enhancement, they can invade the bowel lumen, and they can have digitiform, irregular, or smooth limits. The sliding sign with the uterus and near organs is often negative because the nodule may involve the Douglas pouch or the uterosacral ligaments, or it can be attached to the posterior wall of the uterus.

Figure 4. Appendix dislocated downward and attached to the ovary that may mimic mesorectal endometriosis. (**A,B**) show the clean and the labelled image. Abbreviations: A, appendix; O, Ovary; BPL, broad posterior ligament; C, caecum; MR, mesorectum; RSJ, rectosigmoid junction.

The DD of bowel endometriosis using ultrasound is particularly challenging for gynecologists who are not used to examining lesions other than those of endometriosis. In some cases, bowel disease may resemble endometriosis, and the DD is more difficult [54]. It is important to note that rectosigmoid endometriosis always involves the anterior or the lateral rectosigmoid wall and never the posterior wall that is directed toward the mesorectum/mesosigmoid [54]. The most common bowel diseases that can be mistaken for endometriosis include appendicitis, appendiceal tumors [48], colonic polyps, diverticulosis, and colonic malignancy [54]. Specific factors of the internal surface of the gut should be considered during a DD, such as colonic polyps and malignancies. As we reported in a previous article [54], colon cancer growths typically extend outward and reach the serosa, whereas endometriosis lesions grow inward. A transrectal ultrasound with a radial probe that scans the entire 360 degrees of the rectal lumen is a useful tool to detect and confirm the presence of polyps or malignancies; however, a colonoscopy remains the gold standard for diagnosis. In advanced-stage rectal cancer, there may be infiltration of the entire bowel wall, but the presence of specific symptoms (e.g., rectal bleeding, unexplained weight loss, gas pains or cramps) may help with the correct diagnosis.

It may also be difficult to distinguish bowel endometriosis from colonic diverticula [54]. Diverticula are mainly characterized as outward growths on a thick bowel wall with hyperechoic content, whereas endometriosis is endophytic and hypoechoic. The imaging may even be more complex if inflammation occurs within a closed diverticular abscess. In this case, an undefined oval mass that is growing outward beyond the bowel surface may be identified. Additionally, a transverse section may exhibit intense Doppler positivity in acute diverticulitis. Clinical symptoms (e.g., constant abdominal tenderness, nausea and vomiting, and pyrexia) and inflammatory blood tests may support the sonographic findings and lead to the correct diagnosis and treatment.

3.4. The Bladder and Ureter

Urinary tract endometriosis occurs in 0.3–12% of women with endometriosis [55,56], with an incidence of 43% in women with stage IV endometriosis [17]. Endometriosis of the muscularis propria of the bladder and the ureters are the rarest conditions, with incidences of 4.3% and 9.5%, respectively [17]. The bladder wall can be examined by ultrasound because it is surrounded by a low-echogenic tissue (i.e., perivesical loose connective tissue) and the peritoneum, which appears as a hyperechoic line. In most cases, a hypoechoic lesion that alters the profile of the peritoneum of the bladder and infiltrates into the detrusor muscle indicates bladder endometriosis and originates from uterine adenomyosis [50]. Endometriosis of the bladder is often symptomatic (e.g., urgency, frequency, and pain on passing urine, which worsen days before and during menstruation, and recurrent urinary tract infections) and appears as a consistently solid mass that involves the prevesical space, the serosa (adventitia), and the detrusor muscle, sometimes up to the urothelium [22,42,57]. These lesions always involve the bladder dome on the sagittal plane, and sometimes the nodule may also extend laterally. Additionally, they exhibit color Doppler positivity. The vascularity of these lesions may suggest a malignant origin of the nodule; however, only advanced-stage cancer (either a bladder or cervical carcinoma) invades the prevesical peritoneum. Furthermore, bladder cancer is typically found in postmenopausal women and originates from the internal surface (urothelium) of the lateral wall of the bladder. In cases of advanced-stage cervical cancer, the lesion clearly involves the cervix and quite often the lateral parametrial and paracervical tissues [50,58]. Endometriosis of the bladder may present some uncommon features, such as cystic lesions and multifocal endometriosis. In such cases, it is very difficult to differentiate from bladder cancer that may be both cystic and multifocal [59,60]. Vesical cancer usually presents as a solid papillary mass that projects into the bladder, with a normal thickness of the bladder wall at the site of the lesion [60]. Nevertheless, large carcinomas may exhibit anechoic cystic degeneration within the mass and infiltration of the detrusor muscle [60]. Color Doppler imaging is not useful for this condition because cystic endometriosis of the bladder usually shows no vascularization. When making the DD, the facts that bladder carcinomas typically occur in elderly women and that urinary cytology is the simplest, less-invasive, and least expensive method to obtain a correct diagnosis warrants consideration [50].

We recently reviewed the DD of urinary tract endometriosis [50]. The DD may sometimes be difficult due to the presence of external masses that encroach the bladder dome (i.e., uterine fibroids or an attached small bowel from a previous surgery, such as a cesarean section), an intravesical ureterocele that may resemble deep lesions of endometriosis, or hypertrophic areas of the bladder wall due to a chronic, complete cystocele and recurrent cystitis [50]. In such cases, although bladder endometriosis very often appears as an endophytic lesion, it may sometimes appear flat and may be confused with hypertrophic areas due to chronic mechanical trauma (cystocele) or recurrent cystitis (Figure 5).

Endometriosis of the ureter affects the pelvic segment of the organ as a deepening of foci of the posterior broad ligament. Endometrial tissue may only invade the outer adventitia (extrinsic type) or the mucosal and/or muscular layers of the ureter (intrinsic type) [22,61]. It presents as a nodule along the course of the ureter that causes a dilatation of the ureteral tract proximal to the stenosis. The dilated ureter appears as a blood vessel in the parametrial tissue with negative color Doppler signaling and evidence of peristalsis [47], which is also often associated with hydronephrosis. The presence of ureteric calculi, which cause intense symptoms and appear as solid echogenic masses often with dilatation of the proximal part of the ureter, must be excluded [50].

3.5. Uncommon Endometriosis Locations

Uncommon locations of endometriosis are difficult to detect, and the accuracy of the ultrasound may be significantly reduced due to an inexperienced operator [62]. Endometriosis of the external genitalia (e.g., the perineum and mons pubis) may be easily confused with other conditions (i.e., abscesses, genital Crohn's disease, skin trauma/swollen lesions, and hematomas) [63,64] because it may originate from abdominal wall lesions (i.e., muscular strains, heparin hematomas, muscular tumors, and hernias). In such cases, patient history in addition to the ultrasound findings is useful for identification of any conditions that resemble endometriosis [65–67]. The rarest sites of endometriosis include lesions of the liver, pancreas, kidney, and gallbladder. Hepatic endometriosis appears as superficial hypoechoic lesions and may mimic an abscess, a hematoma, an angioma, or malignancy [62].

Endometriosis of pancreas, kidney, and gallbladder show hypoechoic lesions that can be seen by ultrasound and they require a second evaluation by computerized tomography or magnetic resonance imaging [62]. These lesions do not present pathognomonic features that may differentiate endometriosis from malignancy or adenomas, so the definitive diagnosis relies on histology only [62].

Figure 5. A typical endometriosis nodule (arrow) of the bladder (**A**); figure (**B**) shows a flat nodule of endometriosis (arrow) with a subserosal myoma that distorts the bladder dome; a flat endometriosis nodule (arrow) of the bladder that can be seen at 3D ultrasound only when cut (**C**) while the internal surface of the bladder appears regular (**D**); figure (**E**) shows a thick bladder wall due to cystocele and figure (**F**) in case of recurrent cystitis. Abbreviations: U, uterus; B, bladder; M, myoma.

4. Conclusions

The accuracy of ultrasound for the diagnosis of pelvic endometriosis has greatly improved over recent years, and it is widely regarded as the first-line diagnostic tool, despite a significant interobserver variability has been reported [68]. Certainly, the identification of extra-genitalia lesions requires a specific training [69]; however, ongoing practice is necessary to acquire and maintain competence [70].

DD by ultrasound for patients who have been referred for endometriosis may result in the detection of other gynecological diseases; therefore, it is important to consider other conditions when unusual lesions are detected. A skilled operator is key because his mental reconstruction of the distorted anatomy is necessary to correctly localize and evaluate the lesion of interest. Additional knowledge of the ultrasound appearances of lesions that do not occur within the reproductive system is needed to make a correct diagnosis. however, in such cases, further examinations should be required, or patients should be referred to other experts/specialists. A specific hands-on training for making DDs is not possible, but theoretical courses and off-line scanning sessions for sonographers with experience in gynecological and endometriosis ultrasound help to improve their background and may result in more accurate diagnoses.

Author Contributions: Conceptualization, M.S. and B.A.V.; methodology, S.G.; data curation, M.S., B.A.V., and T.B.; writing—original draft preparation, M.S.; writing—review and editing, A.S.L., N.F., and M.N.; visualization, M.S.; supervision, S.G. All authors have read and agreed to the published version of the manuscript.

References

1. Zondervan, K.T.; Becker, C.M.; Missmer, S.A. Endometriosis. *N. Engl. J. Med.* **2020**, *382*, 1244–1256. [CrossRef] [PubMed]
2. Nnoaham, K.E.; Hummelshoj, L.; Webster, P.; d'Hooghe, T.; de Cicco Nardone, F.; de Cicco Nardone, C.; Jenkinson, C.; Kennedy, S.H.; Zondervan, K.T. World Endometriosis Research Foundation Global Study of Women's Health consortium Impact of endometriosis on quality of life and work productivity: A multicenter study across ten countries. *Fertil. Steril.* **2011**, *96*, 366373.e8. [CrossRef]
3. Burney, R.O.; Giudice, L.C. Pathogenesis and pathophysiology of endometriosis. *Fertil. Steril.* **2012**, *98*, 511–519. [CrossRef] [PubMed]
4. Dunselman, G.A.J.; Vermeulen, N.; Becker, C.; Calhaz-Jorge, C.; D'Hooghe, T.; De Bie, B.; Heikinheimo, O.; Horne, A.W.; Kiesel, L.; Nap, A.; et al. ESHRE guideline: Management of women with endometriosis. *Hum. Reprod.* **2014**, *29*, 400–412. [CrossRef] [PubMed]
5. Schliep, K.; Chen, Z.; Stanford, J.; Xie, Y.; Mumford, S.; Hammoud, A.; Boiman Johnstone, E.; Dorais, J.; Varner, M.; Buck Louis, G.; et al. Endometriosis diagnosis and staging by operating surgeon and expert review using multiple diagnostic tools: An inter-rater agreement study. *BJOG Int. J. Obstet. Gynecol.* **2017**, *124*, 220–229. [CrossRef] [PubMed]
6. Chapron, C.; Marcellin, L.; Borghese, B.; Santulli, P. Rethinking mechanisms, diagnosis and management of endometriosis. *Nat. Rev. Endocrinol.* **2019**, *15*, 666–682. [CrossRef] [PubMed]
7. Collins, B.G.; Ankola, A.; Gola, S.; McGillen, K.L. Transvaginal US of Endometriosis: Looking Beyond the Endometrioma with a Dedicated Protocol. *Radiographics* **2019**, *39*, 1549–1568. [CrossRef]
8. Piessens, S.; Edwards, A. Sonographic Evaluation for Endometriosis in Routine Pelvic Ultrasound. *J. Minim. Invasive Gynecol.* **2020**, *27*, 265–266. [CrossRef] [PubMed]
9. Fraser, M.A.; Agarwal, S.; Chen, I.; Singh, S.S. Routine vs. expert-guided transvaginal ultrasound in the diagnosis of endometriosis: A retrospective review. *Abdom. Imaging* **2015**, *40*, 587–594. [CrossRef]
10. Fratelli, N.; Scioscia, M.; Bassi, E.; Musola, M.; Minelli, L.; Trivella, G. Transvaginal sonography for preoperative assessment of deep endometriosis. *J. Clin. Ultrasound* **2013**, *41*, 69–75. [CrossRef]
11. Guerriero, S.; Condous, G.; van den Bosch, T.; Valentin, L.; Leone, F.P.G.; Van Schoubroeck, D.; Exacoustos, C.; Installé, A.J.F.; Martins, W.P.; Abrao, M.S.; et al. Systematic approach to sonographic evaluation of the pelvis in women with suspected endometriosis, including terms, definitions and measurements: A consensus opinion from the International Deep Endometriosis Analysis (IDEA) group. *Ultrasound Obstet. Gynecol.* **2016**, *48*, 318–332. [CrossRef] [PubMed]
12. Van den Bosch, T.; Van Schoubroeck, D. Ultrasound diagnosis of endometriosis and adenomyosis: State of the art. *Best Pract. Res. Clin. Obstet. Gynaecol.* **2018**, *51*, 16–24. [CrossRef] [PubMed]
13. Deslandes, A.; Parange, N.; Childs, J.T.; Osborne, B.; Bezak, E. Current Status of Transvaginal Ultrasound Accuracy in the Diagnosis of Deep Infiltrating Endometriosis Before Surgery: A Systematic Review of the Literature. *J. Ultrasound Med.* **2020**. [CrossRef] [PubMed]
14. Guerriero, S.; Ajossa, S. Transvaginal ultrasonography in superficial endometriosis. *Aust. N. Z. J. Obstet. Gynaecol.* **2020**, *60*, E5. [CrossRef] [PubMed]

15. Noventa, M.; Scioscia, M.; Schincariol, M.; Cavallin, F.; Pontrelli, G.; Virgilio, B.; Vitale, S.G.; Laganà, A.S.; Dessole, F.; Cosmi, E.; et al. Imaging Modalities for Diagnosis of Deep Pelvic Endometriosis: Comparison between Trans-Vaginal Sonography, Rectal Endoscopy Sonography and Magnetic Resonance Imaging. A Head-to-Head Meta-Analysis. *Diagnostics* **2019**, *9*, 225. [CrossRef]

16. Guerriero, S.; Saba, L.; Pascual, M.A.; Ajossa, S.; Rodriguez, I.; Mais, V.; Alcazar, J.L. Transvaginal ultrasound vs magnetic resonance imaging for diagnosing deep infiltrating endometriosis: Systematic review and meta-analysis. *Ultrasound Obstet. Gynecol.* **2018**, *51*, 586–595. [CrossRef]

17. Scioscia, M.; Bruni, F.; Ceccaroni, M.; Steinkasserer, M.; Stepniewska, A.; Minelli, L. Distribution of endometriotic lesions in endometriosis stage IV supports the menstrual reflux theory and requires specific preoperative assessment and therapy. *Acta Obstet. Gynecol. Scand.* **2011**, *90*, 136–139. [CrossRef]

18. Chamié, L.P.; Ribeiro, D.M.F.R.; Tiferes, D.A.; de Macedo Neto, A.C.; Serafini, P.C. Atypical Sites of Deeply Infiltrative Endometriosis: Clinical Characteristics and Imaging Findings. *RadioGraphics* **2018**, *38*, 309–328. [CrossRef]

19. Van den Bosch, T.; Dueholm, M.; Leone, F.P.G.; Valentin, L.; Rasmussen, C.K.; Votino, A.; Van Schoubroeck, D.; Landolfo, C.; Installé, A.J.F.; Guerriero, S.; et al. Terms, definitions and measurements to describe sonographic features of myometrium and uterine masses: A consensus opinion from the Morphological Uterus Sonographic Assessment (MUSA) group. *Ultrasound Obstet. Gynecol.* **2015**, *46*, 284–298. [CrossRef]

20. Paul, P.G.; Gulati, G.; Shintre, H.; Mannur, S.; Paul, G.; Mehta, S. Extrauterine adenomyoma: A review of the literature. *Eur. J. Obstet. Gynecol. Reprod. Biol.* **2018**, *228*, 130–136. [CrossRef]

21. Testa, A.C.; Di Legge, A.; Bonatti, M.; Manfredi, R.; Scambia, G. Imaging techniques for evaluation of uterine myomas. *Best Pract. Res. Clin. Obstet. Gynaecol.* **2016**, *34*, 37–53. [CrossRef] [PubMed]

22. Exacoustos, C.; Zupi, E.; Piccione, E. Ultrasound Imaging for Ovarian and Deep Infiltrating Endometriosis. *Semin. Reprod. Med.* **2017**, *35*, 005–024. [CrossRef]

23. Na, K.; Park, S.Y.; Kim, H.-S. Clinicopathological Characteristics of Primary Ovarian Adenomyoma: A Single-institutional Experience. *Anticancer Res.* **2017**, *37*, 2565–2574. [CrossRef] [PubMed]

24. Sokalska, A.; Timmerman, D.; Testa, A.C.; Van Holsbeke, C.; Lissoni, A.A.; Leone, F.P.G.; Jurkovic, D.; Valentin, L. Diagnostic accuracy of transvaginal ultrasound examination for assigning a specific diagnosis to adnexal masses. *Ultrasound Obstet. Gynecol.* **2009**, *34*, 462–470. [CrossRef]

25. Valentin, L. Characterising acute gynaecological pathology with ultrasound: An overview and case examples. *Best Pract. Res. Clin. Obstet. Gynaecol.* **2009**, *23*, 577–593. [CrossRef]

26. Sayasneh, A.; Ekechi, C.; Ferrara, L.; Kaijser, J.; Stalder, C.; Sur, S.; Timmerman, D.; Bourne, T. The characteristic ultrasound features of specific types of ovarian pathology (review). *Int. J. Oncol.* **2015**, *46*, 445–458. [CrossRef]

27. Moro, F.; Zannoni, G.F.; Arciuolo, D.; Pasciuto, T.; Amoroso, S.; Mascilini, F.; Mainenti, S.; Scambia, G.; Testa, A.C. Imaging in gynecological disease (11): Clinical and ultrasound features of mucinous ovarian tumors. *Ultrasound Obstet. Gynecol.* **2017**, *50*, 261–270. [CrossRef]

28. Van Holsbeke, C.; Van Calster, B.; Guerriero, S.; Savelli, L.; Paladini, D.; Lissoni, A.A.; Czekierdowski, A.; Fischerova, D.; Zhang, J.; Mestdagh, G.; et al. Endometriomas: Their ultrasound characteristics. *Ultrasound Obstet. Gynecol.* **2010**, *35*, 730–740. [CrossRef]

29. Timmerman, D.; Valentin, L.; Bourne, T.H.; Collins, W.P.; Verrelst, H.; Vergote, I. International Ovarian Tumor Analysis (IOTA) Group Terms, definitions and measurements to describe the sonographic features of adnexal tumors: A consensus opinion from the International Ovarian Tumor Analysis (IOTA) Group. *Ultrasound Obstet. Gynecol.* **2000**, *16*, 500–505. [CrossRef]

30. Van Holsbeke, C.; Van Calster, B.; Guerriero, S.; Savelli, L.; Leone, F.; Fischerova, D.; Czekierdowski, A.; Fruscio, R.; Veldman, J.; Van de Putte, G.; et al. Imaging in gynaecology: How good are we in identifying endometriomas? *Facts Views Vis. ObGyn* **2009**, *1*, 7–17.

31. Timor-Tritsch, I.E.; Lerner, J.P.; Monteagudo, A.; Murphy, K.E.; Heller, D.S. Transvaginal sonographic markers of tubal inflammatory disease. *Ultrasound Obstet. Gynecol.* **1998**, *12*, 56–66. [CrossRef] [PubMed]

32. Van den Bosch, T.; de Bruijn, A.M.; de Leeuw, R.A.; Dueholm, M.; Exacoustos, C.; Valentin, L.; Bourne, T.; Timmerman, D.; Huirne, J.A.F. Sonographic classification and reporting system for diagnosing adenomyosis. *Ultrasound Obstet. Gynecol.* **2019**, *53*, 576–582. [CrossRef] [PubMed]

33. Gründker, C.; Günthert, A.R.; Emons, G. Hormonal heterogeneity of endometrial cancer. *Adv. Exp. Med. Biol.* **2008**, *630*, 166–188. [CrossRef] [PubMed]

34. Yu, O.; Schulze-Rath, R.; Grafton, J.; Hansen, K.; Scholes, D.; Reed, S.D. Adenomyosis incidence, prevalence and treatment: United States population-based study 2006–2015. *Am. J. Obstet. Gynecol.* **2020**, *223*, 94.e1–94.e10. [CrossRef] [PubMed]

35. Chapron, C.; Vannuccini, S.; Santulli, P.; Abrão, M.S.; Carmona, F.; Fraser, I.S.; Gordts, S.; Guo, S.-W.; Just, P.-A.; Noël, J.-C.; et al. Diagnosing adenomyosis: An integrated clinical and imaging approach. *Hum. Reprod. Update* **2020**, *26*, 392–411. [CrossRef]

36. Scioscia, M.; Noventa, M.; Laganà, A.S. Abnormal uterine bleeding and the risk of endometrial cancer: Can subendometrial vascular ultrasound be of help to discriminate cancer from adenomyosis? *Am. J. Obstet. Gynecol.* **2020**, *223*, 605–606. [CrossRef]

37. Guerriero, S.; Ajossa, S.; Gerada, M.; D'Aquila, M.; Piras, B.; Melis, G.B. "Tenderness-guided" transvaginal ultrasonography: A new method for the detection of deep endometriosis in patients with chronic pelvic pain. *Fertil. Steril.* **2007**, *88*, 1293–1297. [CrossRef]

38. Shobeiri, S.A.; Rostaminia, G.; White, D.; Quiroz, L.H.; Nihira, M.A. Evaluation of Vaginal Cysts and Masses by 3-Dimensional Endovaginal and Endoanal Sonography. *J. Ultrasound Med.* **2013**, *32*, 1499–1507. [CrossRef]

39. Testa, A.C.; Ludovisi, M.; Mascilini, F.; Di Legge, A.; Malaggese, M.; Fagotti, A.; Fanfani, F.; Salerno, M.G.; Ercoli, A.; Scambia, G.; et al. Ultrasound evaluation of intra-abdominal sites of disease to predict likelihood of suboptimal cytoreduction in advanced ovarian cancer: A prospective study. *Ultrasound Obstet. Gynecol.* **2012**, *39*, 99–105. [CrossRef]

40. Savelli, L.; Manuzzi, L.; Pollastri, P.; Mabrouk, M.; Seracchioli, R.; Venturoli, S. Diagnostic accuracy and potential limitations of transvaginal sonography for bladder endometriosis. *Ultrasound Obstet. Gynecol.* **2009**, *34*, 595–600. [CrossRef]

41. Chiantera, V.; Petrillo, M.; Abesadze, E.; Sozzi, G.; Dessole, M.; Catello Di Donna, M.; Scambia, G.; Sehouli, J.; Mechsner, S. Laparoscopic Neuronavigation for Deep Lateral Pelvic Endometriosis: Clinical and Surgical Implications. *J. Minim. Invasive Gynecol.* **2018**, *25*, 1217–1223. [CrossRef] [PubMed]

42. Guerriero, S.; Ajossa, S.; Minguez, J.A.; Jurado, M.; Mais, V.; Melis, G.B.; Alcazar, J.L. Accuracy of transvaginal ultrasound for diagnosis of deep endometriosis in uterosacral ligaments, rectovaginal septum, vagina and bladder: Systematic review and meta-analysis. *Ultrasound Obstet. Gynecol.* **2015**, *46*, 534–545. [CrossRef] [PubMed]

43. Mabrouk, M.; Raimondo, D.; Arena, A.; Iodice, R.; Altieri, M.; Sutherland, N.; Salucci, P.; Moro, E.; Seracchioli, R. Parametrial Endometriosis: The Occult Condition that Makes the Hard Harder. *J. Minim. Invasive Gynecol.* **2019**, *26*, 871–876. [CrossRef] [PubMed]

44. Scioscia, M.; Virgilio, B.A.; Scardapane, A.; Pontrelli, G. Fusion Imaging: A Novel Diagnostic Tool for Nerve-sparing Surgery for Deep Infiltrating Endometriosis. *J. Minim. Invasive Gynecol.* **2020**, *27*, 246–247. [CrossRef]

45. Leonardi, M.; Martins, W.P.; Espada, M.; Arianayagam, M.; Condous, G. Proposed technique to visualize and classify uterosacral ligament deep endometriosis with and without infiltration into parametrium or torus uterinus. *Ultrasound Obstet. Gynecol.* **2020**, *55*, 137–139. [CrossRef]

46. Alcazar, J.L.; García, E.; Machuca, M.; Quintana, R.; Escrig, J.; Chacón, E.; Mínguez, J.A.; Chiva, L. Magnetic resonance imaging and ultrasound for assessing parametrial infiltration in cervical cancer. A systematic review and meta-analysis. *Med. Ultrason.* **2020**, *22*, 85–91. [CrossRef]

47. Scioscia, M. Ureteral endometriosis: Correlation between ultrasonography and laparoscopy: Ureteral endometriosis. *Ultrasound Obstet. Gynecol.* **2019**, *53*, 706–708. [CrossRef]

48. Virgilio, B.A.; Pontrelli, G.; Trevisan, P.; Sacchi, D.; Bernardini, T.; Scioscia, M. Incidental diagnosis on transvaginal ultrasound of appendiceal mucocele arising on low-grade appendiceal mucinous neoplasm. *Ultrasound Obstet. Gynecol.* **2019**, *54*, 412–414. [CrossRef]

49. Sima, R.-M.; Radosa, J.C.; Zamfir, R.; Ionescu, C.-A.; Carp, D.; Iordache, I.-I.; Stănescu, A.-D.; Pleş, L. Novel diagnosis of mesenteric endometrioma: Case report. *Medicine (Baltimore)* **2019**, *98*, e16432. [CrossRef]

50. Scioscia, M.; Zanetti, I.; Raspanti, X.; Spoto, E.; Portuese, A.; Noventa, M.; Pontrelli, G.; Greco, P.; Virgilio, B.A. Ultrasound Differential Diagnosis in Deep Infiltrating Endometriosis of the Urinary Tract. *J. Ultrasound Med.* **2020**. [CrossRef]

51. Scardapane, A.; Lorusso, F.; Francavilla, M.; Bettocchi, S.; Fascilla, F.D.; Angelelli, G.; Scioscia, M. Magnetic Resonance Colonography May Predict the Need for Bowel Resection in Colorectal Endometriosis. *BioMed Res. Int.* **2017**, *2017*, 1–7. [CrossRef] [PubMed]

52. Kammann, S.; Menias, C.; Hara, A.; Moshiri, M.; Siegel, C.; Safar, B.; Brandes, S.; Shaaban, A.; Sandrasegaran, K. Genital and reproductive organ complications of Crohn disease: Technical considerations as it relates to perianal disease, imaging features, and implications on management. *Abdom. Radiol.* **2017**, *42*, 1752–1761. [CrossRef] [PubMed]

53. Nezhat, C.; Li, A.; Falik, R.; Copeland, D.; Razavi, G.; Shakib, A.; Mihailide, C.; Bamford, H.; DiFrancesco, L.; Tazuke, S.; et al. Bowel endometriosis: Diagnosis and management. *Am. J. Obstet. Gynecol.* **2018**, *218*, 549–562. [CrossRef] [PubMed]

54. Scioscia, M.; Orlandi, S.; Trivella, G.; Portuese, A.; Bettocchi, S.; Pontrelli, G.; Bocus, P.; Anna Virgilio, B. Sonographic Differential Diagnosis in Deep Infiltrating Endometriosis: The Bowel. *BioMed Res. Int.* **2019**, *2019*, 1–9. [CrossRef] [PubMed]

55. Fujita, M.; Manabe, N.; Honda, K.; Murao, T.; Osawa, M.; Kawai, R.; Akiyama, T.; Shiotani, A.; Haruma, K.; Hata, J. Usefulness of Ultrasonography for Diagnosis of Small Bowel Tumors: A Comparison Between Ultrasonography and Endoscopic Modalities. *Medicine* **2015**, *94*, e1464. [CrossRef] [PubMed]

56. Kołodziej, A.; Krajewski, W.; Dołowy, Ł.; Hirnle, L. Urinary Tract Endometriosis. *Urol. J.* **2015**, *12*, 2213–2217.

57. Pateman, K.; Holland, T.K.; Knez, J.; Derdelis, G.; Cutner, A.; Saridogan, E.; Jurkovic, D. Should a detailed ultrasound examination of the complete urinary tract be routinely performed in women with suspected pelvic endometriosis? *Hum. Reprod.* **2015**, *30*, 2802–2807. [CrossRef]

58. Testa, A.C.; Di Legge, A.; De Blasis, I.; Cristina Moruzzi, M.; Bonatti, M.; Collarino, A.; Rufini, V.; Manfredi, R. Imaging techniques for the evaluation of cervical cancer. *Best Pract. Res. Clin. Obstet. Gynaecol.* **2014**, *28*, 741–768. [CrossRef] [PubMed]

59. Smereczyński, A.; Szopiński, T.; Gołąbek, T.; Ostasz, O.; Bojko, S. Sonography of tumors and tumor-like lesions that mimic carcinoma of the urinary bladder. *J. Ultrason.* **2014**, *14*, 36–48. [CrossRef]

60. Pavlica, P.; Gaudiano, C.; Barozzi, L. Sonography of the bladder. *World J. Urol.* **2004**, *22*, 328–334. [CrossRef]

61. Barra, F.; Scala, C.; Biscaldi, E.; Vellone, V.G.; Ceccaroni, M.; Terrone, C.; Ferrero, S. Ureteral endometriosis: A systematic review of epidemiology, pathogenesis, diagnosis, treatment, risk of malignant transformation and fertility. *Hum. Reprod. Update* **2018**, *24*, 710–730. [CrossRef] [PubMed]

62. Guerriero, S.; Conway, F.; Pascual, M.A.; Graupera, B.; Ajossa, S.; Neri, M.; Musa, E.; Pedrassani, M.; Alcazar, J.L. Ultrasonography and Atypical Sites of Endometriosis. *Diagnostics (Basel)* **2020**, *10*, 345. [CrossRef] [PubMed]

63. Mascilini, F.; Moruzzi, C.; Giansiracusa, C.; Guastafierro, F.; Savelli, L.; De Meis, L.; Epstein, E.; Timor-Tritsch, I.E.; Mailath-Pokorny, M.; Ercoli, A.; et al. Imaging in gynecological disease. 10: Clinical and ultrasound characteristics of decidualized endometriomas surgically removed during pregnancy. *Ultrasound Obstet. Gynecol.* **2014**, *44*, 354–360. [CrossRef] [PubMed]

64. Noventa, M.; Saccardi, C.; Litta, P.; Vitagliano, A.; D'Antona, D.; Abdulrahim, B.; Duncan, A.; Alexander-Sefre, F.; Aldrich, C.J.; Quaranta, M.; et al. Ultrasound techniques in the diagnosis of deep pelvic endometriosis: Algorithm based on a systematic review and meta-analysis. *Fertil. Steril.* **2015**, *104*, 366–383.e2. [CrossRef] [PubMed]

65. Grigore, M.; Socolov, D.; Pavaleanu, I.; Scripcariu, I.; Grigore, A.M.; Micu, R. Abdominal wall endometriosis: An update in clinical, imagistic features, and management options. *Med. Ultrason.* **2017**, *19*, 430. [CrossRef]

66. Morales Martínez, C.; Tejuca Somoano, S. Abdominal wall endometriosis. *Am. J. Obstet. Gynecol.* **2017**, *217*, 701–702. [CrossRef]

67. Ecker, A.M.; Donnellan, N.M.; Shepherd, J.P.; Lee, T.T.M. Abdominal wall endometriosis: 12 years of experience at a large academic institution. *Am. J. Obstet. Gynecol.* **2014**, *211*, 363.e1–363.e5. [CrossRef]

68. Bean, E.; Chaggar, P.; Thanatsis, N.; Dooley, W.; Bottomley, C.; Jurkovic, D. Intra- and interobserver reproducibility of pelvic ultrasound for the detection and measurement of endometriotic lesions. *Hum. Reprod. Open* **2020**, *2020*, hoaa001. [CrossRef]

69. Guerriero, S.; Pascual, M.A.; Ajossa, S.; Rodriguez, I.; Zajicek, M.; Rolla, M.; Rams Llop, N.; Yulzari, V.; Bardin, R.; Buonomo, F.; et al. Learning curve for ultrasonographic diagnosis of deep infiltrating endometriosis using structured offline training program. *Ultrasound Obstet. Gynecol.* **2019**, *54*, 262–269. [CrossRef]

Microbiome Profile of Deep Endometriosis Patients: Comparison of Vaginal Fluid, Endometrium and Lesion

Camila Hernandes [1],*[ID], Paola Silveira [2], Aline Fernanda Rodrigues Sereia [2],
Ana Paula Christoff [2][ID], Helen Mendes [1], Luiz Felipe Valter de Oliveira [2][ID] and Sergio Podgaec [1]

[1] Hospital Israelita Albert Einstein, Av. Albert Einstein 627, Morumbi, São Paulo 05651-901, Brazil;
   helen2002@me.com (H.M.); sergiopodgaec@me.com (S.P.)
[2] BiomeHub, Av. Luiz Boiteux Piazza, 1302, Canasvieiras, Florianópolis 88056-000, Brazil;
   paola@biome-hub.com (P.S.); aline@biome-hub.com (A.F.R.S.); anachff@biome-hub.com (A.P.C.);
   felipe@biome-hub.com (L.F.V.d.O.)
* Correspondence: camila.hernandes@einstein.br

Abstract: This work aimed to identify and compare the bacterial patterns present in endometriotic lesions, eutopic endometrium and vaginal fluid from endometriosis patients with those found in the vaginal fluid and eutopic endometrium of control patients. Vaginal fluid, eutopic endometrium and endometriotic lesions were collected. DNA was extracted and the samples were analyzed to identify microbiome by high-throughput DNA sequencing of the 16S rRNA marker gene. Amplicon sequencing from vaginal fluid, eutopic endometrium and endometriotic lesion resulted in similar profiles of microorganisms, composed most abundantly by the genus *Lactobacillus*, *Gardnerella*, *Streptococcus* and *Prevotella*. No significant differences were found in the diversity analysis of microbiome profiles between control and endometriotic patients; however deep endometriotic lesions seems to present different bacterial composition, less predominant of *Lactobacillus* and with more abundant *Alishewanella*, *Enterococcus* and *Pseudomonas*.

Keywords: vaginal fluid; microbiome; next generation sequencing (NGS); pathogenesis; endometriosis; 16S rRNA

1. Introduction

Endometriosis is a gynecological disorder affecting 10% to 15% of women in reproductive age; up to 70% of the patients have pelvic pain and 48% have fertility problems [1,2]. The disease is characterized by the presence of stromal and/or endometrial glandular epithelium outside the uterus and is classified in three different types: superficial, ovarian and deep endometriosis [3–5]. Endometriosis was first described in the seventeenth century and, despite all research efforts in the last 30 years, its pathogenesis is still unclear [6].

Nowadays the most accepted hypothesis is that the foci of endometriosis originate from retrograde menstruation [7]. According to this theory, initially proposed by Sampson, the retrograde tubal flow seeds menstrual endometrial tissue in the peritoneal cavity and other organs, to which it adheres. However, as around 90% of women have retrograde menstruation, and just only 10% develop the disease, several authors have been proposed that other factors like anatomical, genetic, endocrine, environmental and inflammatory may influence this tissue implantation [8–16].

One of the most described are the inflammatory factors. Several studies have already demonstrated, for example, that the peritoneal fluid of women with endometriosis has high levels of pro-inflammatory cytokines and growth factors, such as TNF-α, IL-1 and IL-6. In previous studies carried out by our research group, we described the role of inflammatory factors presented in peritoneal fluid in the immune balance of patients with endometriosis, showing an increase in the cytokines IL-2, IL-6 and TGF-β, an increase in amyloid protein A (SAA), as well as an increase in CD4(+)CD25(high)Foxp3(+) cells, and a decrease in ICOS+Treg (T regulatory cells) and CD45RO+Treg cells in patients with the disease [10,11,14].

This inflammatory process found in patients with endometriosis has been described because it is possibly related to the presence of microorganisms. Several authors have shown, for example, an increase in the cytokine IL-1β in patients with endometriosis and they correlate this increase with the activation of inflammasomes by stimulating microorganisms, and also correlate the participation of this event in the pathogenesis of the disease [17–19].

Several other studies shown the presence of microorganisms in menstrual blood, peritoneal fluid and vagino-uterine tract [20–24], but no work so far has described the presence of microorganisms in endometriotic lesions, and their correlation with microorganisms found in vaginal secretion and eutopic endometrium.

In this context, the present project aimed to investigate, by using high-throughput DNA sequencing, the microbiome profile present in vaginal fluid, endometrium and deep endometriotic lesions of women with endometriosis in comparison to microbiome profile found in vaginal fluid and endometrium of women without the disease. As there is a lack of understanding of the relationship between them, identifying endometriosis-associated microbiome profiles could help the understanding of pathogenesis and eventually could lead to the development of a noninvasive test for endometriosis.

2. Materials and Methods

2.1. Sample Collection

This case-control study was conducted as a pilot investigation at Hospital Israelita Albert Einstein (HIAE), São Paulo, Brazil, and the protocol was approved on December, 2017 by the Research Ethics Committee of Hospital Israelita Albert Einstein (project number 80280317.5.0000.0071); all patients provided written informed consent.

Twenty-one patients were included in the study according to the inclusion and exclusion criteria outlined below. Patients were assigned to the endometriosis group after lesion(s) identification by laparoscopic surgery, and further confirmation by histopathology analysis. Just women showing deep endometriosis were included. The control group consisted of women who underwent laparoscopic surgery for benign gynecologic diseases or elective tubal ligation in which peritoneal cavity inspection confirmed absence of endometriosis.

Women aged 18–50 years presenting eumenorrheic cycles were included in the study, whether or not under hormonal treatment. Women previously diagnosed with autoimmune, inflammatory and/or neoplastic disease, and who had used antibiotics/antimycotics in the 30 days prior to samples' collection were excluded.

Eutopic endometrium and endometriotic lesion tissue samples were collected by curettage and laparoscopic surgery, respectively. All samples were collected at the operative room to minimize contamination and every care was taken to prevent the swab from touching other tissues adjacent to the target site, not having contact with blood, or any other instrument. Tissue samples were immediately frozen in liquid nitrogen and maintained at −80 °C. Vaginal fluid was sampled with sterile nylon flock swabs (Copan, Murrieta, CA, USA), also did not touched other sites and it was maintained in a microbiome transport solution (BiomeHub, Florianópolis, SC, Brazil) which allows a stable transport at ambient temperatures.

2.2. DNA Extraction and 16S rRNA Amplicon Sequencing

DNA from tissue samples was extracted using the DNeasy Power Soil Kit (QIAGEN). Processing of all samples was carried out under sterile conditions. The tissue fragments were initially minced and submitted to mechanical disruption; the DNA extraction followed the manufacturer's protocol. Vaginal fluid samples in transport solution were extracted using the QIAamp DNA Blood Mini Kit (QIAGEN) according to the manufacturer instructions. Negative control samples were included for the extraction procedures, to evaluate kit reagent DNA background and possible process contaminations.

Preparation of an amplicon sequencing library for bacteria was performed using the V3-V4 16S rRNA gene primers 341F (CCTACGGGRSGCAGCAG) [25] and 806R (GGACTACHV GGGTWTCTAAT) [26], under the following conditions: the first PCR primers contained the Illumina sequences based on TruSeq structure adapter (Illumina, San Diego, CA, USA), allowing the second PCR with indexing sequences. The PCR reactions were always carried out in triplicates using Platinum Taq (Invitrogen, Waltham, MA, USA) with the conditions: 95 °C for 5 min, 25 cycles of 95 °C for 45 s, 55 °C for 30 s and 72 °C for 45s and a final extension of 72 °C for 2 min for PCR 1. In PCR 2 the conditions were 95 °C for 5 min, 10 cycles of 95 °C for 45s, 66 °C for 30 s and 72 °C for 45 s and a final extension of 72 °C for 2 min. Negative control reactions were included to access possible PCR reagent contaminations. The final PCR reactions were cleaned up using AMPureXP beads (Beckman Coulter, Brea, CA, USA) and samples were pooled in the sequencing libraries for quantification. The DNA concentration of the pool amplicon was estimated with Picogreen dsDNA assays (Invitrogen, Waltham, MA, USA), and then the pooled libraries were diluted for accurate qPCR quantification using a KAPA Library Quantification Kit for Illumina platforms (KAPA Biosystems, Woburn, MA, USA). The library pool was adjusted to a final concentration of 11.5 pM and sequenced in a MiSeq system, using the standard Illumina primers provided in the kit. A single-end 300nt run was performed using a V2 × 300 sequencing kit. Original sequencing data are available at NCBI BioProject PRJNA546137.

2.3. Microbiome Profile Evaluation Through Bioinformatics Analysis

After the amplicon sequencing, the EncodeTools Metabarcode Pipeline (BiomeHub, Florianópolis, SC, Brazil) was used [27]. In this pipeline, the sequenced reads were quality filtered and primers trimmed resulting in a read of 283pb. Sequence reads smaller than expected, with remaining adapter sequences or more than one mismatch in the primer were excluded. All the reads that passed this quality assessment were clustered into 100% identity oligotypes and analyzed with Deblur [28] and the VSEARCH [29] packages to remove possible erroneous and chimeric reads. Oligotypes below a frequency of 0.2% in the samples were removed. Additionally, a negative control filter was implemented. If any oligotype was observed in the negative controls, it was checked against the samples and removed from the results.

After all, the oligotypes were used for taxonomical assignment with the BLAST [30] tool against a reference genome database constructed with NCBI and *in-house* bacterial genome sequences. Taxonomy was assigned to each oligotype using a lowest common ancestor (LCA) algorithm. If more than one bacterial reference can be assigned to the same oligotype with equivalent similarity and coverage metrics, the EncodeTools Metabarcode Taxonomy Assignment algorithm leads the taxonomy to the lowest level of possible unambiguous resolution (e.g., genus, family, kingdom) according with the similarity thresholds previously stablished [31].

Microbiome data comparison and diversity analysis were conducted inside the R statistical environment (R version 3.6.0). The Phyloseq R package [32] was used for alpha diversity analysis in the plot_richness function. Raw amplicon sequences were used to construct phylogenetic trees using FastTree 2.1 [33] and these were considered to calculate weighted UniFrac distances [34]. Beta diversity analyses used a proportion-normalized abundances [35,36] to calculate Bray–Curtis dissimilarity and weighted UniFrac using the Phyloseq's distance function. Nonparametric tests, including the Kruskall-Wallis and Wilcoxon tests were used as implemented in base R and in coin R package [37].

DESEq2 R package was used to identify differentially abundant genera with the Generalized Linear Model implemented [38]. The obtained p-values were corrected according to Benjamini and Hochberg procedure [39]. Values were reported as fold-changes in the log2 scale (log2 FC).

Graphical visualizations for the analysis in the boxplots, principal coordinates analysis (PCoA) and heatmap were generated with the ggplot2 R package [40].

3. Results

Twenty-one patients were included in this study, eleven in the control group and ten in endometriotic group. A total of 47 samples were collected and processed for the evaluation of their bacterial profile: 21 samples of vaginal fluid, 18 eutopic endometrium and 8 endometriotic lesion samples.

Considering all collected samples, we were able to identify 51 different bacterial genera, in a total of 414,787.00 reads, with an average of 8465.04 reads per sample.

Microbiome sequencing from vaginal fluid, eutopic endometrium and endometriotic lesions resulted in similar microorganism profiles, which were composed most abundantly by the bacterial genus *Lactobacillus*, *Gardnerella*, *Streptococcus* and *Prevotella* (Figure 1).

Figure 1. Relative abundance of bacterial profiles. Bacterial composition of each sample is reported by color bars relative to a 100% scale. Results are presented by the taxonomic rank of genus. SwV—vaginal fluid (Swab), End—endometrium, CN—negative controls.

Eutopic endometrium, as well as endometriotic lesion samples, had lower amount of detected relative reads in comparison to vaginal fluid samples (Figure 2), on the other hand, these samples showed less diversity, with which showed a marked predominance of *Lactobacillus*.

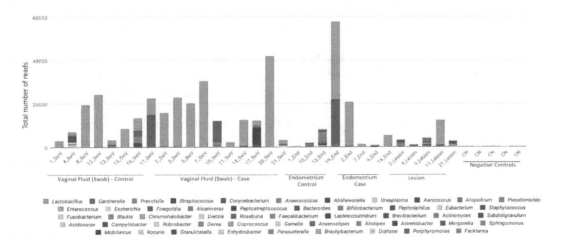

Figure 2. Total reads sequenced for each sample. Bacterial composition of each sample is reported by different color bars and scaled as the total number of reads for each sample. Results are presented by the taxonomic rank of genus. SwV—vaginal fluid (Swab), End—endometrium, CN—negative controls.

We found that endometriotic lesion samples had the most microorganism diversity which included *Lactobacillus, Enterococcus, Gardnerella, Pseudomonas, Alishewanella, Ureaplasma* and *Aerococcus* (Figure 1).

Negative controls (CN) were included in Figures 1 and 2 to demonstrate the lower and different number of reads obtained from kits and reagents background. An average of 66 reads per control was recovered, with a minimum of 45 and a maximum of 204. Negative controls have a totally different bacterial profile from the samples, which demonstrates that there was no contamination of the reagents, and that the presence of microorganisms comes from the studied samples.

A slightly significant difference ($p = 0.036$) among the bacterial composition of lesions (E) compared to other samples was observed when beta-diversity analysis, with weighted UniFrac distances were used, but no differences among samples were observed in Bray-Curtis dissimilarity (Figure 3A).

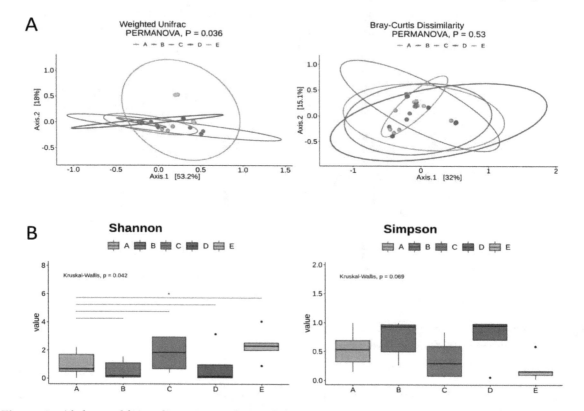

Figure 3. Alpha and beta-diversity analysis. (**A**) Principal coordinates analysis (PCoA) made with weighted UniFrac distances and Bray-Curtis dissimilarity. Sample groups are represented by the letters: A (dark green)-control swab from vaginal fluid; B (orange)-case swab from vaginal fluid; C (purple)-control endometrial tissue; D (pink)-case endometrial tissue; and **E** (light green)-lesion. (**B**) Alpha diversity indexes of Shannon and Simpson are sowed in the boxplots for each collection site group of samples (A, B, C, D and E). Kruskall-Wallis and Wilcoxon tests are showed for group and paired groups comparison, respectively (represented by solid lined above boxplots, only significative comparisons were shown and marked with an *). Black solid points represent outlier samples.

Already when alpha-diversity analysis considering Shannon and Simpson indices was used, we observed highly variable results, but similar diversity levels with the other samples (Figure 3B), despite the tendency to a lower alpha-diversity in endometriotic lesions compared to control vaginal fluid samples.

The most abundant genera detected in the collection sites were plotted (Figure 4A) and it was possible to observe some patterns like the predominance of *Lactobacillus* in vaginal fluid and endometrial samples. The high abundance of *Gardnerella* and *Prevotella* could be observed in the control samples of vaginal fluid and endometrium, while endometriotic lesions showed a higher prevalence of *Alishewanella, Enterococcus* and *Pseudomonas*. This bacterial profile of lesions was also detected in DESeq2 differential abundance analysis, with a significant result (Figure 4B).

Figure 4. Relative and differential abundances. (**A**) Boxplots represent the most abundant genera detected and their distribution in the samples. Swab_ctrl—control swab from vaginal fluid; Swab—case swab from vaginal fluid; Endo_ctrl—control endometrial tissue; Endo—case endometrial tissue; lesion—samples from endometriosis lesion. Black solid points represent outlier samples for each group. (**B**) Differential abundance heatmap comparing all the collection sites from case and control samples. Results are showed as the log2FC for the differentially detected genera. Most abundant genera are showed as red values considering the first sample category in the bottom legend.

555555555555

4. Discussion

In this study, we report the microbiome profile from deep endometriotic lesions in Brazilian women.

We detected the presence of microorganisms of the genus *Lactobacillus, Enterococcus, Gardnerella, Pseudomonas, Alishewanella, Ureaplasma* and *Aerococcus* in deep endometriotic lesions of fifty percent of our endometriosis patient group.

When we compared the microorganism profile from lesions with that found in vaginal fluid and eutopic endometrium of patients with endometriosis, slightly significant differences were found, with a major diversity seen in lesions. Beside this difference, this microbiome data did not reveal a strict bacterial profile specific to the collection sites.

Similar profile between samples derived from 14 women with endometriosis and 14 healthy controls also was observed in a study conduct by Ata et al. [24]. Despite overall similar vaginal, cervical and intestinal microbiota composition between endometriosis and control groups, the authors observed differences at the genus level, with an absence of *Atopobium* in the vaginal and cervical microbiota of the endometriosis group, and enhanced presence of *Gardnerella, Streptococcus, Escherichia, Shigella,* and *Ureaplasma*.

Our results reflect similar profiles of microorganisms as also those obtained by Chen et al. [23] for vaginal and endometrial samples, where the samples collected from endometrium tissue showed a transition profile from the vagina to the upper reproductive tract without sufficient differentiation from other sites of the female reproductive tract. However, the authors still found a change in the microbiota in the peritoneal fluid of women with endometriosis. This alteration found in the peritoneal fluid reinforces our hypothesis that there is an involvement of microorganisms and the immune system in the process of establishment and maintenance of lesions.

Our group investigated the expression of toll-like receptors (TLRs), in T reg cells isolated from peritoneal fluid from patients with and without endometriosis, and we found that there is a change in the activation of TLRs receptors in women with endometriosis, where TLR 1, 2, 3, 4, 5, 6, 7 and 8 were expressed in regulatory T cells isolated from peritoneal fluid from women with endometriosis while only TLR1 and TLR2 receptors were expressed in women without endometriosis [41].

These findings are in line with the findings of this study, which shows that endometriotic lesions have a greater diversity of microorganisms, which consequently cause Treg cells to express a greater number of toll-type receptors, and that there is a relationship between the presence of microorganisms and the inflammatory process.

A retrospective study involving 141.460 patients, out of which 28,292 presented PID (pelvic inflammatory disease) and 113,168 were healthy, showed the correlation between microorganisms and inflammation, suggesting that PID patients were at high risk (three times more) for developing endometriosis than those without PID, suggesting that such bacterial transport in women with PID could facilitate contamination of the upper reproductive tract and pelvic cavity, leading to endometriosis [42]. PID is characterized as a disease caused by the passage of pathogenic bacteria from the vagina to the uterus, fallopian tubes and ovaries.

Present in the plasma membrane or inside vesicles, TLRs are the first receptors to recognize molecular signals of pathogen-associated patterns (PAMPs), triggering a cascade of cellular events. Next, receptors present in the cytosol are activated, via activator protein (AP1) and via interferon regulatory factors (IRFs). These receptors form cytosolic molecular complexes, called inflammasomes, activate caspase- 1 and the production of cytokines, such as IL-1β and IL-18 that induce pyroptosis and apoptosis [43–47]. This process involving TLR receptors, inflammasomes and cytokine production leads to the immune system's response against a wide variety of microorganisms.

These would dampen the natural inflammatory process responsible for the elimination of the retro-flowing uterine endometrial cells during menstruation. As a result, the attachment of ectopic endometrial cells to the peritoneal surfaces would be facilitated. This hypothesis has also been brought forward by other studies related to this topic [48–54].

Our finding of microorganisms in the endometriotic lesions themselves is important as it may advance the hypothesis that one or all of these also ectopically found bacteria may be implicated in the maintenance and survival of the ectopic endometrial cells. The fact that they are also found in the uterine cavity and in the vagina would only be expected.

This was a preliminary evaluation of endometriotic lesions microbiome and there are limitations to the study. A new study with a larger number of patients has to be carried out to confirm the results observed in patients with endometriosis. Moreover, the relation between the presence of these microorganisms and their metabolites in the peritoneal fluid or in the endometriosis lesions should be explored, especially looking into regulation of inflammation and immune responses. As one of the functions of the peritoneal fluid is to remove pathogens the presence of microorganisms in the peritoneal cavity may indicate a poor in situ immune response, one of the possible causes of endometriosis [55].

5. Conclusions

In conclusion, this study revealed that deep endometriotic lesions present a diversity of bacteria as observed in a microbiome analysis using high-throughput DNA sequencing methods. We understand that this result may open new avenues to the study endometriosis and eventually could lead to the development of a noninvasive test for the disease.

Author Contributions: C.H., S.P., A.F.R.S. and L.F.V.d.O. designed the study. C.H., H.M. and S.P. collected the samples. P.S., A.P.C., A.F.R.S. and L.F.V.d.O. conducted the laboratory sample processing. C.H., P.S., A.F.R.S., A.P.C. and L.F.V.d.O. analyzed the results. C.H., S.P., A.F.R.S., P.S. contributed to discussion of results. All authors have read and agree to the published version of the manuscript.

References

1. De Paula Andres, M.; Lopes, L.A.; Baracat, E.C.; Podgaec, S. Dienogest in the treatment of endometriosis: Systematic review. *Arch. Gynecol. Obstet.* **2015**, *292*, 523–529. [CrossRef] [PubMed]

2. Parasar, P.; Ozcan, P.; Terry, K.L. Endometriosis: Epidemiology, Diagnosis and Clinical Management. *Curr. Obstet. Gynecol. Rep.* **2017**, *6*, 34–41. [CrossRef] [PubMed]

3. Nisolle, M.; Donnez, J. Peritoneal endometriosis, ovarian endometriosis, and adenomyotic nodules of the rectovaginal septum are three different entities. *Fertil. Steril.* **1997**, *68*, 585–596. [CrossRef]

4. Bassi, M.A.; Arias, V.; D'Amico, N.; Gueuvoghlanian-Silva, B.Y.; Abrao, M.S.; Podgaec, S. Deep Invasive Endometriosis Lesions of the Rectosigmoid May Be Related to Alterations in Cell Kinetics. *Reprod Sci.* **2015**, *22*, 1122–1128. [CrossRef]

5. Santulli, P.; Tran, C.; Gayet, V.; Bourdon, M.; Maignien, L.; Pocate-Cheriet, K.; Chapron, C.; de Ziegler, D. Oligo-anovulation is not a rarer feature in women with documented endometriosis. *Fertil. Steril.* **2018**, *110*, 941–948. [CrossRef]

6. Klemmt, P.A.B.; Starzinski-Powitz, A. Molecular and Cellular Pathogenesis of Endometriosis. *Curr. Womens Health Rev.* **2018**, *14*, 106–116. [CrossRef]

7. Sampson, J.A. Metastatic or Embolic Endometriosis, due to the Menstrual Dissemination of Endometrial Tissue into the Venous Circulation. *Am. J. Pathol.* **1927**, *3*, 93–110.

8. Silvae, J.C.R.; da Fortunato, G.G.; Barbosa, C.P. Aspectos Gerais da Etiopatogenia da Endometriose. In *Coleção Febrasgo Endometriose*, 1st ed.; Podgaec, S., de Janeiro, R., Eds.; Elsevier: Amsterdam, The Netherlands, 2015; pp. 27–34.

9. Zhang, T.; De Carolis, C.; Man, G.C.W.; Wang, C.C. The link between immunity, autoimmunity and endometriosis: A literature update. *Autoimmun. Rev.* **2018**, *17*, 945–955. [CrossRef]

10. Podgaec, S.; junior, J.A.D.; Chapron, C.; de Oliveira, R.M.; Baracat, E.; Abrao, M.S. Th1 and Th2 immune responses related to pelvic endometriosis. *Rev. Assoc. Med. Bras.* **2010**, *56*, 92–98. [CrossRef]

11. Podgaec, S.; Rizzo, L.V.; Fernandes, L.F.; Baracat, E.C.; Abrao, M.S. CD4$^+$ CD25^{high} Foxp3$^+$ cells increased in the peritoneal fluid of patients with endometriosis. *Am. J. Reprod Immunol.* **2012**, *68*, 301–308. [CrossRef]

12. Sourial, S.; Tempest, N.; Hapangama, D.K. Theories on the pathogenesis of endometriosis. *Int. J. Reprod. Med.* **2014**, *2014*, 1–9. [CrossRef] [PubMed]

13. Khan, K.N.; Fujishita, A.; Hiraki, K.; Kitajima, M.; Nakashima, M.; Fushiki, S.; Kitawaki, J. Bacterial contamination hypothesis: A new concept in endometriosis. *Reprod. Med. Biol.* **2018**, *18*, 125–133. [CrossRef] [PubMed]

14. Gueuvoghlanian-Silva, B.Y.; Bellelis, P.; Barbeiro, F.D.; Hernandes, C.; Podgaec, S. Treg and NK cells related cytokines are associated with deep rectosigmoid endometriosis and clinical symptoms related to the disease. *J. Reprod. Immunol.* **2018**, *126*, 32–38. [CrossRef] [PubMed]

15. Bellelis, P.; Barbeiro, D.F.; Gueuvoghlanian-Silva, B.Y.; Kalil, J.; Abrão, M.S.; Podgaec, S. Interleukin-15 and Interleukin-7 are the Major Cytokines to Maintain Endometriosis. *Gynecol. Obstet. Invest.* **2019**, *84*, 435–444. [CrossRef] [PubMed]

16. Akiyama, K.; Nishioka, K.; Khan, K.N.; Tanaka, Y.; Mori, T.; Nakaya, T.; Kitawaki, J. Molecular detection of microbial colonization in cervical mucus of women with and without endometriosis. *Am. J. Reprod. Immunol.* **2019**, *82*, 1–9. [CrossRef] [PubMed]

17. Bullon, P.; Manuel Navarro, J. Inflammasome as a key pathogenic mechanism in endometriosis. *Curr. Drug Targets* **2017**, *18*, 997–1002. [CrossRef] [PubMed]

18. Chadchan, S.B.; Cheng, M.; Parnell, L.A.; Yin, Y.; Schriefer, A.; Mysorekar, I.U.; Kommagani, R. Antibiotic therapy with metronidazole reduces endometriosis disease progression in mice: A potential role for gut microbiota. *Human Reprod.* **2019**, *34*, 1106–1116. [CrossRef]

19. Campos, G.B.; Marques, L.M.; Rezende, I.S. Mycoplasma genitalium can modulate the local immune response in patients with endometriosis. *Fertil. Steril.* **2018**, *109*, 549–560. [CrossRef]

20. Khan, K.N.; Kitajima, M.; Hiraki, K.; Yamaguchi, N.; Katamine, S.; Matsuyama, T.; Nakashima, M.; Fujishita, A.; Ishimaru, T.; Masuzaki, H. Escherichia coli contamination of menstrual blood and effect of bacterial endotoxin on endometriosis. *Fertil. Steril.* **2010**, *94*, 860–863. [CrossRef]

21. Khan, K.N.; Fujishita, A.; Kitajima, M.; Hiraki, K.; Nakashima, M.; Masuzaki, H. Intra-uterine microbial colonization and occurrence of endometritis in women with endometriosis. *Human Reprod.* **2014**, *29*, 2446–2456. [CrossRef]

22. Khan, K.N.; Fujishita, A.; Masumoto, H.; Muto, H.; Kitajima, M.; Masuzaki, H.; Kitawaki, J. Molecular detection of intrauterine microbial colonization in women with endometriosis. *Eur. J. Obstet. Gynecol. Reprod. Biol.* **2016**, *199*, 69–75. [CrossRef] [PubMed]

23. Chen, C.; Song, X.; Wei, W.; Zhong, H.; Dai, J.; Lan, Z. The microbiota continuum along the female reproductive tract and its relation to uterine-related diseases. *Nat. Commun.* **2017**, *17*, 875–878. [CrossRef] [PubMed]

24. Ata, B.; Yildiz, S.; Turkgeldi, E.; Brocal, V.P.; Dinleyici, E.C.; Moya, A.; Urman, B. The Endobiota Study: Comparison of Vaginal, Cervical and Gut Microbiota between Women with Stage 3/4 Endometriosis and Healthy Controls. *Sci. Rep.* **2019**, *9*, 2204. [CrossRef] [PubMed]

25. Wang, Y.; Qian, P. Conservative Fragments in Bacterial 16S rRNA Genes and Primer Design for 16S Ribosomal DNA Amplicons in Metagenomic Studies. *PLoS ONE* **2009**, *4*, e7401. [CrossRef]

26. Caporaso, J.G.; Christian, L.L.; Walters, W.A.; Berg-lyons, D.; Huntley, J.; Fierer, N.; Owens, S.; Betley, J.; Fraser, L.; Bauer, M.; et al. Ultra-high-throughput microbial community analysis on the Illumina HiSeq and MiSeq platforms. *ISME J.* **2012**, *6*, 1621–1624. [CrossRef] [PubMed]

27. Christoff, A.P.; Cruz, G.F.N.; Sereia, A.F.R.; Yamanaka, L.E.; Silveira, P.P.; Oliveira, L.F.V. End-to-end assessment of fecal bacteriome analysis: From sample processing to DNA sequencing and bioinformatics results. *bioRxiv* **2019**, 646349. [CrossRef]

28. Amir, A.; McDonald, D.; Navas-Molina, J.A.; Kopylova, E.; Morton, J.T.; Xu, Z.Z.; Kightley, E.P.; Thompson, L.R.; Hyde, E.R.; Gonzalez, A.; et al. Deblur Rapidly Resolves Single-Nucleotide Community Sequence Patterns. *mSystems* **2017**, *2*, e00191-16. [CrossRef]

29. Rognes, T.; Flouri, T.; Nichols, B.; Quince, C.; Mahé, F. VSEARCH: A versatile open source tool for metagenomics. *Peerj* **2016**, *4*, e2584. [CrossRef]

30. Altschul, S.; Gish, W.; Miller, W.; Myers, E.; Lipman, D. Basic local alignment search tool. *J. Mol. Biol.* **1990**, *215*, 403–410. [CrossRef]

31. Yarza, P.; Yilmaz, P.; Pruesse, E.; Glöckner, F.O.; Ludwig, W.; Schleifer, K.H.; Whitman, W.B.; Euzéby, J.; Amann, R.; Rosselló-Móra, R. Uniting the classification of cultured and uncultured bacteria and archaea using 16S rRNA gene sequences. *Nat. Rev. Microbiol.* **2014**, *2*, 635–645. [CrossRef]

32. McMurdie, P.; Holmes, S. Phyloseq: An R Package for Reproducible Interactive Analysis and Graphics of Microbiome Census Data. *PLoS ONE* **2013**, *8*, e61217. [CrossRef] [PubMed]

33. Price, M.; Dehal, P.; Arkin, A. FastTree 2—Approximately Maximum-Likelihood Trees for Large Alignments. *PLoS ONE* **2010**, *5*, e9490. [CrossRef] [PubMed]

34. Lozupone, C.; Knight, R. UniFrac: A New Phylogenetic Method for Comparing Microbial Communities. *Appl. Environ. Microbiol.* **2015**, *71*, 8228. [CrossRef] [PubMed]

35. Weiss, S.; Xu, Z.Z.; Peddada, S.; Amir, A.; Bittinger, K.; Gonzalez, A.; Lozupone, C.; Zaneveld, J.R.; Vázquez-Baeza, Y.; Birmingham, A.; et al. Normalization and microbial differential abundance strategies depend upon data characteristics. *Microbiome* **2017**, *5*, 27. [CrossRef]

36. McMurdie, P.; Holmes, S. Waste Not, Want Not: Why Rarefying Microbiome Data Is Inadmissible. *PLoS Comput. Biol.* **2014**, *10*, e1003531. [CrossRef]

37. Hothorn, T.; Hornik, K.; Wiel, M.A.; Zeileis, A. Implementing a class of permutation tests: The coin package. *J. Stat. Softw.* **2008**, *28*, 23. [CrossRef]

38. Love, M.; Huber, W.; Anders, S. Moderated estimation of fold change and dispersion for RNA-seq data with DESeq2. *Genome Biol.* **2014**, *15*, 550. [CrossRef]

39. Benjamini, Y.; Hochberg, Y. Controlling the false discovery rate: A practical and powerful approach to multiple hypothesis testing. *J. R. Stat. Soc. B* **1995**, *57*, 289–300. [CrossRef]

40. Wickham, H. *ggplot2: Elegant Graphics for Data Analysis*; Springer: Berlin/Heidelberg, Germany, 2016.

41. Hernandes, C.; Gueuvoghlanian-Silva, B.Y.; Monnaka, V.U.; Ribeiro, N.M.; Pereira, W.O.; Podgaec, S. Regulatory T cells isolated from endometriotic peritoneal fluid express a different number of Toll-like receptors expressed. *Einstein (São Paulo)* **2020**, *18*, eAO5294.

42. Tai, F.W.; Chang, C.Y.; Chiang, J.H.; Lin, W.C.; Wan, L. Association of Pelvic Inflammatory Disease with Risk of Endometriosis: A Nationwide Cohort Study Involving 141,460 Individuals. *J. Clin. Med.* **2018**, *7*, 379. [CrossRef]

43. Kawai, T.; Akira, S. The roles of TLRs, RLRs and NLRs in pathogen recognition. *Int. Immunol.* **2009**, *21*, 317–337. [CrossRef] [PubMed]

44. Lamkanfi, M.; Dixit, V.M. Mechanisms and functions of inflammasomes. *Cell* **2014**, *15*, 1013–1022. [CrossRef] [PubMed]

45. Broz, P.; Dixit, V.M. Inflammasomes: Mechanism of assembly, regulation and signalling. *Nat. Rev. Immunol.* **2016**, *16*, 407. [CrossRef] [PubMed]

46. Sharma, D.; Kanneganti, T.D. The cell biology of inflammasomes: Mechanisms of inflammasome activation and regulation. *J. Cell Biol.* **2016**, *213*, 617–629. [CrossRef] [PubMed]

47. Webster, S.J.; Goodall, J.C. New concepts in Chlamydia induced inflammasome responses. *Microb. Infect.* **2018**, *20*, 424–431. [CrossRef] [PubMed]

48. Caramalho, I.; Lopes-Carvalho, T.; Ostler, D.; Zelenay, S.; Haury, M.; Demengeot, J. Regulatory T cells selectively express toll-like receptors and are activated by lipopolysaccharide. *J. Exp. Med.* **2003**, *197*, 403–411. [CrossRef] [PubMed]

49. Netea, M.G.; Sutmuller, R.; Hermann, C.; Van der Graaf, C.A.; Van der Meer, J.W.; Van Krieken, J.H.; Hartung, T.; Adema, G.; Kullberg, B.J. Toll-like receptor 2 suppresses immunity against Candida albicans through induction of IL-10 and regulatory T cells. *J. Immunol.* **2004**, *172*, 3712–3718. [CrossRef]

50. Peng, G.; Guo, Z.; Kiniwa, Y.; Voo, K.S.; Peng, W.; Fu, T.; Wang, D.Y.; Li, Y.; Wang, H.Y. Toll-like receptor 8-mediated reversal of CD4+ regulatory T cell function. *Science* **2005**, *309*, 1380–1384. [CrossRef]

51. Liu, G.; Zhao, Y. Toll-like receptors and immune regulation: Their direct and indirect modulation on regulatory CD4+ CD25+ T cells. *Immunology* **2007**, *122*, 149–156. [CrossRef]

52. Van Maren, W.W.; Jacobs, J.F.; de Vries, I.J.; Nierkens, S.; Adema, G.J. Toll-like receptor signalling on Tregs: To suppress or not to suppress? *Immunology* **2008**, *124*, 445–452. [CrossRef]

53. Olivier, A.; Dong, H.; Sparwasser, T.; Majilessi, L.; Leclerc, C. The adjuvant effect of TLR agonists on CD4+ effector T cells is under the indirect control of regulatory T cells. *Eur. J. Immunol.* **2011**, *41*, 2303–2313. [CrossRef] [PubMed]

54.   de Barros, I.B.L.; Malvezzi, H.; Gueuvoghlanian-Silva, B.Y.; Piccinato, C.A.; Rizzo, L.V.; Podgaec, S. Corrigendum to "What do we know about regulatory T cells and endometriosis? A systematic review". *J. Reprod. Immunol.* **2017**, *121*, 48–55. [CrossRef] [PubMed]

55.   Capobianco, A.; Cottone, L.; Monno, A.; Manfredi, A.A.; Rovere-Querini, P. The peritoneum: Healing, immunity, and diseases. *J. Pathol.* **2017**, *243*, 137–147. [CrossRef] [PubMed]

Peritoneal Fluid Cytokines Reveal New Insights of Endometriosis Subphenotypes

Jieliang Zhou [1,†], Bernard Su Min Chern [2,3,†], Peter Barton-Smith [4,‡⦿], Jessie Wai Leng Phoon [3,5], Tse Yeun Tan [5], Veronique Viardot-Foucault [5], Chee Wai Ku [2,3], Heng Hao Tan [3,5], Jerry Kok Yen Chan [3,5] and Yie Hou Lee [1,3,*,§⦿]

[1] Translational 'Omics and Biomarkers group, KK Research Centre, KK Women's and Children's Hospital, Singapore 229899, Singapore; zhou.jieliang@kkh.com.sg

[2] Division of Obstetrics and Gynaecology, KK Women's and Children's Hospital, Singapore 229899, Singapore; bernard.chern.s.m@singhealth.com.sg (B.S.M.C.); gmskcw@nus.edu.sg (C.W.K.)

[3] OBGYN-Academic Clinical Program, Duke-NUS Medical School, Singapore 169857, Singapore; jessie.phoon.w.l@singhealth.com.sg (J.W.L.P.); tan.heng.hao@singhealth.com.sg (H.H.T.); jerry.chan.k.y@singhealth.com.sg (J.K.Y.C.)

[4] Department of Obstetrics and Gynaecology, Singapore General Hospital, Singapore 169608, Singapore; pcbartonsmith@gmail.com

[5] Department of Reproductive Medicine, KKH, Singapore 229899, Singapore; tan.tse.yeun@singhealth.com.sg (T.Y.T.); veronique.viardot@singhealth.com.sg (V.V.-F.)

[*] Correspondence: yiehou.lee@smart.mit.edu

[†] These authors contributed equally to this work.

[‡] Current address: The Princess Grace Hospital, 42-52 Nottingham Place, London W1U 5NY, UK.

[§] Current address: Singapore-MIT Alliance for Research and Technology, 1 CREATE Way, Singapore 138602, Singapore.

Abstract: Endometriosis is a common inflammatory gynecological disorder which causes pelvic scarring, pain, and infertility, characterized by the implantation of endometrial-like lesions outside the uterus. The peritoneum, ovaries, and deep soft tissues are the commonly involved sites, and endometriotic lesions can be classified into three subphenotypes: superficial peritoneal endometriosis (PE), ovarian endometrioma (OE), and deep infiltrating endometriosis (DIE). In 132 women diagnosed laparoscopically with and without endometriosis ($n = 73, 59$ respectively), and stratified into PE, OE, and DIE, peritoneal fluids (PF) were characterized for 48 cytokines by using multiplex immunoassays. Partial-least-squares-regression analysis revealed distinct subphenotype cytokine signatures—a six-cytokine signature distinguishing PE from OE, a seven-cytokine signature distinguishing OE from DIE, and a six-cytokine-signature distinguishing PE from DIE—each associated with different patterns of biological processes, signaling events, and immunology. These signatures describe endometriosis better than disease stages ($p < 0.0001$). Pathway analysis revealed the association of ERK1 and 2, AKT, MAPK, and STAT4 linked to angiogenesis, cell proliferation, migration, and inflammation in the subphenotypes. These data shed new insights on the pathophysiology of endometriosis subphenotypes, with the potential to exploit the cytokine signatures to stratify endometriosis patients for targeted therapies and biomarker discovery.

Keywords: endometriosis; cytokines; peritoneal fluid; microenvironment; precision medicine

---

1. Introduction

Endometriosis inflicts 6–10% of women of reproductive age, with affected women suffering from debilitating pelvic pain, dysmenorrhea, dyspareunia, and painful defecation. The prevalence of subfertility or infertility is higher in the endometriosis population, with up to half of endometriotic women suffering from reduced fecundity [1]. Endometriotic lesions can be classified into three subphenotypes: superficial peritoneal endometriosis (PE), ovarian cysts (ovarian endometrioma; OE), and deep infiltrating endometriosis (DIE) [2]. Superficial peritoneal lesions refer to implants found on the pelvic organs or pelvic peritoneum. They are typically white, red, or blue–black power burns and may be phenotypically progressive over time [3–5]. Endometriomas are formed when endometrial tissue implants on the ovary surface or penetrate into the ovary [6–8]. By contrast, DIE involves nodular lesions which invade the surrounding organs beneath the peritoneum [9]. They are commonly found on the uterosacral ligaments, bladder, vagina, and intestine and are more aggressive in nature [10]. The endometriosis subphenotypes are being recognized as clinicopathologically different from one another and are thought to be separate entities [3,10,11].

Many theories and hypotheses have been proposed to explain the pathogenesis and development of endometriosis [12,13]. The most widely accepted theory to explain the etiology of endometriosis is the retrograde menstrual hypothesis. During menses, viable menstrual fragments of eutopic endometrial origin back-traverse through the fallopian tubes, into the peritoneal cavity, which subsequently leads to these cells being implanted onto extra-uterine ectopic sites. However, this theory is insufficient to explain the presence of the disease in early puberty and in adolescents [14], and it does not address why endometriosis only occurs in a certain subset of the female population. Other theories have been put forth, including the coelomic metaplasia theory, endometrial stem/progenitor cells theory, and Müllerianosis theory. These complementary theories and hypotheses help to generally frame our understanding of plausible mechanisms of the endometriosis pathogenesis and allow for the testing of hypotheses and improvement of the currently existing treatment options and the introduction of new treatments. Recent advances had been made with respect to elucidating partial progestin response based on the progesterone receptor status of endometriosis patients [15], which infers the prospect of precision or targeted medicine for treating endometriosis. In addition, key non-hormonal inflammation or signaling pathways associated with endometriosis subphenotypes could be exploited for therapeutic advantage, particularly in the era of targeted treatment and precision medicine [16].

Ectopic endometriotic lesions secrete chemokines into their surrounding tissues, recruiting immune cells, which in turn secrete cytokines and growth factors, such as TNF-α, IL-1β, IL-6, IL-8, IL-17, EGF, FGF, and VEGF, creating locally specific microenvironments that develop a reciprocal interaction with the peritoneal fluid (PF) [17–19]. The interaction of cytokines constitutes molecular signatures that are used to orchestrate immune and other complex responses in endometriosis development, plausibly in the evolution of lesion subphenotypes [14,20]. With increased appreciation that immunomodulatory proteins are part of an overall signaling network [21,22], significant discoveries of pro-angiogenic, macrophage-derived, and endometriosis-associated infertility cytokine signatures have been made in recent years [23–27]. While these studies provide insight into major pathways involved in disease stages, several outstanding gaps remain in terms of the cytokine relationship with endometriosis subphenotypes [28] and their implications in stratified treatment. Here, in this study, we investigated PF cytokines and their association with the three endometriosis subphenotypes. This allowed us to assemble cytokine signatures, which revealed dysregulated biological processes associated with the pathogenesis/pathophysiology of the three endometriosis subphenotypes. These results might direct new endometriosis therapeutic and diagnostic efforts toward subphenotype clinically relevant cytokine targets.

2. Results

2.1. Peritoneal Fluid Cytokines Inadequately Describe Endometriosis Stages and Their Heterogeneity

PF samples from 132 women (without endometriosis, EM− = 59; with endometriosis, EM+ = 73) (Table 1) were analyzed for 48 cytokines, using a validated multiplex immunoassay platform. Among the cytokines analyzed, 38 (79%) cytokines were detected and compared using univariate analysis

(Tables S1 and S2). Because inflammatory cascades are brought about by the interaction of pro-inflammatory and anti-inflammatory cytokines [21], multivariate analysis such as PLSR provides a powerful way to obtain cytokine signatures to molecularly distinguish the patient groups in relation to disease presence and stages. Using partial least squares regression (PLSR), we identified a cytokine signature comprising IFN-α2, IL-12p70, IL-18, SCGF-β, VEGF-A, IL-3, and HGF that distinguished EM- from EM+ (Figure 1A). Notably, IFN-α2, IL-12p70, IL-18, SCGF-β, and VEGF-A are cytokines previously identified to be significantly altered between EM- from EM+ individuals [29–31]. However, a significant overlap between the EM- and EM+ clusters was observed (cumulative principal component (PC) score: 43%; Figure 1B), congruent with other studies [32]. We used the cumulative PC score as a measure of how well the cytokines could distinguish between EM-, EM+, EM+$_{Mild}$, and EM+$_{Severe}$ patients (perfect separation of patient clusters at 100% cumulative PC score). When EM+$_{Mild}$ and EM+$_{Severe}$ individuals were compared to EM-, the PLSR separations improved slightly, as indicated by higher cumulative PC scores of 51% and 49% (Figure 1C and Figure S1A,B). PLSR modeling of PF cytokines in EM+$_{Mild}$ from EM+$_{Severe}$ separated at 59%, but remains relatively poor as observed in the other models of disease stages (EM- versus EM+$_{Mild}$, EM- versus EM+$_{Severe}$), suggesting heterogeneity of disease stages and subsequent incompleteness to distinguish endometriosis (Figure S1A–F).

Figure 1. Peritoneal fluid cytokines associate with endometriosis stages. (**A**) Partial least squares regression (PLSR) coefficient analysis revealed a signature comprising elevated IL-12p70, IL-18, VEGF-A, and SCGF-β and decreased IFN-α2, IL-3, and HGF that distinguished women with endometriosis (EM+) from women without (EM-). (**B**) Modeling by PLSR scores plot reveals overlap of EM- and EM+, suggesting heterogeneity in the peritoneal fluid environment. PLSR-derived principal component scores of principal component 1 (PC1) and principal component 2 (PC2) of (**C**) stages and (**D**) subphenotypes. Cumulative principal-component scores are shown at the top of each bar.

Table 1. Patient characteristics.

Characteristics	EM- ($n = 59$)	EM+ ($n = 73$)	p-Value [†]
Age, y			0.844
Mean	35	35	
Range	22–51	25–45	
ASRM Stage			
I–II	NA	31	
III–IV	NA	42	
Subtype			
Peritoneal	NA	17	
Endometrioma	NA	30	
Deep infiltrating	NA	14	
Undetermined	NA	12	
Preoperative pain symptoms[a]			<0.0001
Dysmenorrhea	20	56	
Dyspareunia [b]	5	20	
Menstrual phase			0.290
Proliferative	27	41	
Secretory	32	32	
Race			0.650
Chinese	36	46	
Malay	14	13	
Others [c]	9	14	

[†] Student's t-test was performed for age, and Chi square for categorical data in pain, menstrual phase, and race.
[a] 18 patients present with both dysmenorrhea and dyspareunia. [b] 10 patients did not have coitus at time of surgery.
[c] Includes Indians and Filipinos

2.2. Peritoneal Fluid Cytokine Signatures Delineate Endometriosis Subphenotypes

The three subphenotypes of endometriosis, OE, PE, and DIE, present peculiar clinicopathological characteristics, which prompted us to hypothesize that PF cytokines might describe endometriosis better, viz-a-viz capturing molecular variations of the subphenotypes. Based on PF cytokines, PLSR modeling of endometriosis subphenotypes resulted in better models than disease stages (cumulative PC scores: 77% to 92%, $p < 0.0001$; Figures 1D and 2A–C; Table S3). PLSR scores plots revealed clear delineation of OE, PE, and DIE (Figure S2A), suggesting their distinct molecular makeups. In addition, analysis of the subphenotypes with controls showed significant moderate separation (cumulative PC score = 55–69%, $p < 0.001$; Table S4).

DIE has been considered a specific entity in which lesions penetrate more than 5 mm underneath the peritoneum [9,33]. Indeed, PC scores from comparisons of PE with OE (Figure 2A) was smaller than PC scores comparing PE or OE with DIE (Figure 2B,C), suggesting greater distinction of DIE from the superficial subphenotypes. A six-cytokine signature comprising IL-1α, IL-7, IL-8, MCP-1, MIF, and TNF-α distinguished OE from PE was identified (Figure 2D). Comparing OE to DIE, a seven-cytokine signature comprising IL-1α, IL-1RA, IL-8, IL-12p40, IL-12p70, IL-16, and TNF-α was identified (Figure 2E). Comparing DIE to PE, an all-upregulated six-cytokine signature of IL-8, IL-12p70, IL-16, IL-18, MCP-1, and MIP-1α that correlated to DIE was identified (Figure 2F). Cross-correlation and hierarchical clustering of cytokines showed not only intercorrelated inflammatory cytokines (e.g., TNFα, IL-1β, IL-10, and IL-1RA), but also cytokines that are anti-correlated (e.g., IL-12p40 and IL-12p70) [34], affirming the underlying biological information embedded within the PLSR-derived cytokine signatures (Figure 3. Table S3 shows the univariate statistical analysis.

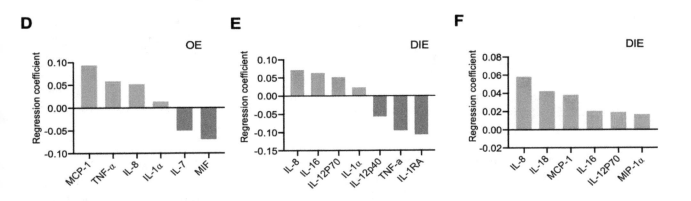

Figure 2. Peritoneal fluid cytokines show distinct delineation of endometriosis subphenotypes. Partial least squares regression (PLSR) models separated (**A**) ovarian endometriomas from peritoneal endometriosis, (**B**) ovarian endometriomas from deep infiltrating endometriosis, and (**C**) peritoneal endometriosis from deep infiltrating endometriosis. The principal component (PC) scores show good separation of endometriosis subphenotypes by using PF cytokines. (**D**–**F**). Corresponding PLSR coefficient analyses reveal cytokine signatures delineating the various subphenotypes. Elevated cytokines associated with a particular endometriosis subphenotype (OE, PE, or DIE) relative to its comparator appear in the same upper or lower half of the plot.

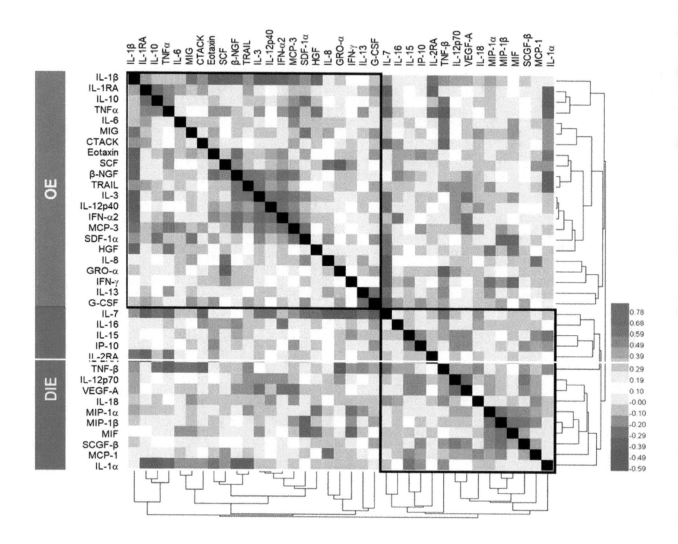

Figure 3. Correlation matrix of peritoneal fluid cytokines. Hierarchical clustering was performed on Spearman *r*-values between the subphenotypes ovarian endometriosis, and deep infiltrating endometriosis revealed consistency in PLSR-derived cytokine signatures that segregated OE from DIE.

2.3. Subphenotype Cytokine Signatures Are Associated with Different Biological Processes.

To examine whether the cytokine signatures associated with different endometriosis subphenotypes showed themes of functional categorization, each signature was investigated by using the gene ontology (GO) classification system (Table 2). In OE relative to PE, enriched biological processes include the following: negative regulation of extrinsic apoptotic signaling pathway; positive regulation of B-cell proliferation; positive regulation of angiogenesis; and positive regulation of ERK1 and ERK2 cascade. In OE relative to DIE, natural-killer-cell-mediated cytotoxicity is directed against tumor-cell target, cell-cycle arrest, and cell migration, and tyrosine phosphorylation of Stat4 protein. Smooth muscle cell metaplasia that is associated with DIE was also identified in our pathway enrichment analysis [35], providing assurance that our cytokine-signature-derived identified meaningful subphenotype biological characteristics. In PE versus DIE, enriched biological processes include the following: positive regulation of interferon-gamma production, protein kinase B (also known as AKT) signaling, and MAPK cascade.

Table 2. Functional enrichment analysis of endometriosis subphenotype cytokine signatures.

(A) OE vs. PE		
Term Identifier	Fold Enrichment	p-Value
immune response	29.9	1.90×10^{-3}
positive regulation of B-cell proliferation	215.3	7.00×10^{-3}
inflammatory response	33.2	1.50×10^{-3}
negative regulation of extrinsic apoptotic signaling pathway in absence of ligand	226.9	6.60×10^{-3}
positive regulation of angiogenesis	73	2.00×10^{-2}
positive regulation of ERK1 and ERK2 cascade	48	3.10×10^{-2}
cell proliferation	22.9	6.40×10^{-2}
negative regulation of apoptotic process	18.5	7.90×10^{-2}

(B) OE vs. DIE		
Term Identifier	Fold Enrichment	p-Value
immune response	31.9	6.10×10^{-5}
positive regulation of natural killer cell activation	1343.4	1.20×10^{-3}
positive regulation of NK T-cell activation	1343.4	1.20×10^{-3}
positive regulation of tyrosine phosphorylation of Stat4 protein	1679.2	9.50×10^{-4}
positive regulation of lymphocyte proliferation	959.5	1.70×10^{-3}
positive regulation of natural killer cell mediated cytotoxicity directed against tumor cell target	959.5	1.70×10^{-3}
positive regulation of mononuclear cell proliferation	2238.9	7.10×10^{-4}
response to UV-B	746.3	2.10×10^{-3}
positive regulation of smooth muscle cell apoptotic process	746.3	2.10×10^{-3}
negative regulation of interleukin-17 production	610.6	2.60×10^{-3}
positive regulation of T-cell-mediated cytotoxicity	516.7	3.10×10^{-3}
defense response to protozoan	353.5	4.50×10^{-3}
negative regulation of smooth muscle cell proliferation	231.6	6.90×10^{-3}
positive regulation of interferon-gamma production	146	1.10×10^{-2}
positive regulation of cell adhesion	156.2	1.00×10^{-2}
positive regulation of T-cell proliferation	111.9	1.40×10^{-2}
cellular response to lipopolysaccharide	59.4	2.70×10^{-2}
cytokine-mediated signaling pathway	51.3	3.10×10^{-2}
cell cycle arrest	47.6	3.30×10^{-2}
cell migration	39.1	4.00×10^{-2}

(C) PE vs. DIE		
Term Identifier	Fold Enrichment	p-Value
immune response	39.9	1.60×10^{-5}
positive regulation of protein kinase B signaling	100	1.50×10^{-2}
positive regulation of inflammatory response	115	1.30×10^{-2}
cellular response to organic cyclic compound	142.3	1.10×10^{-2}
positive regulation of interferon-gamma production	182.5	8.20×10^{-3}
lipopolysaccharide-mediated signaling pathway	262.4	5.70×10^{-3}
MAPK cascade	32	4.60×10^{-2}
cell–cell signaling	33.1	4.50×10^{-2}
inflammatory response	22.2	6.60×10^{-2}

3. Discussion

Reports have long recognized endometriotic lesion heterogeneity in characteristics such as color, size, and location [3–5]. There is increasing evidence that there is marked variation in lesion subphenotypes at the molecular level [36]. Santulli et al. reported that DIE is associated with higher PF advanced oxidation protein products than PE and OE [37]. Immunohistochemical analyses showed a higher prevalence of cyclooxygenase-2 protein expression in OE (78.5%) compared to 11.1% and 13.3% in PE and DIE [38], whereas nerve growth factor is expressed higher in DIE compared to PE and OE [39]. Methylation promotor sites in ectopic lesions are potentially different between the subphenotypes [40]. These reports, collectively, are in strong agreement with our results shown herein, in that OE, PE, and DIE are associated with unique cytokine signatures and corresponding enriched biological pathways.

Our study is likely to have implications for endometriosis therapeutics and biomarker discovery, particularly in the era of targeted treatment and precision medicine [41]. Further interpretation of our observations raises the potentiality of different therapies needed for treating patients with different endometriosis subphenotypes. It is apparent that broad, untargeted usage of therapeutics does not bring about clear clinical benefit across all endometriosis patients [2]. Endometriosis subphenotypes may partly explain these clinical phenomena. While targeted therapies have not been investigated in endometriosis, data from our study offer the possibility of exploiting each subphenotype's unique dependence on critical non-hormonal signaling or inflammation pathways to tailor therapy. Drug side-effect profile and efficacy are two main considerations of treatment choices [42]. Our findings, along with those of others, warrant further deep characterization of cytokine profiles and targeted use of immunomodulators, given the centrality of cytokines cells in the process of establishment and maintenance of this peritoneal disease. Due to often described elevation of peritoneal TNFα in endometriosis by us and others, blockers of TNFα, such as etanercept, leflunomide, and infliximab, were evaluated in preclinical models and in small randomized clinical trials [43–46]. Other immunomodulators, such as levamisole, and IL-12 inhibitors, have also been investigated in experimental models of endometriosis, with certain success [47]. In approved drugs such as infliximab, levamisole, and leflunomide, where safety profiles are established, monotherapeutic efficacy in humans remains untested or uncertain. While larger and more clinical trials are certainly required to test drug efficacy, immunomodulators are not always effective alone and require further development, along with new combination strategies, in order to enhance their efficacy, such as the use of combinatorial therapy or immunotherapy. These combination therapies can be classified based on their strategic targets: firstly, blockage of multiple cytokines based on the abovementioned signatures; secondly, to promote T- or NK-cell priming by enhancing lesion-associated antigen presentation; and thirdly, to target the immunosuppressive environment [48,49]. In the first strategy, choosing the key cytokines is critical, as cytokines are also required physiologically for endometrial growth, decidualization, and implantation [50]. In the second and third strategies, deep phenotyping of peritoneal immune cells and lesion microenvironments in endometriosis is needed before [51,52]. These strategies and their corresponding challenges must be overcome before the promise of an efficacious immunomodulatory therapy can be realized. Our study also has clinical implications on the biomarkers of endometriosis and biomarkers that are predictive of response to treatment. Heterogeneity in endometriosis has had a negative impact on the discovery and validation of predictive biomarkers, insofar that the lack of robust biomarkers is a critical area the community is working toward surmounting [53–55]. While this is not addressed in our study, our study creates the background for future investigations of stratifying patients according to their subphenotypes, prior to investigation of biomarkers.

During endometriosis development, cytokines develop a reciprocal interaction between the lesions and their surroundings, which constitute the modular microenvironment, influencing the evolution of lesion subphenotypes [14,20,56]. In this study, we opted to study the PF as a reflection of the spatial heterogeneity in endometriosis subphenotypes. By doing so, we were able to investigate the dynamic crosstalk between the secreted cytokines of lesions and their juxtaposed microenvironments, and their reciprocal adaptations. Indeed, ovarian endometriomas by growing near or at ovarian tissues with elevated CYP19A1 expressions are exposed to estrogen levels higher than that experienced by lesions implanted in the peritoneum or deep areas [57], creating an ovarian-specific microenvironment. Similarly, the transcriptome of the peritoneum in EM+ women is fundamentally different from that of EM- women [58–60]. The different expressions of inflammatory and adhesion molecules such as ICAM-1, matrix metalloproteases, and IL-6 confer a preferentially adhesive microenvironment for lesion implantation [61]. Elevated peritoneal reactive oxygen species acting through various signaling pathways, such as MAPK, ERK, and AKT, regulate gene expression of cytokines and cell adhesion molecules, which create microenvironments that promote various aspects of endometriosis development and its deleterious effects [62–64]. In DIE, significant fibrotic accumulation and smooth muscle differentiation secondary to the proliferation of stromal cells and inflammation are commonly noted and present yet another kind of microenvironment plausibly enhancing chronic inflammation [65,66]. In addition, the lesion microenvironment and its secreted cytokines plausibly play a key role in therapeutic approach of endometriosis, noting the elicitation of drug resistance by stromal microenvironment surrounding tumors in cancer [67]. Transcriptomic studies, such as those by Suryawanshi et al. [68], would be especially illuminating, had an analysis of the three endometriosis subphenotypes been performed in terms of elucidating each subphenotype's underlying pathogenic/pathophysiological mechanisms and potential "druggability". While additional experiments comparing transcriptome, epigenome, and proteome in PE, OE, and DIE are needed, our results suggest heterogeneity in the subphenotypes, at least in their cytokine levels, is associated with their microenvironments.

We used the GO database to analyze the cytokine signatures for enriched biological processes pertaining to the subphenotypes. Several key themes emerged: OE cytokines centered on proliferation/apoptosis regulation linked to ERK1 and ERK2 signaling, compared to PE; PE cytokines were implicated in MAPK and AKT signaling and highly inflammatory environments, compared to DIE; DIE cytokines were associated with cytotoxicity directed against "tumor cell target" and smooth muscle cell metaplasia, consistent with known outcomes associated with DIE [35]. Further, our analysis identified STAT4 regulation, and so it is congruent with studies by Zamani et al. and Bianco et al., showing *STAT4* polymorphism and susceptibility to endometriosis [69,70]. Increased angiogenesis is linked to the development of maintenance of endometriotic lesions, and our analysis suggests stronger angiogenesis in ovarian endometriomas [71,72], plausibly due to the strong induction of angiogenesis under high levels of ovarian estrogen. The GO analysis also revealed perturbations in immune cells. The positive regulation of natural killer cell activation could be construed as a compensatory mechanism consistent with reduced natural killer cell cytotoxicity [73], facilitating survival of regurgitated menstrual tissues at ectopic sites, probably more so in OE than DIE, as suggested. The combination of reduced IL-17 production and T-cell proliferation suggests exacerbated T-regulatory cells or Tregs activity [74].

Strengths of this study include the use of a carefully phenotyped clinical study population, use of a large, unbiased multiplexed cytokine approach, and advanced biostatistics. Additionally, this study, which was conducted in Singapore, represents a unique strength, as the study population pertains to Asians (Chinese, Malays, Indians, and Filipinos), providing a defined patient background for educated comparison and generalizability of the results when required. Limitations of this study include its observational nature, lack of longitudinal data, and the difficulty in dissecting the specific roles of cytokines within the molecular signatures. It is recognized that findings from this study are preliminary and will need to be validated in other populations, given that cytokine signatures may differ in other study populations. The cellular and molecular mechanisms of endometriosis development are likely to be overlapping (as observed in IL-8) and manifold, and many cytokines are able to induce the pathways. Thus, it is likely that multiple inflammatory pathways induced by a variety of stimuli might lead to endometriosis subphenotype development and endocrine failure. Further experiments will be necessary to define the precise roles of cytokines in the immune regulation of endometriosis. Taken together, the clustering of cytokines into functional groups hints at different pathogenic/pathophysiological mechanisms defining endometriosis subphenotypes. This would have important clinical ramifications, with the prediction that the endometriosis subphenotypes might require different treatment strategies and meet the need of a more personalized approach for endometriosis management [75].

4. Materials and Methods

4.1. Subjects and Sample Collection

Peritoneal fluids (PF) were collected from women participants ($n = 132$), comprising 59 women who are endometriosis-free (EM-) and 73 with endometriosis (EM+) undergoing laparoscopic procedures for suspected endometriosis, infertility, sterilization procedures, and/or pelvic pain recruited in KK Women's and Children's Hospital, Singapore, and Singapore General Hospital, Singapore, under

Centralized Institutional Research Board approval (CIRB 2010-167-D, approved 15 January 2016). Diagnostic laparoscopy was performed on all patients, with careful inspection of the uterus, fallopian tubes, ovaries, pouch of Douglas, and the pelvic peritoneum by gynecologists subspecializing in reproductive endocrinology and infertility. PFs were prepared as previously described [18], in line with Endometriosis Phenome and Biobanking Harmonisation Project Standard Operating Procedures [76]. Presence of endometriosis was systematically recorded and scored according to the revised American Fertility Society classification (rAFS) of endometriosis [77,78]. All patients gave written informed consent. Exclusion criteria included menstruating patients, post-menopausal patients, patients on hormonal therapy (e.g., norethisterone and microgynon) for at least three months before laparoscopy, and other confounding diseases, such as diabetes, adenomyosis, or any other chronic inflammatory diseases (rheumatoid arthritis, inflammatory bowel disease, systemic sclerosis, etc.). Patient characteristics are shown in Table 1. For the subjects undergoing robot-assisted excision of DIE at Singapore General Hospital, all women were preoperatively assessed for pelvic pain, bleeding, or fertility problems by trans-vaginal or trans-rectal ultrasound (if *virgo intacta*), using Voluson ultrasound machines (GE Healthcare). All sonographers were trained in the identification of DIE. All cases had pelvic DIE lesions of >5 mm, as well as evidence of partial or complete obliteration of the POD. In our unit, POD obliteration was taken to be the evidence of bowel involvement, and the use of robot-assisted technology for surgical excision was triggered due to suspected increased surgical complexity. Robot-assisted excision was performed by using the da Vinci Surgical Si™ system (Intuitive Surgical). The possible overlapping of the three lesion subphenotypes led us to classify the patients according to the worst lesion found in each subject, based on endometriosis subphenotype grouping by Chapron et al. [66,79]. Subjects who did not have endometriosis or have benign gynecological presentations, such as uterine fibroids and benign ovarian cysts, were taken as the endometriosis-free control group (EM-). All PFs were stored at −80 °C, until further analysis.

4.2. Multiplex Immunoassay Analysis

Cytokines were detected and measured by using multiplex immunoassay (BioRad, Hercules, CA, USA; Table S1), as previously described [50]. Briefly, 10 μL of PF was mixed with 10 μL of primary antibody-conjugated magnetic beads on in a 96 DropArray plate (Curiox Biosystems, Singapore) and rotated at 450 rpm on a plate shaker for 120 min at 25 °C, while protected from light. Subsequently, the plate was washed three times with wash buffer on the LT210 Washing Station (Curiox), before adding 5 μL of secondary antibody and rotating at 450 rpm for 30 min at 25 °C, protected from light. The plate was washed three times with wash buffer, and 10 μL of streptavidin-phycoerythrin was added and rotated at 450 rpm for 30 min at 25 °C, protected from light. The plate was again washed thrice with wash buffer. Then, 60 μL of reading buffer was added and transferred to a 96-conical-well microtiter plate, and the samples were read by using the Bio-Plex Luminex 200 (BioRad). The beads are classified by the red classification laser (635 nm) into its distinct sets, while a green reporter laser (532 nm) excites the phycoerythrin, a fluorescent reporter tag bound to the detection antibody. Quantitation of the 48 cytokines in each sample was then determined by extrapolation to a six- or seven-point standard curve, using five-parameter logistic regression modeling. Assay CV averaged <12%. When samples were detected in less than 50% of patients or below the lower limit of quantitation, they were considered undetected. Calibrations and validations were performed prior to runs and on a monthly basis, respectively.

4.3. Sample Size Calculation

We estimated the sample size before commencing the study: We assumed a 95% sensitivity of the cytokine signatures in distinguishing the subphenotypes, and a 95% confidence interval (CI) of approximately ±10.0% would need 18 cases of one endometriosis subphenotype and the same number of another subphenotype. This statistical analysis, assuming the sensitivity of the signature cutoff is p = # test positive/N, where the sample size (n), number of women diagnosed with a particular endometriosis subtype (DIE, OE, PE), necessary to estimate p with precision $\pm$ L is given by the formula n = $Z^*Zp(1-p)/(L^*L)$, where Z corresponds to the correct percentile of the standard normal distribution [80]. Our clinical experience noted a 1:2:1 PE:OE:DIE ratio, and hence we targeted 36 OE cases, and the patient numbers were rounded to fall within the estimated sensitivity.

4.4. Statistical Analysis

GraphPad Prism 6 (GraphPad Software Inc., San Diego, CA, USA) was used for statistical analyses. Data were checked for normal distribution, using the Kolmogorov–Smirnov test. Unpaired or paired Student's t-test was performed, as appropriate, to determine statistical significance between groups for normally distributed data. Mann–Whitney U test was used for non-normally distributed data. For comparing three or more groups, the data were analyzed by using one-way ANOVA, followed by the Student's t-test with Bonferroni adjustment for pairwise comparisons. A p-value <0.05 was deemed to be statistically significant. A two-tailed Pearson correlation matrix was first performed with a confidence interval of 95%, followed by hierarchical clustering and the results plotted as heatmap 1.0 (GPS HemI 1.0 Heatmap Illustrator), using the clustering method of Average linkage and similarity metric of Pearson distance. Cytokines were further analyzed and signatures obtained by partial least squares regression (PLSR) modeling (Unscrambler X version 10.1) after the normalization of data by performing log2 transformation. Full cross-validation was applied in PLSR to increase model performance and for the calculation of coefficient regression values. PLSR models were compared by using Q-residuals obtained from the best principal components.

4.5. Pathway Enrichment Analysis

PLSR coefficient-derived cytokines were imputed into the Database for Annotation, Visualization and Integrated Discovery (DAVID) and cross-referenced against Gene Ontology (GO), for biological-process-enrichment analysis [81]. The p-values <0.05, based on Fisher Exact analysis and fold change >10 were imposed as enriched pathways. Bonferroni and Benjamini adjusted p-values are reported in Table S5. As a result of these corrections, the adjusted p-values get larger, and it could hurt the sensitivity of discovery if overemphasizing them [81,82]. Furthermore, these commonly used multiple testing-adjustment methods assume independence of tests, which in cytokines studies translates to a questionable assumption that all cytokines operate independently; instead, cytokines form biological networks [21,22].

5. Conclusions

Taken together, this study suggests that women with endometriosis subphenotypes can be stratified molecularly. Although the determination of lesion heterogeneity has not yet formed part of the clinical decision-making process in endometriosis, subphenotype-specific cytokine signatures suggest that suitable targeted therapeutic approaches specific to each individual patient's lesion and peritoneal heterogeneity composition may be tailored, and also the consideration of endometriosis subphenotypes for biomarker discovery studies. We anticipate our results to stimulate further studies, with accompanying detailed anatomical locations, and the use of genomic, proteomic, and metabolomic studies to evaluate the subphenotype molecular characteristics.

Author Contributions: P.B.-S., V.V.-F., J.K.Y.C., H.H.T., T.Y.T., and J.W.L.P. recruited patients and provided patient samples. J.Z. performed cytokine analysis and analyzed data. Y.H.L., C.W.K., and J.Z. wrote and revised the paper. Y.H.L. conceived of the study and supervised the study. Y.H.L., B.S.M.C., and J.K.Y.C. provided research resources. All authors have read and agreed to the published version of the manuscript.

Abbreviations

ASRM   American Society for Reproductive Medicine
DIE   Deep infiltrating endometriosis
EM-   Control without endometriosis
EM+   Case with endometriosis
OE   Ovarian endometriosis
PC   Principal Component
PE   Peritoneal endometriosis
PF   Peritoneal fluid
PLSR   Partial least squares regression

References

1.   Practice Committee of the American Society for Reproductive Medicine. Endometriosis and infertility. *Fertil. Steril.* **2006**, *86*, S156–S160. [CrossRef] [PubMed]
2.   Bulun, S.E. Endometriosis. *N. Engl. J. Med.* **2009**, *360*, 268–279. [CrossRef] [PubMed]
3.   Nisolle, M.; Donnez, J. Peritoneal endometriosis, ovarian endometriosis, and adenomyotic nodules of the rectovaginal septum are three different entities. *Fertil. Steril.* **1997**, *68*, 585–596. [CrossRef]
4.   Stegmann, B.J.; Sinaii, N.; Liu, S.; Segars, J.; Merino, M.; Nieman, L.K.; Stratton, P. Using location, color, size, and depth to characterize and identify endometriosis lesions in a cohort of 133 women. *Fertil. Steril.* **2008**, *89*, 1632–1636. [CrossRef] [PubMed]
5.   Burney, R.O.; Giudice, L.C. Pathogenesis and pathophysiology of endometriosis. *Fertil. Steril.* **2012**, *98*, 511–519. [CrossRef] [PubMed]
6.   van Langendonckt, A.; Casanas-Roux, F.; Donnez, J. Oxidative stress and peritoneal endometriosis. *Fertil. Steril.* **2002**, *77*, 861–870. [CrossRef]
7.   Yamaguchi, K.; Mandai, M.; Toyokuni, S.; Hamanishi, J.; Higuchi, T.; Takakura, K.; Fujii, S. Contents of endometriotic cysts, especially the high concentration of free iron, are a possible cause of carcinogenesis in the cysts through the iron-induced persistent oxidative stress. *Clin. Cancer Res.* **2008**, *14*. [CrossRef]
8.   Guo, S.W.; Ding, D.; Shen, M.; Liu, X. Dating endometriotic ovarian cysts based on the content of cyst fluid and its potential clinical implications. *Reprod. Sci.* **2015**, *22*, 873–883. [CrossRef]
9.   Koninckx, P.R.; Meuleman, C.; Demeyere, S.; Lesaffre, E.; Cornillie, F.J. Suggestive evidence that pelvic endometriosis is a progressive disease, whereas deeply infiltrating endometriosis is associated with pelvic pain. *Fertil. Steril.* **1991**, *55*, 759–765. [CrossRef]
10. Chapron, C.; Fauconnier, A.; Vieira, M.; Barakat, H.; Dousset, B.; Pansini, V.; Vacher-Lavenu, M.C.; Dubuisson, J.B. Anatomical distribution of deeply infiltrating endometriosis: Surgical implications and proposition for a classification. *Hum. Reprod.* **2003**, *18*, 157–161. [CrossRef]
11. Koninckx, P.R.; Kennedy, S.H.; Barlow, D.H. Endometriotic disease: The role of peritoneal fluid. *Hum. Reprod. Update* **1998**, *4*, 741–751. [CrossRef] [PubMed]
12. Laganà, A.S.; Garzon, S.; Götte, M.; Viganò, P.; Franchi, M.; Ghezzi, F.; Martin, D.C. The Pathogenesis of Endometriosis: Molecular and Cell Biology Insights. *Int. J. Mol. Sci.* **2019**, *20*, 5615. [CrossRef] [PubMed]
13. Riemma, G.; Laganà, A.S.; Schiattarella, A.; Garzon, S.; Cobellis, L.; Autiero, R.; Licciardi, F.; della Corte, L.; la Verde, M.; de Franciscis, P. Ion Channels in The Pathogenesis of Endometriosis: A Cutting-Edge Point of View. *Int. J. Mol. Sci.* **2020**, *21*, 1114. [CrossRef] [PubMed]
14. Gordts, S.; Koninckx, P.; Brosens, I. Pathogenesis of deep endometriosis. *Fertil. Steril.* **2017**, *108*, 872–885. [CrossRef]
15. Flores, V.A.; Vanhie, A.; Dang, T.; Taylor, H.S. Progesterone Receptor Status Predicts Response to Progestin Therapy in Endometriosis. *J. Clin. Endocrinol. Metab.* **2018**, *103*, 4561–4568. [CrossRef]
16. Zondervan, K.T.; Becker, C.M.; Missmer, S.A. Endometriosis. *N. Engl. J. Med.* **2020**, *382*, 1244–1256. [CrossRef]
17. Herington, J.L.; Bruner-Tran, K.L.; Lucas, J.A.; Osteen, K.G. Immune interactions in endometriosis. *Expert Rev. Clin. Immunol.* **2011**, *7*, 611–626. [CrossRef]

18. Lee, Y.H.; Tan, C.W.; Venkatratnam, A.; Tan, C.S.; Cui, L.; Loh, S.F.; Griffith, L.; Tannenbaum, S.R.; Chan, J.K.Y. Dysregulated sphingolipid metabolism in endometriosis. *J. Clin. Endocrinol. Metab.* **2014**, *99*, E1913–E1921. [CrossRef]

19. Lee, Y.H.; Cui, L.; Fang, J.; Chern, B.S.M.; Tan, H.H.; Chan, J.K.Y. Limited value of pro-inflammatory oxylipins and cytokines as circulating biomarkers in endometriosis—A targeted 'omics study. *Sci. Rep.* **2016**, *6*, 26117. [CrossRef]

20. Bhat, R.; Bissell, M.J. Of plasticity and specificity: Dialectics of the microenvironment and macroenvironment and the organ phenotype, Wiley Interdiscip. *Rev. Dev. Biol.* **2014**, *3*, 147–163. [CrossRef]

21. Schmitz, M.L.; Weber, A.; Roxlau, T.; Gaestel, M.; Kracht, M. Signal integration, crosstalk mechanisms and networks in the function of inflammatory cytokines. *Biochim. Biophys. Acta Mol. Cell Res.* **2011**, *1813*, 2165–2175. [CrossRef] [PubMed]

22. Pinheiro, M.B.; Martins-Filho, O.A.; Mota, A.P.L.; Alpoim, P.N.; Godoi, L.C.; Silveira, A.C.O.; Teixeira-Carvalho, A.; Gomes, K.B.; Dusse, L.M. Severe preeclampsia goes along with a cytokine network disturbance towards a systemic inflammatory state. *Cytokine* **2013**, *62*, 165–173. [CrossRef] [PubMed]

23. Siedentopf, F.; Tariverdian, N.; Rücke, M.; Kentenich, H.; Arck, P.C. Immune Status, Psychosocial Distress and Reduced Quality of Life in Infertile Patients with Endometriosis. *Am. J. Reprod. Immunol.* **2008**, *60*, 449–461. [CrossRef] [PubMed]

24. Khan, K.N.; Masuzaki, H.; Fujishita, A.; Kitajima, M.; Sekine, I.; Ishimaru, T. Differential macrophage infiltration in early and advanced endometriosis and adjacent peritoneum. *Fertil. Steril.* **2004**, *81*, 652–661. [CrossRef]

25. Beste, M.T.; Pfäffle-Doyle, N.; Prentice, E.A.; Morris, S.N.; Lauffenburger, D.A.; Isaacson, K.B.; Griffith, L.G. Molecular network analysis of endometriosis reveals a role for c-Jun-regulated macrophage activation. *Sci. Transl. Med.* **2014**, *6*, 222ra16. [CrossRef]

26. Gottschalk, P.G.; Dunn, J.R. The five-parameter logistic: A characterization and comparison with the four-parameter logistic. *Anal. Biochem.* **2005**, *343*, 54–65. [CrossRef]

27. Rakhila, H.; Al-Akoum, M.; Bergeron, M.-E.; Leboeuf, M.; Lemyre, M.; Akoum, A.; Pouliot, M. Promotion of angiogenesis and proliferation cytokines patterns in peritoneal fluid from women with endometriosis. *J. Reprod. Immunol.* **2016**, *116*, 1–6. [CrossRef]

28. Vercellini, P.; Viganò, P.; Somigliana, E.; Fedele, L. Endometriosis: Pathogenesis and treatment. *Nat. Rev. Endocrinol.* **2013**, *10*, 261–275. [CrossRef]

29. Bersinger, N.A.; Dechaud, H.; McKinnon, B.; Mueller, M.D. Analysis of cytokines in the peritoneal fluid of endometriosis patients as a function of the menstrual cycle stage using the Bio-Plex® platform. *Arch. Physiol. Biochem.* **2012**, *118*, 210–218. [CrossRef]

30. Jørgensen, H.; Hill, A.S.; Beste, M.T.; Kumar, M.P.; Chiswick, E.; Fedorcsak, P.; Isaacson, K.B.; Lauffenburger, D.A.; Griffith, L.G.; Qvigstad, E. Peritoneal fluid cytokines related to endometriosis in patients evaluated for infertility. *Fertil. Steril.* **2017**, *107*, 1191–1199. [CrossRef]

31. Mahnke, J.L.; Dawood, M.Y.; Huang, J.C. Vascular endothelial growth factor and interleukin-6 in peritoneal fluid of women with endometriosis. *Fertil. Steril.* **2000**, *73*, 166–170. [CrossRef]

32. Knific, T.; Fishman, D.; Vogler, A.; Gstöttner, M.; Wenzl, R.; Peterson, H.; Rižner, T.L. Multiplex analysis of 40 cytokines do not allow separation between endometriosis patients and controls. *Sci. Rep.* **2019**, *9*, 16738. [CrossRef] [PubMed]

33. Cornillie, F.J.; Oosterlynck, D.; Lauweryns, J.M.; Koninckx, P.R. Deeply infiltrating pelvic endometriosis: Histology and clinical significance. *Fertil. Steril.* **1990**, *53*, 978–983. [CrossRef]

34. Sun, L.; He, C.; Nair, L.; Yeung, J.; Egwuagu, C.E. Interleukin 12 (IL-12) family cytokines: Role in immune pathogenesis and treatment of CNS autoimmune disease. *Cytokine* **2015**, *75*, 249–255. [CrossRef]

35. van Kaam, K.J.A.F.; Schouten, J.P.; Nap, A.W.; Dunselman, G.A.J.; Groothuis, P.G. Fibromuscular differentiation in deeply infiltrating endometriosis is a reaction of resident fibroblasts to the presence of ectopic endometrium. *Hum. Reprod.* **2008**, *23*, 2692–2700. [CrossRef]

36. Carmona, F.; Chapron, C.; Martínez-Zamora, M.-Á.; Santulli, P.; Rabanal, A.; Martínez-Florensa, M.; Lozano, F.; Balasch, J. Ovarian endometrioma but not deep infiltrating endometriosis is associated with increased serum levels of interleukin-8 and interleukin-6. *J. Reprod. Immunol.* **2012**, *95*, 80–86. [CrossRef]

37. Santulli, P.; Chouzenoux, S.; Fiorese, M.; Marcellin, L.; Lemarechal, H.; Millischer, A.E.; Batteux, F.; Borderie, D.; Chapron, C. Protein oxidative stress markers in peritoneal fluids of women with deep infiltrating endometriosis are increased. *Hum. Reprod.* **2015**, *30*, 49–60. [CrossRef]

38. Fagotti, A. Analysis of cyclooxygenase-2 (COX-2) expression in different sites of endometriosis and correlation with clinico-pathological parameters. *Hum. Reprod.* **2004**, *19*, 393–397. [CrossRef]

39. Anaf, V.; Simon, P.; el Nakadi, I.; Fayt, I.; Simonart, T.; Buxant, F.; Noel, J.-C. Hyperalgesia, nerve infiltration and nerve growth factor expression in deep adenomyotic nodules, peritoneal and ovarian endometriosis. *Hum. Reprod.* **2002**, *17*, 1895–1900. [CrossRef]

40. Borghese, B.; Barbaux, S.; Mondon, F.; Santulli, P.; Pierre, G.; Vinci, G.; Chapron, C.; Vaiman, D. Research Resource: Genome-Wide Profiling of Methylated Promoters in Endometriosis Reveals a Subtelomeric Location of Hypermethylation. *Mol. Endocrinol.* **2010**, *24*, 1872–1885. [CrossRef]

41. Bedaiwy, M.A.; Alfaraj, S.; Yong, P.; Casper, R. New developments in the medical treatment of endometriosis. *Fertil. Steril.* **2017**, *107*, 555–565. [CrossRef] [PubMed]

42. Dunselman, G.A.J.; Vermeulen, N.; Becker, C.; Calhaz-Jorge, C.; D'Hooghe, T.; de Bie, B.; Heikinheimo, O.; Horne, A.W.; Kiesel, L.; Nap, A.; et al. ESHRE guideline: Management of women with endometriosis. *Hum. Reprod.* **2014**, *29*, 400–412. [CrossRef] [PubMed]

43. Altintas, D.; Kokcu, A.; Kandemir, B.; Cetinkaya, M.B.; Tosun, M. Efficacy of imiquimod, an immunomodulatory agent, on experimental endometriosis. *Fertil. Steril.* **2008**, *90*, 401–405. [CrossRef] [PubMed]

44. Uygur, D.; Aytan, H.; Zergeroglu, S.; Batioglu, S. Leflunomide—An Immunomodulator—Induces Regression of Endometrial Explants in a Rat Model of Endometriosis. *J. Soc. Gynecol. Investig.* **2006**, *13*, 378–383. [CrossRef]

45. Barrier, B.F.; Bates, G.W.; Leland, M.M.; Leach, D.A.; Robinson, R.D.; Propst, A.M. Efficacy of anti-tumor necrosis factor therapy in the treatment of spontaneous endometriosis in baboons. *Fertil. Steril.* **2004**, *81*, 775–779. [CrossRef]

46. Koninckx, P.R.; Craessaerts, M.; Timmerman, D.; Cornillie, F.; Kennedy, S. Anti-TNF-treatment for deep endometriosis-associated pain: A randomized placebo-controlled trial. *Hum. Reprod.* **2008**, *23*, 2017–2023. [CrossRef]

47. Itoh, H.; Sashihara, T.; Hosono, A.; Kaminogawa, S.; Uchida, M. Interleukin-12 inhibits development of ectopic endometriotic tissues in peritoneal cavity via activation of NK cells in a murine endometriosis model. *Cytotechnology* **2011**, *63*, 133–141. [CrossRef]

48. Oosterlynck, D.J.; Meuleman, C.; Waer, M.; Koninckx, P.R.; Vandeputte, M. Immunosuppressive activity of peritoneal fluid in women with endometriosis. *Obstet. Gynecol.* **1993**, *82*, 206–212.

49. Ścieżyńska, A.; Komorowski, M.; Soszyńska, M.; Malejczyk, J. NK Cells as Potential Targets for Immunotherapy in Endometriosis. *J. Clin. Med.* **2019**, *8*, 1468. [CrossRef]

50. Durairaj, R.R.P.; Aberkane, A.; Polanski, L.; Maruyama, Y.; Baumgarten, M.; Lucas, E.S.; Quenby, S.; Chan, J.K.Y.; Raine-Fenning, N.; Brosens, J.J.; et al. Deregulation of the endometrial stromal cell secretome precedes embryo implantation failure. *MHR Basic Sci. Reprod. Med.* **2017**, *23*, 478–487. [CrossRef]

51. Symons, L.K.; Miller, J.E.; Kay, V.R.; Marks, R.M.; Liblik, K.; Koti, M.; Tayade, C. The Immunopathophysiology of Endometriosis. *Trends Mol. Med.* **2018**, *24*, 748–762. [CrossRef] [PubMed]

52. Vallvé-Juanico, J.; Houshdaran, S.; Giudice, L.C. The endometrial immune environment of women with endometriosis. *Hum. Reprod. Update* **2019**, *25*, 565–592. [CrossRef] [PubMed]

53. Ahn, S.H.; Singh, V.; Tayade, C. Biomarkers in endometriosis: Challenges and opportunities. *Fertil. Steril.* **2017**, *107*, 523–532. [CrossRef] [PubMed]

54. May, K.E.; Villar, J.; Kirtley, S.; Kennedy, S.H.; Becker, C.M. Endometrial alterations in endometriosis: A systematic review of putative biomarkers. *Hum. Reprod. Update* **2011**, *17*, 637–653. [CrossRef] [PubMed]

55. Anastasiu, C.V.; Moga, M.A.; Neculau, A.E.; Bălan, A.; Scârneciu, I.; Dragomir, R.M.; Dull, A.-M.; Chicea, L.-M. Biomarkers for the Noninvasive Diagnosis of Endometriosis: State of the Art and Future Perspectives. *Int. J. Mol. Sci.* **2020**, *21*, 1750. [CrossRef]

56. Wimalachandra, D.; Yang, J.X.; Zhu, L.; Tan, E.; Asada, H.; Chan, J.Y.K. Lee, Y.H. Long-chain glucosylceramides crosstalk with LYN mediates endometrial cell migration. *Biochim. Biophys Acta. Mol. Cell Biol. Lipids.* **2018**, *1863*, 71–80. [CrossRef]

57. Huhtinen, K.; Desai, R.; Ståhle, M.; Salminen, A.; Handelsman, D.J.; Perheentupa, A.; Poutanen, M. Endometrial and Endometriotic Concentrations of Estrone and Estradiol Are Determined by Local Metabolism Rather than Circulating Levels. *J. Clin. Endocrinol. Metab.* **2012**, *97*, 4228–4235. [CrossRef]

58. Kyama, C.; Overbergh, L.; Debrock, S.; Valckx, D.; Vanderperre, S.; Meuleman, C.; Mihalyi, A.; Mwenda, J.; Mathieu, C.; Dhooghe, T. Increased peritoneal and endometrial gene expression of biologically relevant cytokines and growth factors during the menstrual phase in women with endometriosis. *Fertil. Steril.* **2006**, *85*, 1667–1675. [CrossRef]

59. Kyama, C.M.; Overbergh, L.; Mihalyi, A.; Meuleman, C.; Mwenda, J.M.; Mathieu, C.; D'Hooghe, T.M. Endometrial and peritoneal expression of aromatase, cytokines, and adhesion factors in women with endometriosis. *Fertil. Steril.* **2008**, *89*, 301–310. [CrossRef]

60. Young, V.J.; Brown, J.K.; Saunders, P.T.K.; Horne, A.W. The role of the peritoneum in the pathogenesis of endometriosis. *Hum. Reprod. Update* **2013**, *19*, 558–569. [CrossRef]

61. Tani, H.; Sato, Y.; Ueda, M.; Miyazaki, Y.; Suginami, K.; Horie, A.; Konishi, I.; Shinomura, T. Role of Versican in the Pathogenesis of Peritoneal Endometriosis. *J. Clin. Endocrinol. Metab.* **2016**, *101*, 4349–4356. [CrossRef] [PubMed]

62. Scutiero, G.; Iannone, P.; Bernardi, G.; Bonaccorsi, G.; Spadaro, S.; Volta, C.A.; Greco, P.; Nappi, L. Oxidative Stress and Endometriosis: A Systematic Review of the Literature. *Oxid. Med. Cell. Longev.* **2017**, *2017*, 1–7. [CrossRef] [PubMed]

63. Vitale, S.G.; Capriglione, S.; Peterlunger, I.; la Rosa, V.L.; Vitagliano, A.; Noventa, M.; Valenti, G.; Sapia, F.; Angioli, R.; Lopez, S.; et al. The Role of Oxidative Stress and Membrane Transport Systems during Endometriosis: A Fresh Look at a Busy Corner. *Oxid. Med. Cell. Longev.* **2018**, *2018*, 1–14. [CrossRef] [PubMed]

64. Lee, Y.H.; Yang, J.X.; Allen, J.C.; Tan, C.S.; Chern, B.S.M.; Tan, T.Y.; Tan, H.H.; Mattar, C.N.Z.; Chan, J.K.Y. Elevated peritoneal fluid ceramides in human endometriosis-associated infertility and their effects on mouse oocyte maturation. *Fertil. Steril.* **2018**, *110*, 767–777. [CrossRef]

65. Leconte, M.; Nicco, C.; Ngô, C.; Arkwright, S.; Chéreau, C.; Guibourdenche, J.; Weill, B.; Chapron, C.; Dousset, B.; Batteux, F. Antiproliferative Effects of Cannabinoid Agonists on Deep Infiltrating Endometriosis. *Am. J. Pathol.* **2010**, *177*, 2963–2970. [CrossRef]

66. Chapron, C.; Souza, C.; de Ziegler, D.; Lafay-Pillet, M.-C.; Ngô, C.; Bijaoui, G.; Goffinet, F.; Borghese, B. Smoking habits of 411 women with histologically proven endometriosis and 567 unaffected women. *Fertil. Steril.* **2010**, *94*, 2353–2355. [CrossRef]

67. Straussman, R.; Morikawa, T.; Shee, K.; Barzily-Rokni, M.; Qian, Z.R.; Du, J.; Davis, A.; Mongare, M.M.; Gould, J.; Frederick, D.T.; et al. Tumour micro-environment elicits innate resistance to RAF inhibitors through HGF secretion. *Nature* **2012**, *487*, 500–504. [CrossRef]

68. Suryawanshi, S.; Huang, X.; Elishaev, E.; Budiu, R.A.; Zhang, L.; Kim, S.; Donnellan, N.; Mantia-Smaldone, G.; Ma, T.; Tseng, G.; et al. Complement Pathway Is Frequently Altered in Endometriosis and Endometriosis-Associated Ovarian Cancer. *Clin. Cancer Res.* **2014**, *20*, 6163–6174. [CrossRef]

69. Zamani, M.R.; Salmaninejad, A.; Asbagh, F.A.; Masoud, A.; Rezaei, N. STAT4 single nucleotide gene polymorphisms and susceptibility to endometriosis-related infertility. *Eur. J. Obstet. Gynecol. Reprod. Biol.* **2016**, *203*, 20–24. [CrossRef]

70. Bianco, B.; Fernandes, R.F.M.; Trevisan, C.M.; Christofolini, D.M.; Sanz-Lomana, C.M.; Bernabe, J.V.; Barbosa, C.P. Influence of STAT4 gene polymorphisms in the pathogenesis of endometriosis. *Ann. Hum. Genet.* **2019**, *83*, 249–255. [CrossRef]

71. Fasciani, A. High concentrations of the vascular endothelial growth factor and interleukin-8 in ovarian endometriomata. *Mol. Hum. Reprod.* **2000**, *6*, 50–54. [CrossRef] [PubMed]

72. Jana, S.; Chatterjee, K.; Ray, A.K.; DasMahapatra, P.; Swarnakar, S. Regulation of Matrix Metalloproteinase-2 Activity by COX-2-PGE2-pAKT Axis Promotes Angiogenesis in Endometriosis. *PLoS ONE* **2016**, *11*, e0163540. [CrossRef] [PubMed]

73. Thiruchelvam, U.; Wingfield, M.; O'Farrelly, C. Natural Killer Cells: Key Players in Endometriosis. *Am. J. Reprod. Immunol.* **2015**, *74*, 291–301. [CrossRef] [PubMed]

74. Tanaka, Y.; Mori, T.; Ito, F.; Koshiba, A.; Takaoka, O.; Kataoka, H.; Maeda, E.; Okimura, H.; Mori, T.; Kitawaki, J. Exacerbation of Endometriosis Due to Regulatory T-Cell Dysfunction. *J. Clin. Endocrinol. Metab.* **2017**, *102*, 3206–3217. [CrossRef]

75. Ferrero, S.; Evangelisti, G.; Barra, F. Current and emerging treatment options for endometriosis. *Expert Opin. Pharmacother.* **2018**, *19*, 1109–1125. [CrossRef]

76. Rahmioglu, N.; Fassbender, A.; Vitonis, A.F.; Tworoger, S.S.; Hummelshoj, L.; D'Hooghe, T.M.; Adamson, G.D.; Giudice, L.C.; Becker, C.M.; Zondervan, K.T.; et al. World Endometriosis Research Foundation Endometriosis Phenome and Biobanking Harmonization Project: III. Fluid biospecimen collection, processing, and storage in endometriosis research. *Fertil. Steril.* **2014**, *102*, 1233–1243. [CrossRef]

77. ASRM. Revised American Society for Reproductive Medicine classification of endometriosis: 1996. *Fertil Steril.* **1997**, *67*, 817–821. [CrossRef]

78. AFS. Revised American Fertility Society classification of endometriosis: 1985. *Fertil. Steril.* **1985**, *43*, 351–352. [CrossRef]

79. Somigliana, E.; Infantino, M.; Candiani, M.; Vignali, M.; Chiodini, A.; Busacca, M.; Vignali, M. Association rate between deep peritoneal endometriosis and other forms of the disease: Pathogenetic implications. *Hum. Reprod.* **2004**, *19*, 168–171. [CrossRef]

80. Cochran, W.G. Methodological problems in the study of human populations. *Ann. N. Y. Acad. Sci.* **2006**, *107*, 476–489. [CrossRef]

81. Huang, D.W.; Sherman, B.T.; Lempicki, R.A. Systematic and integrative analysis of large gene lists using DAVID bioinformatics resources. *Nat. Protoc.* **2009**, *4*, 44–57. [CrossRef] [PubMed]

82. Yoav, B.; Daniel, Y. The control of the false discovery rate in multiple testing under dependency. *Ann. Stat.* **2001**, *29*, 1165–1188.

8

A Prospective Study Comparing Three-Dimensional Rectal Water Contrast Transvaginal Ultrasonography and Computed Tomographic Colonography in the Diagnosis of Rectosigmoid Endometriosis

Fabio Barra [1,2], Ennio Biscaldi [3], Carolina Scala [4], Antonio Simone Laganà [5],
Valerio Gaetano Vellone [6], Cesare Stabilini [6], Fabio Ghezzi [5] and Simone Ferrero [1,2,*]

1   Academic Unit of Obstetrics and Gynecology, IRCCS Ospedale Policlinico San Martino, 16132 Genoa, Italy;
    fabio.barra@icloud.com
2   Department of Neurosciences, Rehabilitation, Ophthalmology, Genetics, Maternal and Child
    Health (DiNOGMI), University of Genoa, 16132 Genoa, Italy
3   Department of Radiology, Galliera Hospital, 16142, Genoa, Italy; ennio.biscaldi@gmail.com
4   Unit of Obstetrics and Gynecology, Gaslini Institute, 16147 Genova, Italy; carolinascala@icloud.com
5   Department of Obstetrics and Gynecology, "Filippo Del Ponte" Hospital, University of Insubria,
    21100 Varese, Italy; antoniosimone.lagana@uninsubria.it (A.S.L.); fabio.ghezzi@uninsubria.it (F.G.)
6   Department of Surgical and Diagnostic Sciences, IRCCS Ospedale Policlinico San Martino, 16132 Genoa,
    Italy; vgvellone@gmail.com (V.G.V.); cesare.stabilini@unige.it (C.S.)
*   Correspondence: simoneferrero@me.com

Abstract: (1) Objectives: In patients with symptoms suggestive of rectosigmoid endometriosis, imaging techniques are required to confirm the presence and establish the extent of the disease. The objective of the current study was to compare the performance of three-dimensional rectal water contrast transvaginal ultrasonography (3D-RWC-TVS) and computed tomographic colonography (CTC) in predicting the presence and characteristics of rectosigmoid endometriosis. (2) Methods: This prospective study included patients with suspicion of rectosigmoid endometriosis who underwent both 3D-RWC-TVS and CTC and subsequently were surgically treated. The findings of imaging techniques were compared with surgical and histological results. (3) Results: Out of 68 women included in the study, 37 (48.9; 95% C.I. 38.2–59.7%) had rectosigmoid nodules and underwent bowel surgery. There was no significant difference in the accuracy of 3D-RWC-TVS and CTC in diagnosing the presence of rectosigmoid endometriotic nodules ($p = 0.118$), although CTC was more precise in diagnosing endometriosis located in the sigmoid ($p = 0.016$). 3D-RWC-TVS and CTC had similar precision in estimating the largest diameter of the main endometriotic nodule ($p = 0.099$) and, in patients undergoing segmental resection, the degree of the stenosis of the bowel lumen ($p = 0.293$). CTC was more accurate in estimating the distance between the lower margin of the intestinal nodule and the anal verge ($p = 0.030$) but was less tolerated than 3D-RWC-TVS ($p < 0.001$). (4) Conclusion: This was the first study comparing the performance of 3D-RWC-TVS and CTC in the diagnosis of rectosigmoid endometriosis. Both techniques allowed for the evaluation of the profile of the bowel lumen in a pseudoendoscopic fashion and had a similar performance for the diagnosis of rectosigmoid endometriosis, although CTC was more accurate in diagnosing and characterizing sigmoid nodules.

Keywords: rectosigmoid endometriosis; three-dimensional rectal water contrast transvaginal ultrasonography; computed colonography; bowel stenosis; bowel endometriosis; intestinal segmental resection

1. Introduction

Rectosigmoid endometriosis is one of the most severe forms of endometriosis, and it is defined by the presence of endometriotic glands and stroma infiltrating at least the muscularis propria of the rectosigmoid colon. Besides pain symptoms, this disease may cause several intestinal complaints that often worsen during the menstrual cycle (such as painful bowel movements, abdominal bloating, cyclical diarrhea or constipation, passage of mucus with the stools and rectal bleeding) [1]. An accurate preoperative diagnostic workup of rectosigmoid endometriosis is necessary to provide the patient with informed consent on the benefits and risks of the potential treatments (hormonal therapies or surgical approach) and to obtain adequate informed consent in case of surgery [2,3]. Furthermore, knowing the presence of bowel endometriosis preoperatively allows planning surgery with an appropriate multidisciplinary team, including the colorectal surgeon. Finally, the features of intestinal nodules may be relevant for some surgeons to choose the technique used to excise rectosigmoid nodules (shaving, discoid excision, or segmental bowel resection) [4,5].

Several ultrasonographic and radiological techniques (such as transvaginal ultrasonography (TVS), magnetic resonance imaging (MR), and rectal endoscopic ultrasonography) have been used for diagnosing rectosigmoid endometriosis [6]. In most of these techniques, the intestinal lumen is not distended, and, therefore, it is not possible to reliably estimate the degrees of stenosis caused by rectosigmoid nodules. This parameter is relevant for patients undergoing surgery, as it may affect the surgical technique. In addition, the degree of stenosis of the intestinal lumen is important for patients undergoing hormonal therapies in order to predict the risk of stenosis and occlusive symptoms during treatment. Finally, this parameter is relevant for patients desiring to conceive to minimize the risk of intestinal occlusion during pregnancy [7–11].

TVS is the first-line imaging technique in patients with suspicion of rectosigmoid endometriosis and, when performed by expert ultrasonographers in referral centers specializing in the diagnosis of endometriosis, it may provide most of the information useful to the clinicians [6]. Over the last ten years, several ultrasonographic techniques based on the distention of the vagina and/or rectosigmoid with saline solution and/or ultrasonographic gel have been proposed with the aim of improving the diagnosis of deep infiltrating endometriosis [12]. Among the others, rectal water contrast transvaginal ultrasonography (RWC-TVS) has been employed in this setting, demonstrating a high accuracy in ruling out the presence of rectosigmoid endometriosis [13–15].

Three-dimensional (3D) reconstructions convert standard 2D grayscale acquisitions into a volumetric dataset. 3D ultrasound has been employed for the evaluation of many gynecological diseases, including uterine shape abnormalities (e.g., Mullerian duct abnormalities), uterine intracavitary pathology (submucous uterine fibroids or endometrial polyps) [16]. The use of 3D-TVS has also been proposed for the diagnosis of deep endometriosis [17–19].

In general, radiological techniques can be used to establish the presence and extent of rectosigmoid endometriosis, particularly when there is suspicion of disease despite negative ultrasonographic findings and/or of the presence of multifocal disease with sigmoid or upper intestinal nodules. Moreover, in order to plan surgery, nowadays the role of radiologic imaging still remains relevant and many patients with clinical suspicion of rectosigmoid endometriosis are routinely referred to radiologists for the diagnosis of intestinal endometriosis [20,21].

Computed colonography (CTC) is used worldwide for the screening of colorectal cancer. Over the last ten years, several studies showed that CTC has high diagnostic performance in the diagnosis of rectosigmoid endometriosis [22–26]; this exam is as accurate as TVS in diagnosing rectosigmoid endometriosis and has the advantage of investigating the whole colon [27]. Image post-processing is performed using workstations suitable for 3D data management and reconstruction. The evaluation of CTC also includes the anatomic reconstruction by 3D images; in case of large bowel evaluation, 3D review typically refers to an optical colonoscopy-like endoluminal fly-through (FT) of a 3D reconstructed colon.

At the best of our knowledge, no previous study has compared the diagnostic performance of 3D-rectal water contrast transvaginal ultrasonography (3D-RWC-TVS) and CTC in the diagnosis of rectosigmoid endometriosis. As both techniques are based on the distention of the rectosigmoid and allow the evaluation of the profile of the bowel lumen in a pseudoendoscopic fashion, the objective of the current study was to compare the diagnostic performance of 3D-RWC-TVS and CTC in predicting the presence and characteristics of rectosigmoid endometriosis.

2. Materials and Methods

The primary objective of the study was to compare the performance of 3D-RWC-TVS and CTC in the diagnosis of rectosigmoid endometriosis. The secondary objectives were to compare the precision of the two techniques in estimating the length (mid-sagittal diameter) of the intestinal nodules, the presence of multifocal disease (presence of one or more lesions affecting the sigmoid colon that are associated with a colorectal primary lesion) and the distance between the lower margin of the nodules and the anal verge.

This was a prospective study performed between March 2017 and September 2019. Subjects of the study were recruited among patients referred to our institution because of pain and intestinal symptoms suggestive of rectosigmoid endometriosis. Some patients had histological diagnosis of pelvic endometriosis during previous surgery. Previous surgical diagnosis of intestinal endometriosis, previous radiological diagnosis of intestinal endometriosis (based on MR or double-contrast barium enema), history of colorectal surgery (except appendectomy), contraindications to bowel preparation or CTC (such as non-compliant patients), previous bilateral ovariectomy, or psychiatric disorders were exclusion criteria for this study.

Study patients underwent 3D-RWC-TVS performed by an ultrasonographer highly skilled in the diagnosis of deep endometriosis. CTC was done within the following three months by a radiologist expert in the diagnosis of deep endometriosis, blinded to the results of the previous ultrasonographic exam.

As described in the consensus opinion from the International Deep Endometriosis Analysis (IDEA) group, intestinal nodules located below the level of the insertion of the uterosacral ligaments on the cervix were defined as "anterior lower rectal nodules", those above this level were defined as "anterior upper rectal nodules", those at the level of the uterine fundus were defined as "rectosigmoid junction nodules" and those above the level of the uterine fundus were defined as "anterior sigmoid nodules" [6]. Bowel stenosis was defined as a reduction in lumen, by measuring the smallest stricture diameter and comparing it with the closest healthy bowel lumen diameter.

Patients underwent surgery within six months from the performance of 3D-RWC-TVS. The results of CTC and 3D-RWC-TVS were compared with surgical and histological findings.

The local ethics committee approved the study protocol (CE2439PRNO161219-24/2020). Patients participating in the study provided written informed consent. This study was registered in Clinicaltrial.gov (NCT04295343).

2.1. Three-Dimensional Rectal Water Contrast Transvaginal Sonography

A sonographer (S.F.) with extensive experience in the diagnosis of intestinal endometriosis (>500 exams every year) performed all the exams. 3D-RWC-TVS was performed by Voluson E6 and E10 machines equipped with transvaginal transducers (GE Healthcare Ultrasound, Milwaukee, WI, USA). Patients received a rectal enema (133 mL of monobasic sodium phosphate anhydrous; Clisma Lax; Sofar, Milan, Italy) a few hours before TVS. A total of 300–400 mL of saline solution was employed to distend the rectosigmoid under ultrasonographic control, by using a catheter connected to a 100 mL syringe introduced in the anus [14,28].

During the ultrasonographic scan, acquisitions of images by 3D rendering were made in the sagittal and coronal planes. Two specific quality enhancement tools (GE Healthcare Ultrasound, Milwaukee, WI, USA) were applied during 3D rendering: advanced Speckle Reduction Imaging (SRI), which helps heighten the visibility of lesions with high-definition contrast resolution and CrossXBeamCRI^{TM}, which improves the enhancement of tissue and border differentiation. On the 3D rendering, rectosigmoid lesions typically appear as spiculated lesions with a retracting line all around the nodule (Figure 1) [18].

Multiple acquisitions were performed to characterize the endometriotic nodules, in particular, measuring their largest diameter and their distance from the anal verge. When the volume acquisition was completed, the data file was sent via Digital Imaging and Communication in Medicine (DICOM) to a personal computer and stored in order to be analysed by the use of an appropriate software (4Dview 5.0; GE Healthcare Ultrasound, Milwaukee, WI, USA). All the acquisitions were examined by another sonographer who has performed over 1000 analysis of 3D imaging related to deep endometriosis in his life (F.B.). This sonographer was blinded to the results of the 2D-RWC-TVS. For estimating the stenosis, at least three measurements of the diameter of rectosigmoid lumen were performed above and below the nodule (mean of all measurements) in a healthy bowel; close to the nodule surface, at least one measurement every 5 mm was performed (mean of the three lower measurements).

Figure 1. Same rectal endometriotic nodule (arrowheads) is shown in three-dimensional rectal water contrast transvaginal ultrasonography (3D-RWC-TVS) (**A**) and computed tomographic colonography (CTC) (**B**, sagittal plane). The asterisk indicates the same rectal Houston's valve. The nodule has largest diameter of 2.6 cm.

2.2. Computed Colonography

Patients underwent a low residue diet and a liquid diet on the three days before and in the 24 h before CTC, respectively. On the afternoon and the evening of the day before the exam, the patients had an intestinal preparation, which consisted in sodium picosulfate (10.0 mg), light magnesium oxide (3.5 g) and anhydrous citric acid (10.97 g) (CitraFleet, CasenRecordati SL, Zaragoza, Spain). Patients were asked to drink a dose of diatrizoatemeglumine and diatrizoate sodium solution (Gastrografin; Schering, Berlin, Germany) diluted 1:1 with tap water at 6 p.m. on the day before the exam.

A radiologist (E.B.) with extensive experience in the diagnosis of intestinal endometriosis (>500 exams every year) performed all the exams.

The scans were performed by using a 64-section multidetector CT scanner (LightSpeed, GE Healthcare, Milwaukee, WI, USA) according to a standardized protocol [27]. A 12F Foley catheter was introduced into the distal rectum before the scan on the CT bed, and 2.5–3 L of room air were introduced in the colon, calculating the same number of manual pomp inflations in all the distensions. The patients were scanned in the supine and prone positions. No intravenous injection of iodinated contrast medium was employed. The abdomen was scanned as in conventional CTC performed for rectal cancer screening.

The DLP (dose length product) of CTC depended on the length of the abdominal surface of the women that is related to her height. The estimated radiation dose was in the range of 6 mSv. The adaptive statistical iterative reconstruction (ASIR; GE Healthcare) was used to decrease the x-ray dose without a significant loss of image quality.

A weight-based automated tube-current modulation technique was employed with a tube current range of 130–150 mA for patients weighing less than 70 kg in order to decrease the effective radiation dose (abdominal volume acquisition wCTDi = 6–7 mSv). Collimation was 1.25 mm with a helical pitch of 1.375; the reconstruction interval (overlap) was 1 mm. The raw data were transferred to a workstation having a dedicated CTC software package (General Electric ADW 4.2.4, General Electric Medical System, Milwaukee, WT, USA).

Post-processing image editing was performed, being the scans evaluated by various reconstructions: the 3D endo-luminal FT and virtual dissection reconstructions allowed for the visualization of the lumen of the rectum, sigmoid, and the other parts of the colon. 3D images were always used in case of problem solving; the diagnosis was performed on the basis of axial images and multiplanar reconstructions (MPRs).

Rectosigmoid endometriotic nodules appear on CTC as strictures usually involving a variable part of the circumference of the bowel wall (Figure 1); the site of these findings is constant on both the supine and prone scans and stenosis may be highlighted by the 3D endo-luminal FT reconstructions (Figure 2). The MPRs sometimes allow for the detection of a transmural involvement of the endometriotic nodule [27].

For estimating the stenosis, at least one measurement of the diameter of rectosigmoid lumen was performed every 10 mm in the 50 mm above and below the nodule (mean of all measurements) in healthy bowel; on the nodule surface, at least one measurement every 5 mm was performed (mean of the three lower measurements).

Figure 2. *Cont.*

Figure 2. Rectal endometriotic nodule. (**A**) CTC: 3D reconstruction of dilated colon, showing rectal stenosis (arrow) by an endometriotic nodule. (**B**) CTC: sagittal 2D image, the rectal nodule (asterisk) causes stenosis of the intestinal lumen. (**C**) CTC: pseudoendoscopic view and 3D endoluminal fly-through reconstruction, showing normal rectal lumen. (**D**) CTC: pseudoendoscopic view and 3D endoluminal fly-through reconstruction, showing rectal stenosis by the endometriotic nodule. (**E**) 3D-RWC-TVS showing the rectal nodule (asterisk). The nodule has a largest diameter of 2.8 cm; the distance between the lower margin of the nodule and the anal verge is 10 cm.

2.3. Tolerability of Radiological Exams

After each exam, the intensity of the pain perceived was rated by each patient by using a 100-mm visual analogue scale (VAS) scale. Furthermore, patients were asked to qualitatively rate the discomfort perceived during the exam by a 5-point Likert scale (very tolerable, tolerable, neutral, painful, very painful).

2.4. Surgical Procedures

The surgeons were aware of the findings of the 3D-RWC-TVS and CTC. A team of gynecological and colorectal surgeons performed all the procedures by laparoscopy. The rectosigmoid nodules were excised by shaving (excision of the nodule with cold scissor or monopolar hook without entering the intestinal lumen), discoid excision (removal of the nodule with opening of the intestinal wall and suture of the bowel) or by segmental bowel resection. The retrieval of surgical specimens was done through laparoscopic accesses by using an endo-bag (the laparoscopic accesses may have been enlarged in case of large specimen). The morcellation of surgical specimens was always avoided. During laparoscopy, the distance between the main rectosigmoid endometriotic nodule and the anal verge was estimated by introducing a 20-F soft rectal catheter within the rectum up to the level of the intestinal lesion. In case of laparoscopic shaving, a rectal probe was employed for exposing better the endometriotic lesion. In patients who underwent segmental bowel resection, the stenosis of bowel lumen caused by endometriosis was evaluated.

2.5. Statistical Analysis

Accuracy, sensitivity, specificity, positive predictive value (PPV) and negative predictive value (NPV) were evaluated for 3D-RWC-TVS and CTC. The diagnostic value of each technique was also assessed by calculating the positive likelihood ratio and negative likelihood ratio. Efficacy parameters were calculated with 95% confidence intervals (CIs). The accuracy of 3D-RWC-TVS and CTC in the diagnosis of intestinal endometriosis was compared by using the McNemar's test with the Yates continuity correction. The precision of the measurements of nodule size and distance from the anal verge by imaging techniques was calculated by subtracting the size of the nodule, as measured by the imaging techniques, from the size of the nodule, as measured at histology. The limits of agreement were calculated as mean difference ± 2 standard deviations of the difference. Correlations between nominal categories were estimated by phi coefficient. The normality of distribution of continuous variables was evaluated by the Kolmogorov–Smirnov normality test. The pain intensity experienced by the patients during both exams was evaluated by the nonparametric Mann–Whitney test. The data were analyzed using the SPSS software version 24.0 (SPSS Science, Chicago, IL, USA). p values < 0.05 was considered statistically significant.

3. Results

3.1. Characteristics of the Study Population

Table 1 shows the demographic characteristics and Supplementary Table S1 presents the main symptoms complained by the study population. Out of the 68 women included in the study, 37 (48.9; 95% C.I. 38.2–59.7%) had rectosigmoid nodules and underwent bowel surgery. The main nodules were located on the sigmoid in 16 (43.2%) patients, on the rectosigmoid junction in four (10.8%) patients, on the upper rectum in 10 (27.0%) patients and on the lower rectum in seven patients (18.9%). Twelve patients (32.4%) underwent shaving of the colorectal nodules; nine (24.3%) underwent discoid excision; 16 patients (43.2%) underwent segmental colorectal resection; in this last group of patients, the mean (± SD) length of the resected bowel specimen was 11.5 ± 1.9 cm. Concerning the depth of infiltration of endometriosis in the intestinal wall, at histology, the disease infiltrated only the muscularis mucosae in 33 patients (75.0%), the submucosa in eight patients (18.2%) and the mucosa in three patients (6.8%). Seven patients (15.9%) had multifocal disease.

Table 1. Demographic characteristics of the study population ($n = 68$).

Age (years; mean ± SD)	**35.4 ± 6.0**
Body mass index (kg/m^2; mean ± SD)	24.7 ± 3.2
Race (n, %) • Caucasian • African • Asiatic	64 (94.1%) 3 (4.4%) 1 (1.5%)
Previous live birth (n, %)	19 (27.9%)
Previous surgery for endometriosis (n, %)	30 (44.1%)
Concomitant endometriomas (n, %)	32 (47.1%)
Use of hormonal therapies at the time of study inclusion and surgical approach (n, %) - oral estroprogestin pill - contraceptive vaginal ring - desogestrel - norethindrone acetate - dienogest - etonogestrel-releasing implant - levonorgestrel-releasing intrauterine device - gonadotropin-releasing hormone analogue	50 (73.5%) 13 2 5 15 9 3 2 1

3.2. Diagnostic Performance of 3D-RTW-TVS and CTC

3D-RTW-TVS and CTC detected 26 (70.3%) and 35 (94.6%) rectosigmoid endometriotic nodules out of 37 confirmed during surgery (Figure 2 and Table 2). There was no significant difference in the accuracy of 3D-RWC-TVS and CTC in diagnosing the presence of rectosigmoid endometriotic nodules ($p = 0.118$). However, a subgroup analysis demonstrated that CTC was more precise than 3D-RWC-TVS in diagnosing endometriosis located in the sigmoid ($p = 0.016$). In fact, 3D-RWC-TVS did not identify the presence of eight sigmoid nodules, whereas CTC did not identify only one sigmoid endometriotic nodule. The presence of an endometrioma with diameter >4 cm was positively statistically correlated to the lack of identification of sigmoid endometriotic nodules (phi coefficient 0.516; p = 0.039) during 3D-RWC-TVS, but not during CTC (phi coefficient 0.333; p = 0.182).

Table 2. Diagnostic performance of 3D-RWC-TVS and CTC in the diagnosis of rectosigmoid endometriosis.

	3D-RWC-TVS	**CTC**
Sensitivity [a]	70.27% (53.02% to 84.13%)	94.59% (81.81% to 99.34%)
Specificity [a]	96.55% (82.24% to 99.91%)	93.10% (77.23% to 99.15%)
Positive likelihood ratio [b]	20.38 (2.94 to 141.42)	13.72 (3.59 to 52.36)
Negative likelihood ratio [b]	0.31 (0.19 to 0.51)	0.06 (90.02 to 0.22)
Positive predictive value [a]	96.30% (78.93% to 99.45%)	94.59% (82.09% to 98.53%)
Negative predictive value [a]	71.79% (60.69% to 80.76%)	93.10% (77.75% to 98.12%)
Accuracy [a]	81.82% (70.39% to 90.24%)	93.94% (85.20% to 98.32%)

[a] Values presented as percentage and 95% confidence interval; [b] Values presented as ratio and 95% confidence interval; 3D-RWC-TVS: Three-dimensional rectal water contrast transvaginal ultrasonography; CTC: Computed colonography.

The mean (±SD) largest diameter of the main endometriotic nodule at histology was 22.3 (±8.7) mm. 3D-RWC-TVS and CTC estimated the largest diameter of the main endometriotic nodules (p = 0.099) similarly, independent of their location. The mean difference was −3.2 (±7.4) mm (95% CI, −6.0 to −0.3 mm; limits of agreement, −17.3 to 11.1 mm) at 3D-RWC-TVS and −1.0 (±2.7) mm (95% CI, −2.1 to 0.1 mm; limits of agreement, −6.4 to 4.5 mm) at CTC when compared with histology (Table 3).

Table 3. Difference between the size of the largest nodule estimated by imaging techniques and that measured on histopathology.

Location	Length on Histology (mm; Mean ±SD)	3D-RWC-TVS		CTC		p [c]
		Difference (mm; mean, 95% CI) [a]	LA [b]	Difference (mm; Mean, 95% CI) [a]	LA [b]	
All (n = 37)	22.3 ± 8.7	−3.2 (−6.0 to −0.3)	−17.3 to 11.1	−1.0 (−2.1 to 0.1)	−6.4 to 4.5	0.099
Anterior lower rectum (n = 7)	22.1 ± 12.4	−1.0 (−3.3 to 1.4)	−5.5 to 3.3	−1.0 (−3.7 to 1.7)	−6.0 to 4.0	1.000
Anterior upper rectum (n = 13)	26.9 ± 11.3	−1.0 (−3.2 to 1.2)	−6.2 to 4.2	−1.3 (−2.7 to 0.2)	−4.4 to 1.7	0.836
Rectosigmoid junction (n = 4)	20.3 ± 3.1	1.6 (−3.5 to 6.8)	−2.4 to 5.7	1.0 (−1.5 to 3.5)	−3.1 to 3.6	0.728
Sigmoid (n = 17)	22.0 ± 6.4	−7.2 (−15.4 to −3.2)	−16.4 to 9.1	−1.4 (−3.8 to 1.1)	−8.2 to 6.3	0.060

[a] Mean difference calculated by subtracting the size of the nodule measured by the imaging technique from the size of the nodule measured on histology; [b] Limits of agreement (LA) calculated as a mean difference ±2 SDs of the difference. [c] Comparison of the mean difference of 3D-RWC-TVS with that of CTC. 3D-RWC-TVS: Three-dimensional rectal water contrast transvaginal ultrasonography; CTC: Computed colonography

At surgery, the mean (±SD) distance between the more distal rectosigmoid nodule and the anal verge was 142.7 (±45.3) mm. CTC was more accurate than 3D-RWC-TVS in estimating the distance between the lower margin of the intestinal nodule and the anal verge (p = 0.030). The mean difference was −16.5 (±30.1) mm (95% CI, −28.7 to −4.2 mm; limits of agreement, −75.7 to 43.4) for 3D-RWC-TVS and 3.3 (±2.0) mm (95% CI, −10.1 to 16.7 mm; limits of agreement, −57.3 to 62.1) for CTC when compared with surgery (Table 4).

Table 4. Difference between the lower margin of the lowest rectosigmoid nodule and the anal verge estimated by imaging techniques and that measured on histopathology.

Location	Distance at Surgery (mm; mean ±SD)	3D-RWC-TVS		CTC		p [c]
		Difference (mm; Mean, 95% CI) [a]	LA [b]	Difference (mm; Mean, 95% CI) [a]	LA [b]	
All (n = 37)	142.7 ± 45.3	−16.5 (−28.7 to −4.2)	−75.7 to 43.4	3.3 (−10.1 to 16.7)	−57.3 to 62.1	0.030
Anterior lower rectum (n = 7)	90.7 ± 10.9	3.1 (−14.1 to 20.4)	−28.7 to 32.1	6.6 (−0.1 to 13.4)	−5.9 to 19.2	0.653
Anterior upper rectum (n = 13)	131.3 ± 16.5	−25.6 (−58.2 to 7.1)	−34.8 to 11.0	13.8 (−30.3 to 58.1)	−91.0 to 11.2	0.125
Rectosigmoid junction (n = 4)	138.3 ± 7.6	−6.6 (−32.5 to 19.1)	−27.1 to 13.7	−11.7 (−30.6 to 7.3)	−27.0 to 0.4	0.667
Sigmoid (n = 17)	165.7 ± 47.5	−23.8 (−43.1 to −4.4)	−73.1 to 16.8	−4.5 (−13.4 to 4.5)	−26.3 to 23.0	0.048

[a] Mean difference calculated by subtracting distance between the nodule and anal verge measured by imaging technique from distance between the nodule and anal verge measured at surgery. [b] Limits of agreement (LA) calculated as mean difference ±2 SDs of the difference. [c] Comparison of the mean difference of 3D-RWC-TVS with that of CTC. 3D-RWC-TVS: Three-dimensional rectal water contrast transvaginal ultrasonography; CTC: Computed colonography.

In patients undergoing colorectal segmental resection, at pathological examination, the degree of the stenosis of the bowel lumen was 65.1 (±21.4) %. CTC and 3D-RWC-TVS similarly estimated the degree of the stenosis of the bowel lumen (p = 0.293), although 3D-RWC-TVS was less accurate than CTC in determining this parameter in endometriotic nodules located in the sigmoid (p = 0.005). The mean difference was 17.3 (±13.8) % for 3D-RWC-TVS and 13.8 (±10.0) % for CTC in comparison to surgery (Figure 3).

CTC only identified all the cases (6/6) of multifocal disease; in one patient, 3D-RWC-TVS did not diagnose the presence of multifocal disease that was diagnosed at surgery (1/6; 16.6%). There was no significant difference in the performance of 3D-RWC-TVS and CTC in diagnosing multifocal disease (p = 1.000) (Supplementary Table S2).

The mean (±SD) intensity of pain experienced during CTC was higher than that perceived during RWC-TVS (VAS, 29 ± 57 vs. 15 ± 05 mm; p < 0.001). A higher proportion of patients complained of pain during CTC than RWC-TVS (the % of patients experiencing a painful/very painful exam was 7.5% vs. 44.1%; p < 0.001).

Figure 3. *Cont.*

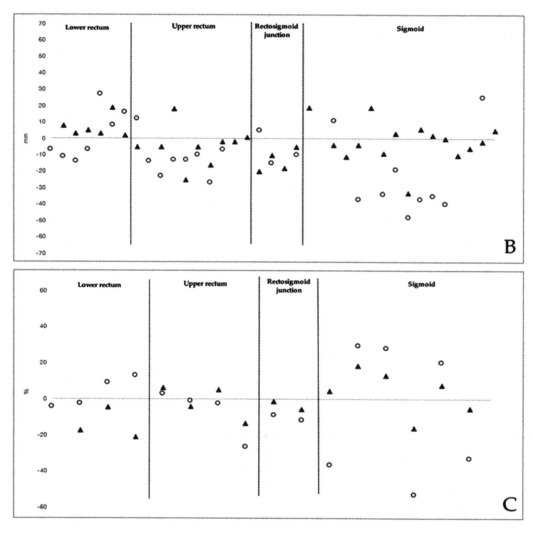

Figure 3. (**A**) Difference (mm) between imaging methods and surgery in estimating the largest diameter of endometriotic rectosigmoid nodules; (**B**) difference (mm) between imaging methods and surgery in estimating the distance from the lowest endometriotic rectosigmoid nodule and the anal verge; (**C**) Difference (%) between imaging methods and surgery in estimating the stenosis of bowel lumen due to the endometriotic nodules (calculated in patients undergoing colorectal segmental resection). White circles: 3D-RWC-TVS; black triangles: CTC.

4. Discussion

This is the first study comparing the performance of 3D-RWC-TVS and CTC in the diagnosis of rectosigmoid endometriosis. Both techniques are based on the distention of the rectosigmoid (with either saline solution or air/CO_2) and allow for the evaluation of the profile of the bowel lumen in a pseudoendoscopic fashion. Moreover, 3D-RWC-TVS and CTC enable the acquisition of ultrasonographic volumetric data with unrestricted access to an infinite number of viewing planes; thus, further images can be obtained even after the first acquisition.

Our data demonstrate that 3D-RWC-TVS and CTC have similar accuracy in the diagnosis of rectosigmoid endometriosis (81.82% vs. 93.94%). However, CTC is more accurate than 3D-RWC-TVS in assessing the presence of sigmoid nodules. In fact, most of the nodules (8/11; 72.7%) not detected by 3D-RWC-TVS were located in the sigmoid; nevertheless, 62.5% of patients (6/10) had ovarian endometriotic cysts with a diameter >4 cm that may have hampered the detection of these upper intestinal nodules. Overall, thirteen false negatives procedures occurred in our study; however, in twelve cases (92.3%), the detection of endometriotic nodules was done by at least one of the two imaging techniques. These data may justify the combined use of both CTC and 3D-RWC-TVS for the workup of patients with suspicion of rectosigmoid endometriosis.

CTC was more precise than 3D-RWC-TVS in estimating the distance between the lower margin of the intestinal nodule and the anal verge: in particular, both techniques equally estimated this parameter in patients with lower, upper rectum, and rectosigmoid junction endometriotic nodules, but not in those with sigmoid nodules. Furthermore, these diagnostic exams were equally precise in estimating the largest diameter of the main rectosigmoid nodule and detecting the presence of multifocal disease.

According to IDEA consensus opinion [6], TVS should be considered the first-line imaging technique for investigating women with suspicion of rectosigmoid endometriosis, in particular, whenever performed by expert ultrasonographers in referral centers specializing in diagnosis of endometriosis. Recently, it has been reported that the need for segmental resection in patients with bowel-infiltrating nodules depends on the degree of muscular layer infiltration and corresponding thickness (muscularis rule) in addition to nodule length and can be accurately identified by preoperative ultrasonographic investigation [5]. Nevertheless, until now, nodule features and threshold values for the choice and timing of either conservative or radical surgical approach for rectosigmoid endometriosis have not been well defined [21]. In current practice, the choice of optimal surgical technique should not depend on only rectosigmoid nodule features, but also on patients' symptoms, age, desire of conception and intention to undergo postoperative hormonal treatment for reducing the risk of disease recurrence. However, the preoperative estimation of the stenosis of rectosigmoid lumen may be helpful in the decision to plan surgery, particularly in infertile patients that may be at risk of bowel occlusion during ovarian stimulation and pregnancy [1]. In our study, CTC and 3D-RWC-TVS similarly estimated the degree of the stenosis of the bowel lumen in patients with rectosigmoid nodules undergoing segmental resection. However, 3D-RWC-TVS was again less accurate than CTC in assessing this parameter in endometriotic nodules located above the rectosigmoid junction.

CTC can characterize endometriotic rectosigmoid nodules and precisely assess the distance between their localization and the anal verge. Colonic distension with air provides a better estimation of digestive tract narrowness than that of any other imaging techniques and allows for an accurate investigation of the whole colon and, in particular, of the intestinal nodules located above the sigmoid colon (such as those on the transverse colon and the cecum) [27]. These nodules cannot be diagnosed by TVS because they are beyond the field of view of the transvaginal probe. In addition, they can also be difficult to detect when performing MR, even in the case of rectal enema (which allows for a less extended retrograde colorectal distension in comparison to CTC) [29]. Considering that more than one-third of cases of bowel lesions are multifocal [30], a complete assessment of the colon is essential to detect all endometriotic lesions for planning the surgical management; in fact, multiple endometriotic nodules on the digestive tract may require multiple segmental bowel resections or disc excisions. Furthermore, CTC is a quick outpatient exam characterized by high spatial resolution, and it allows for scanning the entire abdominal volume within seconds; this may rule out some macroscopic visceral findings (such as cysts, or calcifications) that may be relevant in the differential diagnosis of abdominal pain in patients of reproductive age. Nevertheless, CTC should not be considered as an alternative to TVS or MR, because these imaging techniques can offer a better assessment of deep pelvic endometriosis, ovarian endometriotic cysts, and uterine adenomyosis [31].

Previous studies investigated the performance of CTC in the diagnosis of bowel endometriosis [25,27,32–35]. In a prospective study including 92 women undergoing surgery for deep infiltrating endometriosis, Baggio et al. compared the diagnostic value of TVS, serum Ca125 and CTC [33]. Forty-nine subjects had rectosigmoid endometriosis. CTC had the highest accuracy in detecting bowel involvement with a sensitivity of 68% and a specificity of 67%. However, both TVS and CTC had lower performance than that previously reported by other authors, possibly because of the limited experience of the gynecologists and radiologists in the diagnosis of deep endometriosis. Zannoni et al. compared the performance of TVS and CTC in the diagnosis of rectosigmoid endometriosis in a prospective study including 47 patients with suspicion of rectosigmoid endometriosis [34]. The study showed that TVS has higher accuracy in the diagnosis of intestinal deep infiltrating endometriosis in the rectovaginal septum, rectum and sigma. In contrast, the two techniques had similar accuracy for the diagnosis of overall intestinal deep infiltrating endometriosis. Recently, a systematic review with meta-analysis investigated the performance of CTC by meta-regression, showing a global sensitivity of 93% (95% CI 84–100%) and a specificity of 91% (95% CI 81–100%) [36]. In a prospective study by our academic group, CTC was compared to RWC-TVS in 70 patients with suspicion of rectosigmoid endometriosis, obtaining a similar accuracy in diagnosing endometriotic nodules (sensitivity 90.0% and 94.3%; specificity 92.5% and 92,5%, respectively) [27]. The diagnostic performance of 3D-RWC-TVS reported in the current study is lower than that observed with RWC-TVS. In our experience, obtaining good quality 3D acquisition was more difficult in the sigmoid than in the rectum. Similar to the current data, CTC was previously found to be more precise than RWC-TVS in estimating the distance between the lower margin of the rectosigmoid nodule and the anal verge, but it was less tolerated than RWC-TVS [27].

In our prospective study, CTC was performed without the use of iodinated contrast medium in order to reduce the invasiveness of the exam. For this reason, an accurate estimation of the depth of infiltration of endometriosis in the intestinal wall was not feasible; otherwise, 3D-RWC-TVS reliably estimates this parameter [12].

Ultrasonographic study with 3D modalities has increasingly been employed for the evaluation of many gynecological diseases, being in recent years also investigated for the diagnosis of deep endometriosis [17–19,37]. Two previous studies prospectively compared the performance of 3D-RWC-TVS and MR with colorectal enema in the diagnosis of rectosigmoid endometriosis, finding similar accuracy parameters, nevertheless stating the advantage of an accurate visualization and characterization of the nodules by performing the 3D evaluation [38,39]. In particular, 3D-RWC-TVS is characterized by a wide spatial orientation by providing the observer with a range of different displays of the images in the three orthogonal planes. Moreover, all the acquisitions can be selected and rotated or scrolled through in fascinating virtual navigation and they can be easily assessed off-line. In our study, this advantage let us avoid a 3D real-time evaluation, which would have been subjected to the risk of bias due to 2D-RWC-TVS scan performed at the same consultation; thus, after being stored, the images acquired were interpreted by another expert ultrasonographer blinded to the results of conventional RWC-TVS and CTC imaging. Otherwise, a learning curve has to be considered because the sonographer acquired optimal expertise in 3D acquisitions and interpretation. Notably, the comparison of accuracy of 3D-RWC-TVS versus conventional 2D-RWC-TVS in the detection or characterization of rectosigmoid endometriotic nodules would be of interest. Until now, only a study published in the abstract form performed a preliminary comparison between the two ultrasonographic techniques. This study included 36 women of reproductive age with pain symptoms and intestinal complaints suggestive of rectosigmoid endometriosis. 3D-RWC-TVS and 2D-RWC-TVS had similar performance in the diagnosis of rectosigmoid endometriosis ($p = 0.50$). In particular, for the 3D-RWC-TVS, the sensitivity, specificity, positive and negative predictive values were 86.4%, 85.7%, 90.5% and 80.0%. The two techniques similarly estimated the volume of the largest intestinal nodule and the distance between the lower endometriotic bowel nodule and the anus [40].

In a similar way to the conventional 2D scan, 3D-RWC-TVS is better tolerated and less expensive than CTC. Our data show that patients experienced more discomfort during CTC than during 3D-RWC-TVS. This may be in primis due to the air distension of the colon employed during the radiologic exam, but also to the intestinal cleansing required prior to the exam, less tolerable than that employed for 3D-RWC-TVS. Another not negligible disadvantage related to the use of CTC is the exposure to X-rays; this limit is relevant since women with symptomatic endometriosis are in their fertile age and do not have an oncological pathology that would justify the radiation dose. Nevertheless, in current CTC protocols, the radiation dose has been decreased, and the average radiation administered to the patient is around 6–7 mSv that is lower than that usually used for a barium enema.

This study has some limitations. Indeed, the extensive experience of the radiologist and the gynecologist performing CTC and 3D-RWC-TVS, respectively, may have influenced the accuracy of these techniques in diagnosing rectosigmoid endometriosis. Moreover, we did not perform a power calculation for determining the sample size. As this study was based on a population of symptomatic patients with a high prevalence of intestinal symptoms, a high prevalence of rectosigmoid endometriosis was observed in this sample; subsequently, this issue may potentially have influenced the diagnostic performance of CTC and 3D-RWC-TVS. Nevertheless, the use of these diagnostic exams is justified only in symptomatic patients at high risk of having rectosigmoid endometriosis. The positive, but not statistically significative, trend in favor of CTC with regard to diagnostic parameters may be partly due to limited sample size of our study.

5. Conclusions

In conclusion, 3D-RWC-TVS and CTC can be used to screen the presence of rectosigmoid endometriosis, as they have comparable diagnostic accuracy. However, we deem that symptomatic patients in case of negative findings at 3D-RWC-TVS and patients undergoing surgery should also be investigated using other techniques, aiming to study the presence of sigmoid or upper intestinal nodules. Nevertheless, CTC should not be considered as an alternative to TVS or MR, because these imaging techniques provide a better assessment of deep pelvic endometriosis, ovarian endometriotic cysts, and uterine adenomyosis. In this perspective, CTC may be combined with 3D-RWC-TVS because of the high diagnostic performance in detecting rectosigmoid endometriosis and the ability to diagnose endometriotic nodules located above the sigmoid.

Author Contributions: Conceptualization, F.B. and S.F.; methodology, F.B., F.G. and C.S.(Carolina Scala); software, C.S. (Carolina Scala) and E.B.; validation, F.B., A.S.L.; formal analysis, V.G.V., C.S.(Cesare Stabilini); investigation, E.B., V.G.V., F.B. and S.F.; writing—original draft preparation, F.B.; writing—review and editing, S.F. All authors have read and agreed to the published version of the manuscript.

References

1.   Remorgida, V.; Ferrero, S.; Fulcheri, E.; Ragni, N.; Martin, D.C. Bowel endometriosis: Presentation, diagnosis, and treatment. *Obstet. Gynecol. Surv.* **2007**, *62*, 461–470. [CrossRef]

2.   Abrao, M.S.; Petraglia, F.; Falcone, T.; Keckstein, J.; Osuga, Y.; Chapron, C. Deep endometriosis infiltrating the recto-sigmoid: Critical factors to consider before management. *Hum. Reprod. Update* **2015**, *21*, 329–339. [CrossRef]

3.   Ferrero, S.; Camerini, G.; Ragni, N.; Venturini, P.L.; Biscaldi, E.; Seracchioli, R.; Remorgida, V. Letrozole and norethisterone acetate in colorectal endometriosis. *Eur. J. Obs. Gynecol. Reprod. Biol.* **2010**, *150*, 199–202. [CrossRef]

4.   Ferrero, S.; Camerini, G.; Leone Roberti Maggiore, U.; Venturini, P.L.; Biscaldi, E.; Remorgida, V. Bowel endometriosis: Recent insights and unsolved problems. *World. J. Gastrointest. Surg.* **2011**, *3*, 31–38. [CrossRef]

5.   Malzoni, M.; Casarella, L.; Coppola, M.; Falcone, F.; Iuzzolino, D.; Rasile, M.; Di Giovanni, A. Preoperative Ultrasound Indications Determine Excision Technique for Bowel Surgery for Deep Infiltrating Endometriosis: A Single, High-Volume Center. *J. Minim. Invasive. Gynecol.* **2020**. [CrossRef]

6.   Guerriero, S.; Condous, G.; van den Bosch, T.; Valentin, L.; Leone, F.P.; Van Schoubroeck, D.; Exacoustos, C.; Installe, A.J.; Martins, W.P.; Abrao, M.S.; et al. Systematic approach to sonographic evaluation of the pelvis in women with suspected endometriosis, including terms, definitions and measurements: A consensus opinion from the International Deep Endometriosis Analysis (IDEA) group. *Ultrasound. Obs. Gynecol.* **2016**, *48*, 318–332. [CrossRef]

7.   Takeuchi, H.; Kuwatsuru, R.; Kitade, M.; Sakurai, A.; Kikuchi, I.; Shimanuki, H.; Kinoshita, K. A novel technique using magnetic resonance imaging jelly for evaluation of rectovaginal endometriosis. *Fertil. Steril.* **2005**, *83*, 442–447. [CrossRef]

8.   Kikuchi, I.; Takeuchi, H.; Kuwatsuru, R.; Kitade, M.; Kumakiri, J.; Kuroda, K.; Takeda, S. Diagnosis of complete cul-de-sac obliteration (CCDSO) by the MRI jelly method. *J. Magn. Reson. Imaging.* **2009**, *29*, 365–370. [CrossRef]

9.   Loubeyre, P.; Petignat, P.; Jacob, S.; Egger, J.F.; Dubuisson, J.B.; Wenger, J.M. Anatomic distribution of posterior deeply infiltrating endometriosis on MRI after vaginal and rectal gel opacification. *Ajr. Am. J. Roentgenol.* **2009**, *192*, 1625–1631. [CrossRef]

10.   Chassang, M.; Novellas, S.; Bloch-Marcotte, C.; Delotte, J.; Toullalan, O.; Bongain, A.; Chevallier, P. Utility of vaginal and rectal contrast medium in MRI for the detection of deep pelvic endometriosis. *Eur. Radiol.* **2010**, *20*, 1003–1010. [CrossRef]

11.   Biscaldi, E.; Ferrero, S.; Leone Roberti Maggiore, U.; Remorgida, V.; Venturini, P.L.; Rollandi, G.A. Multidetector computerized tomography enema versus magnetic resonance enema in the diagnosis of rectosigmoid endometriosis. *Eur. J. Radiol.* **2014**, *83*, 261–267. [CrossRef]

12.   Ferrero, S.; Leone Roberti Maggiore, U.; Barra, F.; Scala, C. Modified ultrasonographic techniques. In *How to Perform Ultrasonography in Endometriosis*; Guerriero, S., Condous, G., Alcazar, J.L., Eds.; Springer: Berlin, Germany, 2018; pp. 133–145.

13.   Ferrero, S.; Scala, C.; Stabilini, C.; Vellone, V.G.; Barra, F.; Leone Roberti Maggiore, U. Transvaginal sonography with vs. without bowel preparation in diagnosis of rectosigmoid endometriosis: Prospective study. *Ultrasound. Obs. Gynecol.* **2019**, *53*, 402–409. [CrossRef]

14.   Ferrero, S.; Biscaldi, E.; Morotti, M.; Venturini, P.L.; Remorgida, V.; Rollandi, G.A.; Valenzano Menada, M. Multidetector computerized tomography enteroclysis vs. rectal water contrast transvaginal ultrasonography in determining the presence and extent of bowel endometriosis. *Ultrasound. Obstet. Gynecol.* **2011**, *37*, 603–613. [CrossRef]

15.   Leone Roberti Maggiore, U.; Biscaldi, E.; Vellone, V.G.; Venturini, P.L.; Ferrero, S. Magnetic resonance enema vs. rectal water-contrast transvaginal sonography in diagnosis of rectosigmoid endometriosis. *Ultrasound. Obs. Gynecol.* **2017**, *49*, 524–532. [CrossRef]

16.   Armstrong, L.; Fleischer, A.; Andreotti, R. Three-dimensional volumetric sonography in gynecology: An overview of clinical applications. *Radiol. Clin. N. Am.* **2013**, *51*, 1035–1047. [CrossRef]

17.   Guerriero, S.; Alcazar, J.L.; Pascual, M.A.; Ajossa, S.; Perniciano, M.; Piras, A.; Mais, V.; Piras, B.; Schirru, F.; Benedetto, M.G.; et al. Deep Infiltrating Endometriosis: Comparison Between 2-Dimensional Ultrasonography (US), 3-Dimensional US, and Magnetic Resonance Imaging. *J. Ultrasound. Med.* **2018**, *37*, 1511–1521. [CrossRef]

18.   Guerriero, S.; Saba, L.; Ajossa, S.; Peddes, C.; Angiolucci, M.; Perniciano, M.; Melis, G.B.; Alcazar, J.L. Three-dimensional ultrasonography in the diagnosis of deep endometriosis. *Hum. Reprod.* **2014**, *29*, 1189–1198. [CrossRef]

19.   Grasso, R.F.; Di Giacomo, V.; Sedati, P.; Sizzi, O.; Florio, G.; Faiella, E.; Rossetti, A.; Del Vescovo, R.; Zobel, B.B. Diagnosis of deep infiltrating endometriosis: Accuracy of magnetic resonance imaging and transvaginal 3D ultrasonography. *Abdom. Imaging* **2010**, *35*, 716–725. [CrossRef]

20.   Mabrouk, M.; Raimondo, D.; Altieri, M.; Arena, A.; Del Forno, S.; Moro, E.; Mattioli, G.; Iodice, R.; Seracchioli, R. Surgical, Clinical, and Functional Outcomes in Patients with Rectosigmoid Endometriosis in the Gray Zone: 13-Year Long-Term Follow-up. *J. Minim. Invasive. Gynecol.* **2019**, *26*, 1110–1116. [CrossRef]

21.   Donnez, O.; Roman, H. Choosing the right surgical technique for deep endometriosis: Shaving, disc excision, or bowel resection? *Fertil. Steril.* **2017**, *108*, 931–942. [CrossRef]

22.   Tzambouras, N.; Katsanos, K.H.; Tsili, A.; Papadimitriou, K.; Efremidis, S.; Tsianos, E.V. CT colonoscopy for obstructive sigmoid endometriosis: A new technique for an old problem. *Eur. J. Intern. Med.* **2002**, *13*, 274–275.

23.   Van der Wat, J.; Kaplan, M.D. Modified virtual colonoscopy: A noninvasive technique for the diagnosis of rectovaginal septum and deep infiltrating pelvic endometriosis. *J. Minim. Invasive Gynecol.* **2007**, *14*, 638–643. [CrossRef]

24.   Koutoukos, I.; Langebrekke, A.; Young, V.; Qvigstad, E. Imaging of endometriosis with computerized tomography colonography. *Fertil. Steril.* **2011**, *95*, 259–260. [CrossRef]

25.   Jeong, S.Y.; Chung, D.J.; Myung Yeo, D.; Lim, Y.T.; Hahn, S.T.; Lee, J.M. The usefulness of computed tomographic colonography for evaluation of deep infiltrating endometriosis: Comparison with magnetic resonance imaging. *J. Comput. Assist. Tomogr.* **2013**, *37*, 809–814. [CrossRef]

26. Van der Wat, J.; Kaplan, M.D.; Roman, H.; Da Costa, C. The use of modified virtual colonoscopy to structure a descriptive imaging classification with implied severity for rectogenital and disseminated endometriosis. *J. Minim. Invasive. Gynecol.* **2013**, *20*, 543–546. [CrossRef]

27. Ferrero, S.; Biscaldi, E.; Vellone, V.G.; Venturini, P.L.; Leone Roberti Maggiore, U. Computed tomographic colonography vs. rectal water—Contrast transvaginal sonography in diagnosis of rectosigmoid endometriosis: A pilot study. *Ultrasound. Obs. Gynecol.* **2017**, *49*, 515–523. [CrossRef]

28. Valenzano Menada, M.; Remorgida, V.; Abbamonte, L.H.; Nicoletti, A.; Ragni, N.; Ferrero, S. Does transvaginal ultrasonography combined with water-contrast in the rectum aid in the diagnosis of rectovaginal endometriosis infiltrating the bowel? *Hum. Reprod.* **2008**, *23*, 1069–1075. [CrossRef]

29. Biscaldi, E.; Barra, F.; Ferrero, S. Magnetic Resonance Enema in Rectosigmoid Endometriosis. *Magn. Reson. Imaging Clin. N. Am.* **2020**, *28*, 89–104. [CrossRef]

30. Chapron, C.; Fauconnier, A.; Vieira, M.; Barakat, H.; Dousset, B.; Pansini, V.; Vacher-Lavenu, M.C.; Dubuisson, J.B. Anatomical distribution of deeply infiltrating endometriosis: Surgical implications and proposition for a classification. *Hum. Reprod.* **2003**, *18*, 157–161. [CrossRef]

31. Exacoustos, C.; Manganaro, L.; Zupi, E. Imaging for the evaluation of endometriosis and adenomyosis. *Best. Pr. Res. Clin. Obs. Gynaecol.* **2014**, *28*, 655–681. [CrossRef]

32. Roman, H.; Carilho, J.; Da Costa, C.; De Vecchi, C.; Suaud, O.; Monroc, M.; Hochain, P.; Vassilieff, M.; Savoye-Collet, C.; Saint-Ghislain, M. Computed tomography-based virtual colonoscopy in the assessment of bowel endometriosis: The surgeon's point of view. *Gynecol. Obs. Fertil.* **2016**, *44*, 3–10. [CrossRef]

33. Baggio, S.; Zecchin, A.; Pomini, P.; Zanconato, G.; Genna, M.; Motton, M.; Montemezzi, S.; Franchi, M. The Role of Computed Tomography Colonography in Detecting Bowel Involvement in Women With Deep Infiltrating Endometriosis: Comparison With Clinical History, Serum Ca125, and Transvaginal Sonography. *J. Comput. Assist. Tomogr.* **2016**, *40*, 886–891. [CrossRef]

34. Zannoni, L.; Del Forno, S.; Coppola, F.; Papadopoulos, D.; Valerio, D.; Golfieri, R.; Caprara, G.; Paradisi, R.; Seracchioli, R. Comparison of transvaginal sonography and computed tomography-colonography with contrast media and urographic phase for diagnosing deep infiltrating endometriosis of the posterior compartment of the pelvis: A pilot study. *Jpn. J. Radiol.* **2017**, *35*, 546–554. [CrossRef]

35. Mehedintu, C.; Brinduse, L.A.; Bratila, E.; Monroc, M.; Lemercier, E.; Suaud, O.; Collet-Savoye, C.; Roman, H. Does Computed Tomography-Based Virtual Colonoscopy Improve the Accuracy of Preoperative Assessment Based on Magnetic Resonance Imaging in Women Managed for Colorectal Endometriosis? *J. Minim. Invasive Gynecol.* **2018**. [CrossRef]

36. Woo, S.; Suh, C.H.; Kim, H. Diagnostic performance of computed tomography for bowel endometriosis: A systematic review and meta-analysis. *Eur. J. Radiol.* **2019**, *119*, 108638. [CrossRef]

37. Pascual, M.A.; Guerriero, S.; Hereter, L.; Barri-Soldevila, P.; Ajossa, S.; Graupera, B.; Rodriguez, I. Diagnosis of endometriosis of the rectovaginal septum using introital three-dimensional ultrasonography. *Fertil. Steril.* **2010**, *94*, 2761–2765. [CrossRef]

38. Sandre, A.; Philip, C.A.; De-Saint-Hilaire, P.; Maissiat, E.; Bailly, F.; Cortet, M.; Dubernard, G. Comparison of three-dimensional rectosonography, rectal endoscopic sonography and magnetic resonance imaging performances in the diagnosis of rectosigmoid endometriosis. *Eur. J. Obs. Gynecol. Reprod. Biol.* **2019**, *240*, 288–292. [CrossRef]

39. Philip, C.A.; Prouvot, C.; Cortet, M.; Bisch, C.; de Saint-Hilaire, P.; Maissiat, E.; Huissoud, C.; Dubernard, G. Diagnostic Performances of Tridimensional Rectosonography and Magnetic Resonance Imaging in Rectosigmoid Endometriosis: A Prospective Cohort Study on 101 Patients. *Ultrasound. Med. Biol.* **2019**. [CrossRef]

40. Barra, F.S.; Vellone, V.G.; Ferrero, S. Bidimensional rectal-water contrast-transvaginal ultrasonography (2D-RWC-TVS) versus 3D-RWC-TVS in the diagnosis of rectosigmoid endometriosis: A pilot prospective comparative study. In Proceedings of the ESHRE Annual Meeting, Vienna, Austria, 26–29 June 2019.

Impaired Expression of Ectonucleotidases in Ectopic and Eutopic Endometrial Tissue is in Favor of ATP Accumulation in the Tissue Microenvironment in Endometriosis

Carla Trapero [1,2], August Vidal [1,2,3], Maria Eulàlia Fernández-Montolí [2,4],
Buenaventura Coroleu [5], Francesc Tresserra [5], Pere Barri [5], Inmaculada Gómez de Aranda [1],
Jean Sévigny [6,7], Jordi Ponce [2,4], Xavier Matias-Guiu [2,3] and Mireia Martín-Satué [1,2,*]

[1] Departament de Patologia i Terapèutica Experimental, Facultat de Medicina i Ciències de la Salut, Campus Bellvitge, Universitat de Barcelona, 08907 Barcelona, Spain; ctrapero@idibell.cat (C.T.); avidal@bellvitgehospital.cat (A.V.); igomezdearanda@ub.edu (I.G.d.A.)

[2] Oncobell Program, CIBERONC, Institut d'Investigació Biomèdica de Bellvitge (IDIBELL), 08908 Barcelona, Spain; mefernandez@bellvitgehospital.cat (M.E.F.-M.); jponce@bellvitgehospital.cat (J.P.); fjmatiasguiu.lleida.ics@gencat.cat (X.M.-G.)

[3] Servei d'Anatomia Patològica, Hospital Universitari de Bellvitge, 08907 Barcelona, Spain

[4] Servei de Ginecologia, Hospital Universitari de Bellvitge, 08907 Barcelona, Spain

[5] Salud de la Mujer Dexeus, Hospital Universitari Quiron Dexeus, 08028 Barcelona, Spain; VENCOR@dexeus.com (B.C.); francesc.tresserra@quironsalud.es (F.T.); barper@dexeus.com (P.B.)

[6] Centre de Recherche du CHU de Québec - Université Laval, Québec City, QC G1V 4G2, Canada; jean.sevigny@crchudequebec.ulaval.ca

[7] Départment de Microbiologie-Infectiologie et d'Immunologie, Faculté de Médecine, Université Laval, Quebec City, QC G1V 4G2, Canada

* Correspondence: martinsatue@ub.edu

Abstract: Endometriosis is a prevalent disease defined by the presence of endometrial tissue outside the uterus. Adenosine triphosphate (ATP), as a proinflammatory molecule, promotes and helps maintain the inflammatory state of endometriosis. Moreover, ATP has a direct influence on the two main symptoms of endometriosis: infertility and pain. Purinergic signaling, the group of biological responses to extracellular nucleotides such as ATP and nucleosides such as adenosine, is involved in the biology of reproduction and is impaired in pathologies with an inflammatory component such as endometriosis. We have previously demonstrated that ectonucleotidases, the enzymes regulating extracellular ATP levels, are active in non-pathological endometria, with hormone-dependent changes in expression throughout the cycle. In the present study we have focused on the expression of ectonucleotidases by means of immunohistochemistry and in situ activity in eutopic and ectopic endometrial tissue of women with endometriosis, and we compared the results with endometria of women without the disease. We have demonstrated that the axis CD39-CD73 is altered in endometriosis, with loss of CD39 and CD73 expression in deep infiltrating endometriosis, the most severe, and most recurring, endometriosis subtype. Our results indicate that this altered expression of ectonucleotidases in endometriosis boosts ATP accumulation in the tissue microenvironment. An important finding is the identification of the nucleotide pyrophophatase/phosphodiesterase 3 (NPP3) as a new histopathological marker of the disease since we have demonstrated its expression in the stroma only in endometriosis, in both eutopic and ectopic tissue. Therefore, targeting the proteins directly involved in ATP breakdown could be an appropriate approach to consider in the treatment of endometriosis.

Keywords: endometriosis; endometrium; uterus; purinergic signaling; ATP

1. Introduction

Endometriosis is a chronic gynecological estrogen-dependent disease characterized by the presence of endometrial tissue, both glands and stroma, outside the uterus. There are multiple possible locations for this ectopic tissue which may be grouped into three endometriosis subtypes: peritoneal, ovarian, with ovarian cysts called endometriomas, and deeply infiltrative. It is a debilitating disorder affecting around 10% of women of reproductive age [1], with pelvic pain and infertility as the two main symptoms. The etiology and physiopathology of this disease remain unknown and there are no clinical biomarkers; in consequence, there is no cure and a long delay in the diagnosis. Studies focused on the discovery of diagnostic tools for endometriosis to help to design effective treatments that preserve fertility are of great interest.

Inflammation is necessary for the establishment and maintenance of endometrial cells in ectopic locations [2–5]. Purinergic signaling, the group of biological effects mediated by extracellular nucleotides, such as adenosine triphosphate (ATP), and nucleosides, such as adenosine, is involved in a wide range of physiological and pathological inflammatory conditions [6]. Extracellular ATP is mostly a proinflammatory molecule released during tissue stress situations, such as necrosis or apoptosis, hypoxia, and inflammation. Purinergic signaling is also studied in the context of human reproduction [7–11]; for instance, ATP is involved in the initiation and maintenance of myometrium and oviduct contractions. It increases the oviductal ciliary beat frequency [12] and contributes to the regulation of the uterine fluid microenvironment [9]. Moreover, adenosine, an ATP hydrolysis product, is necessary for sperm capacitation [10]. ATP is also a pain-related molecule, and some of the pharmacological treatments used to relieve pain in endometriosis do indeed affect ATP levels or their effects. Moreover, extracellular ATP and its derivative adenosine influence cell migration, proliferation and survival—three necessary events for the establishment of ectopic endometrial foci.

Extracellular ATP and adenosine levels are controlled by the ecto-nucleotidases, which are broadly expressed enzymes that, acting alone or sequentially, hydrolyze ATP into adenosine. There are four families of ectonucleotidases: (i) the ecto-nucleoside triphosphate diphosphohydrolase (E-NTPDase) family, also known as CD39 family, which hydrolyzes the ATP, and adenosine diphosphate (ADP), to adenosine monophosphate (AMP); (ii) the ecto-nucleotide pyrophophatase/phosphodiesterase (E-NPP) family, which mainly hydrolyzes ATP to AMP; (iii) the 5′-nucleotidase (5′-NT) (known as CD73) that dephosphorylates AMP to adenosine; and, (iv) the alkaline phosphatases family that hydrolyzes nucleoside triphosphates and diphosphates to monophosphates [6]. Adenosine deaminase (ADA) inactivates adenosine. This is a soluble enzyme often associated with CD26/dipeptidyl peptidase IV, expressed at the cell membrane [13]. Ectonucleotidases and CD26 are well characterized in human cyclic and postmenopausal endometria, showing differences in its expression and distribution throughout the cycle [8,14]. The presence of ectonucleotidases in the contents of endometrioma had previously been described [15,16] but no studies had yet to be conducted on eutopic and ectopic endometrial tissue from women with endometriosis.

With the present study, we aimed to characterize the expression of ectonucleotidases in the eutopic and ectopic endometrial tissue of women with endometriosis and compare it with the eutopic endometrium of women without this pathology. We believe that assessing the participation of these proteins directly involved in ATP breakdown in endometriosis could contribute to facilitating the diagnosis and ameliorating the treatment status of this pathology.

2. Results

Protein expression of NTPDase1 (CD39 from here on), NTPDase2, NTPDase3, NPP3, 5′-NT (CD73 from here on), and CD26 was detected in the eutopic and ectopic endometrial tissue of women with endometriosis. Results are compared with endometria from women without the disease whose data was previously published [8,14]. Staining distribution and intensity scores were recorded for each protein by double blinded observation. In situ nucleotidase activity, in the presence or absence of specific inhibitors, was also detected. The most relevant findings in eutopic endometria and endometrial lesions are described for each protein hereafter, and compiled in detail in Tables 1 and 2. The proportion of positive tissues stained in the immunolabeling assays is commented on in the text and compiled in Appendix A (Table A1).

Table 1. Summary of the ectoenzyme expression in the eutopic endometrium from women with endometriosis.

	NTPDase1 (CD39)	NTPDase2	NTPDase3	NPP3	5'-NT (CD73)	CD26
Proliferative endometrium						
Surface epithelium	-	+++	+	++	++	-
Glandular epithelium						
Functional layer	-	+++	++	++	+++	++/- [1]
Basal layer	-	+++	+	+	+++	+++
Endometrial stromal cells	-	+++	-	+++	++	-
Spiral arteries	+++	-	-	+	-	-
Secretory endometrium						
Surface epithelium	-	+++	+/- [1]	+++	+++	+
Glandular epithelium						
Functional layer	-	+++	+++	+++	++	+++
Basal layer	-	+++	+++	+++	+++	++
Endometrial stromal cells	-	+++	-	+	++	-
Spiral arteries	+++	-	-	+	-	-
Atrophic endometrium						
Surface epithelium	-	+++	-	+	+	++/- [1]
Glandular epithelium	-	+++	-	++	++	-
Endometrial stromal cells	++	+++	-	++	-	-
Vessels	++	-	-	+	-	-

Semi-quantitative analysis independently evaluated by two observers. Label is recorded as: (-) negative, (+) weak, (++) moderate, (+++) strong. [1] 50% of tissues studied had each of these staining intensities.

Table 2. Summary of the ectoenzyme expression in the ectopic endometrial tissue (peritoneal, ovarian, and deep infiltrative lesions) from women with endometriosis.

	NTPDase1 (CD39)	NTPDase2	NTPDase3	NPP3	5'-NT (CD73)	CD26
Peritoneal endometriosis						
Endometrial epithelial cells	-	+++	+	+++	+++	+++
Endometrial stromal cells	+++	++	-	++	++	-
Vessels of the lesion	+++	-	-	-	-	-
Ovarian endometriosis						
Endometrial epithelial cells	-	+++	+++	+++	+++	+++
Endometrial stromal cells	++	-	-	+	-	-
Vessels of the lesion	+++	-	-	-	-	-
Deep endometriosis						
Endometrial epithelial cells	-	+++	-	++	+++	+++
Endometrial stromal cells	-	++	-	+	-	-
Vessels of the lesion	-	-	-	-	-	-

Semi-quantitative analysis independently evaluated by two observers. Label is recorded as: (-) negative, (+) weak, (++) moderate, (+++) strong.

2.1. CD39 Expression in the Eutopic and Ectopic Endometrial Tissues

CD39 staining was detected in stromal cells and in endothelial cells from blood vessels of endometria from women without endometriosis (Figure 1), coinciding with previously published findings [8]. In the eutopic cyclic endometria from women with endometriosis, CD39 label in the stroma was absent in 65% of cases although it was always present in endothelial cells (Figure 1). However, atrophic endometria from women with endometriosis maintained the CD39 expression in the stromal component (Figure S1).

Figure 1. Immunolocalization of CD39 in eutopic (**A–C**) and ectopic (**D–F**) endometrial tissue. CD39 was expressed in blood vessels (arrowheads) of eutopic endometria from women without (NON ENDOMETRIOSIS, (**A**) or with endometriosis (ENDOMETRIOSIS, (**B,C**), and in peritoneal (**D**), ovarian (**E**), and deep infiltrating (**F**) lesions. CD39 was immunodetected in the stroma (asterisk) of endometrium of women without the disease (**A**), but not in endometria of women with endometriosis (**B,C**). Stroma is also labelled in the peritoneal (**D**) and ovarian (**E**) ectopic tissues of women with endometriosis. Inset in (**F**) is a detail of a deep lesion (oviductal infiltrating nodule) showing the absence of CD39 in the endometrial stroma. Scale bars are 100 μm (**A–F**) and 10 μm (**F** inset).

In endometriotic lesions, CD39 was immunodetected with strong labeling in the stroma of the peritoneal (86% of cases) and ovarian (59%) lesions, but not in the deep ones, where this label was only in 36% of the samples. Moreover, 54% of deeply infiltrative lesions lost the expression of CD39 in blood vessels. ADPase activity was seen at the same locations where the protein was immunodetected. The activity was inhibited by the E-NTPDase inhibitor POM 1 (Figure 2).

Figure 2. Nucleotidase in situ histochemistry in superficial peritoneal endometriosis lesions. Dark brown deposits correspond to enzyme activity. ATPase activity was detected in the epithelial cells (arrows) and stroma (asterisk) of the lesion (**A**). ADPase activity was strongly detected in the stroma (asterisks) of the lesion and, remarkably, in blood vessels (arrowheads) (**C**). ATPase and ADPase activities were abrogated in the presence of the NTPDase inhibitor POM 1 (**B,D**, respectively). In situ AMPase activity was detected in the epithelial (arrows) and stromal (asterisk) components of the lesion (**E**). The AMPase was inhibited in the presence of α,β-meADP (**F**). Insets in (**B,D,F**) correspond to the activity experiments performed in the absence of substrate (no ATP, no ADP, and no AMP, respectively). TPPase activity was distributed in the stroma (asterisks), including the blood vessels (arrowheads) of lesions (**G**). As a control, TPPase activity was also performed without substrate (no TPP, **H**). Scale bars are 100 μm.

2.2. NTPDase2 Expression in the Eutopic and Ectopic Endometrial Tissues

NTPDase2 label in endometria of women with endometriosis was found in basal stroma and cilia of epithelial ciliated cells (Figure 3), coinciding with the recently described expression in non-pathological endometria [14]. All types of ectopic lesions displayed cilia staining, except three deeply infiltrative lesions localized in oviducts that did not display NTPDase2 staining in the cilia. However, the rest of the deep lesions with another ectopic location showed NTPDase2 labeling in their ciliated cells. Stroma was labeled in peritoneal (100% of the cases) and deep lesions (65%), but much less so in ovarian lesions (37%). In situ ATPase activity was detected in the same locations where NTPDase2 was expressed, and it was inhibited by the E-NTPDase inhibitor POM 1 (Figure 2).

Figure 3. Immunolocalization of NTPDase2 in the eutopic (**A**–**C**) and ectopic (**D**–**F**) endometrial tissue. NTPDase2 was detected in the stroma of the basal layer (asterisks) in cyclic endometria from women without (**A**) and with (**B,C**) endometriosis. It was also present in the stromal component (asterisks) of the superficial peritoneal (**D**) and deep infiltrating lesions (**F**, vaginal nodule). NTPDase2 was also found in eutopic and ectopic epithelial ciliated cells in the cilia (arrows) (detail in the inset in **E**). Scale bars are 200 μm (**A,C**), 100 μm (**B,D**–**F**), and 10 μm (inset in **E**).

Interestingly, we observed the NTPDase2 label in the connective tissue that surrounds the lesions clearly defining the limits of the ectopically located endometrial tissue in a large number of cases (Figure S2).

Perivascular NTPDase2+ cells were also found in eutopic and ectopic endometrial tissue. We confirmed that these cells were also positive for the endometrial mesenchymal stem cell (eMSC) marker Sushi Domain Containing 2 (SUSD2). Double immunolabeling for NTPDase2 and SUSD2 revealed that both proteins were expressed by the same perivascular cells (Figure S3). This coincides with recently published results in non-pathological endometria [14]. Nevertheless, NTPDase2+ SUSD2+ perivascular cells were not present in all the endometriotic lesions.

2.3. NTPDase3 Expression in the Eutopic and Ectopic Endometrial Tissues

In endometrium, NTPDase3 was immunolocalized apically in the epithelial glandular cells. The expression varied during the cycle, being maximal in the secretory phase, as previously described for non-pathological endometria [8]. Ciliated cells were also apically labeled with the label accumulated at the base of the cilia (Figure 4). In addition, NTPDase3 was not detected in atrophic endometria in endometriosis (Figure S1) while it is expressed in atrophic endometria of women without the disease.

Figure 4. Immunolocalization of NTPDase3 in the eutopic (**A–C**) and ectopic (**D–F**) endometrial tissue. NTPDase3 was immunodetected in ciliated and non-ciliated cells of cyclic endometrium from women without (**A**) and those with (**B,C**) endometriosis (arrows), with changes in expression along the menstrual cycle, reaching a maximum at the secretory phase (**C**). Moreover, NTPDase3 was present in the endothelial cells of spiral arteries of women without endometriosis (inset in **A**) but not in the cyclic endometria from women with the disease (inset in **B**). In ectopic endometrial tissue, NTPDase3 was weakly expressed in the epithelial cells (arrows) of peritoneal lesions (**D**) and highly expressed in the epithelium (arrows) of the ovarian endometriomas (**E**). NTPDase3 was absent in the deep infiltrating lesions (**F**, vaginal nodule) (arrows). Insets in images (**D–F**) are details of the epithelium of the three different ectopic lesions. Scale bars are 100 μm (**A–F**), 20 μm (inset in **A**), and 10 μm (insets in **B,D–F**).

The only, but not negligible, difference between endometria from women with and those without endometriosis is the lack of NTPDase3 staining in spiral arteries in endometriosis. It was previously reported that NTPDase3 was a marker of spiral arteries, displaying a perivascular smooth muscle actin (SMA)+ labeling [8].

In endometriotic lesions, NTPDase3 expression was found in the epithelial component. And while in ovarian lesions labeling was intense, in deep infiltrating lesions labeling was sparse and it was only present in 44% of lesions (Figure 4).

2.4. NPP3 Expression in the Eutopic and Ectopic Endometrial Tissues

NPP3 was expressed in epithelial cells of endometria from women with endometriosis with changes in expression throughout the cycle, being maximal in the secretory phase, similar to the features described in a non-endometriosis condition [8].

Remarkably, de novo NPP3 expression was seen in the stroma of endometrial tissue, both eutopic (including atrophic) and ectopic, from women with endometriosis (Figure 5 and Figure S1). Thiamine pyrophosphatase (TPPase) in situ activity, a functional assay for E-NPPs, was also seen in the stroma of eutopic endometrium and endometriotic lesions (Figure 2).

Figure 5. Immunolocalization of NPP3 in the eutopic (**A–C**) and ectopic (**D–F**) endometrial tissue. NPP3 is present in the luminal and glandular epithelial cells of endometrium from women without (**A**) or with (**B,C**) endometriosis (arrows), with changes in expression along the menstrual cycle, reaching a maximum at the secretory phase (**C**). NPP3 was expressed by the stroma (asterisks) only in endometriosis condition, including eutopic endometrium (**B,C**), and ectopic lesions: peritoneal (**D**), ovarian (**E**), and deep infiltrating (**F**, intestinal nodule). NPP3 is also present in the endometrial epithelial cells of lesions (arrows). Scale bars are 200 µm (**A**) and 100 µm (**B–F**).

2.5. CD73 Expression in the Eutopic and Ectopic Endometrial Tissues

CD73 was expressed in ciliated cells from the surface epithelium. The label is apical and comprised the entire length of the cilia. CD73 was also immunodetected in glands.

Moreover, CD73 was detected in the stromal cells in both proliferative and secretory phases, mainly in the functional layer. CD73 was, however, absent in the stromal cells of the atrophic endometria from women with endometriosis, in contrast to the atrophic endometria of women without endometriosis (Figure 6). The ectopic endometrial tissue also displayed CD73 epithelial label; however, the endometriotic lesions with stromal CD73 label decreased in relation to the severity of the lesion. In fact, 71% of peritoneal lesions presented CD73 in the endometrial stromal cells versus 48% of the ovarian endometriomas and 22% of deep infiltrating lesions.

Figure 6. Immunolocalization of CD73 in the eutopic (**A**–**C**) and ectopic (**D**–**F**) endometrial tissue. CD73 was detected in the stroma (asterisks) of the cyclic endometrium from women without (**A**) or with (**B,C**) endometriosis and in the superficial peritoneal lesions (**D**). CD73 labelling was absent in the stroma (asterisks) of the ovarian (**E**) and deep infiltrating lesions (**F**, vaginal nodule). CD73 was also present in the ciliated and non-ciliated epithelial cells in the eutopic and ectopic endometrial tissue (arrows). Insets in images E and F correspond to the epithelium of ovarian and deep lesions, respectively. Scale bars are 100 μm (**A,B,D**), 50 μm (**C,E**), 10 μm (**E** inset), 200 μm (**F**), and 15 μm (**F** inset).

In situ AMPase activity was detected in the same locations where CD73 was expressed and it was inhibited by the specific inhibitor α, β-methylene-ADP (α, β-meADP) (Figure 2).

2.6. Enzyme Dipeptidyl Peptidase IV/CD26 Expression in the Eutopic and Ectopic Endometrial Tissues

CD26 was immunodetected in endometria from women with and without endometriosis. CD26 was only detected in the epithelial cells of endometrium with the already described changes in the level of expression throughout the cycle (Figure 7). CD26 staining was very weak in atrophic endometria, and only 33% of cases presented CD26 labeling in the glandular epithelium (Figure S1).

Figure 7. Immunolocalization of CD26 in the eutopic (**a–c**) and ectopic (**d–f**) endometrial tissue. CD26 was detected in epithelial cells (arrows) of the cyclic endometria of women without (**a**) or with (**b,c**) endometriosis. CD26 was also expressed by the endometrial epithelial cells (arrows) of peritoneal (**d**), ovarian (**e**), and deep infiltrating lesions (**F**, vesical nodule). Inset in (**e**) shows a detail of the CD26 labelling at the apical membrane of epithelial non-ciliated cells of an ovarian lesion. Scale bars are 100 μm (**a–d,f**), 50 μm (**e**), and 10 μm (**e** inset).

CD26 was expressed in the epithelial component of all types of endometriotic lesions (Figure 7).

3. Discussion

Purinergic signaling plays a role in reproduction, and changes in its elements have been described in the pathology of endometriosis. Extracellular ATP may be involved in two of the major symptoms of endometriosis, which are infertility and pain [9,15,16]. In the present study we characterized the expression in eutopic and ectopic endometrial tissue of different ectonucleotidases involved in the regulation of ATP levels in tissue microenvironment. We have compared the results with those previously published in non-pathological endometria [8,14]. Tissue distribution in endometriosis coincides with the control condition except in the case of NPP3 which is present in stroma only in endometriosis. Ciliated cells of endometria display the same expression pattern as in control fallopian tubes. Changes in expression and activity are consistently recorded, the greatest being in the stroma (Figure 8). These findings provide information to elucidate the cellular and molecular mechanism as well as the etiology and the progression of the disease, which might help to identify new diagnostic and therapeutic targets.

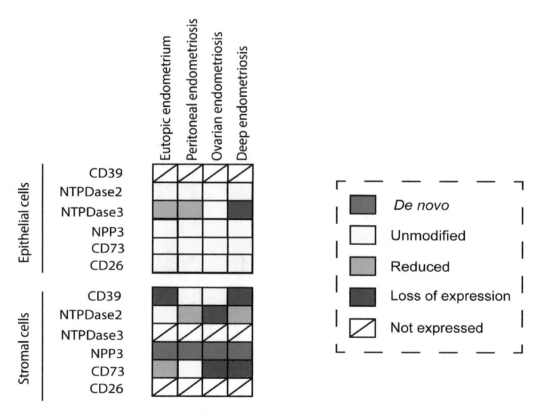

Figure 8. Color representation of changes of ectonucleotidase expression in the eutopic and ectopic endometrial tissue in endometriosis in comparison to the endometria of women without endometriosis. De novo, in red, indicates that this is the first time the label is detected in this cell type; unmodified; in yellow, indicates no changes in label between endometriosis and non-endometriosis; reduced, in green, indicates that the label is diminished in the endometriosis condition; loss of expression, in blue, indicates lack of expression in endometriosis; not expressed indicates that the label is never reported in this particular cell type in any condition.

The CD39-adenosinergic axis, with CD39 and CD73 acting sequentially to hydrolyze ATP to adenosine, is considered the main duo responsible for metabolizing extracellular ATP, generating an immunosuppressive adenosine-rich microenvironment in physiological and pathophysiological conditions [17]. In endometrium, the expression pattern of these ectonucleotidases and their changes throughout the cycle are well studied. Under physiological conditions, endometrial stromal cells express both CD39 and CD73. While CD39 expression is constant throughout the cycle, CD73 fluctuates [8,18], thus determining variations in adenosine level in the microenvironment. In the present study we note that eutopic endometrium of women with endometriosis displays the same already known expression pattern of CD73 but mostly loses CD39 stromal expression. A plausible consequence of the concomitant unbalanced ATP hydrolysis is the accumulation of extracellular ATP in the endometrial stromal microenvironment. This might well play a role in the generation and maintenance of the chronic inflammatory state of endometria of women with endometriosis. Moreover, extracellular ATP is closely related to various immune and inflammatory factors that are known to be involved in the infertility of women with endometriosis, by reducing the quality of gametes and their rates of transport and implantation, and by increasing the pregnancy loss rate [19].

This situation could explain the de novo stromal expression of NPP3 in endometriosis throughout the cycle and in atrophic endometrium, as a cellular tool to offset the loss of ATPase activity due to the lack of CD39. However, NPP3 action would not be sufficient to replace ATPase activity because NPP3 has a lower affinity for ATP than CD39 [6]; moreover stromal NPP3 expression is not coordinated with CD73 expression throughout the cycle.

Changes in the CD39-CD73 pathway were also found in endometriotic lesions. Our findings indicate that the changes in ATP hydrolysis resulting from CD39 and CD73 activity are related to the severity of endometriosis since their expression is lost in deep infiltrating lesions. These changes of expression would lead to an extracellular ATP accumulation that would in turn promote the secretion of cytokines and growth factors into the ectopic milieu, with a concomitant increase in survival and growth rates of endometrial cells [20,21]. Unfortunately, the exact function of extracellular ATP in endometriosis is not clear. While ATP signaling seems to be closely related to the origin and progression of endometriosis, intramuscular injection of ATP in a rat model of endometriosis was found to reduce the size of the ectopic induced lesions [22]. Our results are in line with previous studies that showed differing expression of the protein ATPase Na+/K+ Transporting Family Member Beta 4 (ATP1B4) between patients with and without endometriosis, in favor of a decrease of the hydrolysis of ATP in the endometriosis patients [23,24]. The authors stated that ATP was clearly related with the formation and development of endometriosis disease. Moreover, pain is a characteristic symptom of endometriosis, and ATP is a pain factor mainly acting through the purinoreceptor P2X3 that has also been studied in endometriosis. P2X3 has been found in the epithelial and some stromal cells of eutopic and ectopic endometrial tissue as well as on sensory nerve fibers in endometriotic lesions. Its expression levels correlate with the severity of pain in women with endometriosis [25]. Moreover, the use of A-317491, a selective P2X3 receptor antagonist, relieved pain with a prolonged antinociceptive effect in rats [26], and the receptor is thus a target for the pharmacological approach of endometriosis pain relief. Therefore, the increased levels of extracellular ATP might well be related to the endometriosis-associated pain. These results parallel the difference in CD73 and CD39 expression between the three entities of endometriosis, where the most extreme change has been detected in the deep infiltrating lesions, an important indicator of the severity of pain in endometriosis [27]. Additionally, the downregulation of CD73 has been described in poorly differentiated and advanced-stage endometrial carcinoma. Adenosine generated by the activity of CD73 located in the areas of cell-cell contacts regulates cell-cell adhesions by the regulation of the primary component of filopodia (F-actin). In fact, cell migration and invasion in high-grade and advanced-stage endometrial carcinomas is dependent on the loss of the adenosine generated by CD73 [28]. According to Sampson's theory of retrograde menstruation, endometrial tissue detached during menses has to travel through the fallopian tubes to the ectopic site of implantation, such as the ovarian surface or the peritoneal wall, and must then invade and adhere to the self-tissue of the new localization, proliferating and evading the immune response to form the endometriotic lesion [29]. For this reason, the loss of CD73 in the two most severe entities of endometriosis, ovarian and deep endometriosis, as well as its implication in the inflammatory state of endometriosis, might also play a role in the migration and invasive properties of ectopic cells needed to generate the lesion.

An important finding is the identification of NPP3 label as a new histopathological marker of the disease since we have demonstrated its expression and activity in the stroma only in endometriosis, in both eutopic and ectopic tissues. NPP3 has already been identified in endometrial epithelial cells, a fact that is also confirmed in the case of endometriosis without any variation. A previous study by our group also demonstrated the presence of NPP3 in the contents of endometriomas although the levels did not differ from those of the simple ovarian cysts used as controls and therefore its presence was not exclusive of endometriosis [16]. The relevance of the study reported here is its presence in eutopic endometria which discriminates between endometriosis and non-endometriosis conditions, which might allow its use as a histopathological diagnostic tool. To our knowledge, NPP3 has been identified in epithelial cell types, in cells of the immune system, mainly mast cells, and in tumor cells with an epithelial or myeloid origin [8,30–34]. The specific detection of NPP3 in the endometrial stromal cells of eutopic endometria and in all three entities of endometriosis can be used as a histopathologic marker of endometriosis disease. In addition to its role in the control of extracellular ATP levels, NPP3 might well play a role in the invasive capacity of the stromal endometrial cells in endometriosis since it is known that overexpression of NPP3 in murine fibroblasts stimulates the motility and the invasiveness of these cells [35]. Our finding of de novo NPP3 in stromal cells, with greater expression in the functional layer which is shed during menses, and the relation of NPP3 with the cell motility and invasion, suggest involvement of NPP3 in the formation and progression of endometriotic lesions based on the retrograde menstruation theory [29]. Besides the importance of NPP3 as histopathological marker, additional studies are needed to determine the precise role of NPP3 in the pathogenesis and progression of endometriosis. It might well be a new target for pharmacological therapy of endometriosis. Indeed, targeting NPP3 is feasible since phase 1 trials using an antibody drug conjugate targeting this protein have been completed in patients with advanced metastatic renal cell carcinoma with promising antitumor results [36].

We found NTPDase2 expression in the same cell types and structures as in the non-endometriosis condition. Moreover, NTPDase2 was expressed by perivascular cells in some lesions with colocalization with the eMSCs marker SUSD2. Functional studies are needed to determinate whether NTPDase2+ SUSD2+ cells are eMSCs as in the eutopic endometrium. Retrograde shedding of stem cells into the pelvic cavity without immune clearance is thought to be lesion-initiating. Therefore, it would be of interest to compare lesions containing the NTPDase2+ SUSD2+ cell population with lesions without it.

NTPDase3 was described in epithelial cells and spiral arteries in healthy endometria. In fact, NTPDase3 has been considered a spiral artery marker [8]. But we did not find NTPDase3 labeling in spiral arteries of women with endometriosis. Spiral artery remodeling plays a central role in establishing and maintaining a normal pregnancy, and impaired remodeling is involved in common pregnancy disorders. This might be also one of the mechanisms underlying the decreased pregnancy rates in women with endometriosis. It is important to highlight the loss of NTPDase3 in the epithelial cells of deep infiltrating lesions. Although NTPDase3 has been little explored in pathological conditions, a decrease in *ntpdase3* expression has been described during the induction of mouse bladder cancer, suggesting its participation in cancer establishment and progression [37]. This result, together with the loss of NTPDase3 in the epithelial cells of the most severe form of endometriosis, provides further evidence of the need to study its role in the pathophysiology of endometriosis and cancer.

CD26 or dipeptidyl peptidase IV (DPPIV) is a membrane glycoprotein that binds, among other peptides, the ectoenzyme ADA in humans. It is involved in the protection of the tissue against local inflammation and in intracellular signaling. CD26 has been described as a cancer stem cell marker and tumor suppressor protein in certain types of cancer. By contrast, CD26 overexpression promotes cell proliferation, invasion, and tumorigenesis in endometrial carcinoma cells [38]. In endometriosis, Tan et al. [39] described the increase of endometrial stromal cell migration and invasion in part by reduced expression of CD26 under hypoxia conditions and also by CD26 inhibition. Other studies performed in tissue, including ours, have not matched these in vitro results with cell culture since we were not able to detect CD26 in endometrial stroma, but only in epithelial glandular cells. This might be due to the differing behavior of cells in vitro or even to technical reasons. Here, we show high expression of CD26 in the epithelial cells of eutopic endometrium and in ectopic tissue. The difference with the endometrial expression in women without endometriosis is that CD26 expression in endometriosis is constant throughout the cycle. It would be interesting to see whether the high expression of CD26 in ectopic epithelial cells has a similar effect to that of endometrial carcinoma cells on cell migration and invasion ability. In relation to the ATP metabolism, knowing the levels of ADA, the soluble enzyme that hydrolyses the extracellular adenosine to control the immunosuppressive milieu, is key to understanding what is happening in endometriosis. In a previous study, high levels of ADA were found in the contents of ovarian endometriomas [16]. We were, however, unable to detect ADA by immunostaining due to the technical limitations of the antibodies available, and we cannot be certain whether high levels of CD26 in tissue is related to an increase in ADA activity.

The changes in the expression of the ectonucleotidases described here in eutopic and ectopic endometrium argue for extracellular ATP accumulation. The greatest loss of ectonucleotidase expression was found in the deep infiltrating endometriosis, the most severe endometriosis subtype [40,41]. Our results, together with the role of ATP in pain [25,42], lend support to the involvement of ectonucleotidase expression changes with the severity of endometriosis. Moreover, our results reinforce the relevance of the stroma and tissue microenvironment in the etiopathology and progression of endometriosis disease. Future studies on the role of purinergic signaling in endometriosis are needed to identify biomarkers of the disease and to develop new therapeutic strategies that would allow for earlier detection and respect for the reproductive wishes of women with endometriosis. However, unlike in cancer, where ectonucleotidase blockade is a therapeutic tool, in endometriosis the use of inhibitors of ectonucleotidases does not seem to represent an appropriate strategy. On the contrary, increasing the ATPase activity would combat the eventual ATP accumulation of endometrial microenvironment. In line with this, the use of A-317491, an antagonist of the ATP receptor P2X3, relieves pain in endometriosis [26]. Administration of soluble CD39 is known to be safe and is well studied in the context of cardiovascular diseases where it is known to prevent thrombus formation (reviewed in [43]).

4. Materials and Methods

4.1. Samples

The ethical principles of this study adhere to the Helsinki Declaration, and all the procedures were approved by the ethics committee for clinical investigation of Bellvitge Hospital (project identification code PR090/15, Acta 21/16, 12/2016). All the patients included gave written informed consent. Fifty-seven patients with endometriotic lesions (ectopic endometrial tissue) were recruited for the study by the Gynecology Service of Bellvitge Hospital (Barcelona, Spain) between March 2016 and July 2019, and by the Gynecology Service of Dexeus Institute (Barcelona, Spain) between October 2016 and March 2018. Thirty-four endometrium samples were obtained by the Gynecology Service of Bellvitge Hospital from women without endometriosis or endometrial malignancy as a control group (including 10 proliferative, 4 secretory, and 20 atrophic endometria; age mean of patients = 55.03 years, standard derivation = 11.83).

Human endometrial samples from women with endometriosis ($n = 25$) were obtained from hysterectomy specimens without endometrial malignancy at the pathology services of Bellvitge Hospital and Dexeus Hospital. Peritoneal endometriosis ($n = 7$), ovarian endometriosis ($n = 27$), and/or deep endometriosis ($n = 28$) were surgically removed in the gynecology services of the same hospitals. Demographic description of the samples from the women with endometriosis are summarized in Table 3. Endometrial dating was carried out by the pathology services.

Table 3. Demographics of patients with endometriosis.

Type of Endometrium	Number of Cases	Age (years) ± Standard Deviation	Average (Range)
Proliferative	12	44.33 ± 3.11	39–51
Secretory	10	45.00 ± 5.21	38–53
Atrophic	3	43.00 ± 4.00	39–47
Type of Lesion			
Peritoneal	7	40.29 ± 4.96	35–46
Ovarian	27	43.42 ± 8.36	23–57
Deep	21	38.00 ± 5.73	27–47

Excised tissue samples were fixed with 4% paraformaldehyde, cryoprotected by introducing them into a 30% (w/v) sucrose solution at 4 °C for 24 h, and then embedded in O.C.T freezing media (Tissue-Tek®; Sakura Finetk, Zoeterwoude, Netherlands). Fifteen µm sections were obtained using a Cryostat Leica CM1950 (Leica, Wetzlar, Germany). Sections were put onto poly-L-lysine coated glass slides and stored at −20 °C until use. Routine haematoxylin and eosin staining was performed.

4.2. Antibodies

Primary antibodies used in this study are listed in Table 4. Secondary antibodies used for immunohistochemistry were horseradish peroxidase (HRP)-conjugated goat anti-mouse (EnVision™ + System; DAKO, Carpinteria, CA, USA) and HRP-conjugated goat anti-rabbit (EnVision™ + System).

Table 4. List of primary antibodies used for immunolabeling experiments.

Antibody Specificity	Name/Clone	Source	Supplier	Dilution
NTPDase1 (CD39)	BU-61	Mouse	Ancell (188-820)	1:500
NTPDase2	-	Rabbit	Enzo (ALX-215-045)	1:100
NTPDase2	H9s	Mouse	http://ectonucleotidases-ab.com	1:400
NTPDase3	B_3S_{10}	Mouse	http://ectonucleotidases-ab.com	1:500
NPP3	NP4D6	Mouse	Abcam (ab90754)	1:100
5'-nucleotidase (CD73)	4G4	Mouse	Abcam (ab81720)	1:50
CD26	202-36	Mouse	Abcam (ab3154)	1:100
CD26	202-36	Mouse	NovusBio (NBP2-44571)	1:100
SUSD2	-	Rabbit	Abcam (ab121214)	1:400

Secondary antibodies used for immunofluorescence assays were Alexa Fluor 488 goat anti-mouse and Alexa Fluor 647 goat anti-rabbit (Thermo Fisher Scientific, Rockford, Illinois, USA). Secondary antibodies were used at 1:500 and dilutions were made in PBS.

4.3. Immunolabeling Experiments

Slices were washed twice with PBS to remove the O.C.T freezing media and then pre-incubated for 1 h at room temperature (RT) with PBS containing 20% normal goat serum (NGS, Gibco, Paisley, UK), 0.2% Triton and 0.2% gelatin (Merck, Darmstadt, Germany). For immunohistochemistry experiments a previous blocking of endogenous peroxidase activity was performed with 10% methanol (*v/v*) and 2% H2O2 (*v/v*) in PBS for 30 min. Slices were then incubated overnight (O/N) at 4 °C with the primary antibodies (listed in Table 2) diluted in PBS. After three washes in PBS, tissue sections were incubated with the appropriate secondary antibodies for 1 h at RT, except HRP-goat anti-mouse and HRP-goat anti-rabbit, which were incubated for 30 min at RT. Secondary antibodies alone were routinely included as controls for the experiments.

For immunohistochemistry, the peroxidase reaction was performed in a solution containing 0.6 mg/mL 3, 3'-diaminobenzidine substrate (DAB; D-5637, Sigma-Aldrich, Saint Louis, MO, USA) and 0.5 µL/mL H2O2 in PBS for 10 min, and stopped with PBS. Nuclei were counterstained with haematoxylin and slides were then dehydrated and mounted with DPX mounting medium. Samples were observed under light Nikon Eclipse E200 and photographed under a light Leica DMD 108 microscope. In fluorescence assays, for nuclei labeling, slides were mounted with aqueous mounting medium with DAPI (ProLong™ Gold antifade reagent with DAPI, Life Technologies, Paisley, UK). Samples were then observed and photographed under a Zeiss LSM 880 Confocal Laser Scanning Microscope. Fluorescence images were processed with the software ZEN 2.3 SP1 (Zeiss, Oberkochen, Germany).

Immunohistochemical staining was independently evaluated by two observers. Staining distribution was recorded. Label intensity was scored as negative (-), weak (+), intermediate (++), or strongly positive (+++).

4.4. In situ ATPase, ADPase, AMPase, and TPPase Activity Experiments

A protocol based on the Wachstein/Meisel lead phosphate method was used [8,11,44,45]. The sections were washed twice with 50 mM Tris-maleate buffer pH 7.4 and pre-incubated for 30 min at RT with 50 mM Tris-maleate buffer pH 7.4 containing 2 mM MgCl2 and 0.25 mM sucrose. The enzymatic reaction was carried out by incubating tissue sections for 1 h at 37 °C with 50 mM

Tris-maleate buffer pH 7.4 supplemented with 0.25 mM sucrose, 2 mM $MgCl_2$, 5 mM $MnCl_2$, 3 % Dextran, 2 mM $Pb(NO_3)_2$, and 2 mM $CaCl_2$. All experiments were performed in the presence of 2.5 mM levamisole, as an inhibitor of alkaline phosphatase (AP) activity, and in the presence of 1 mM AMP, ADP, ATP, or TPP as a substrate. TPP is a false substrate, which can be cleaved by the pyrophosphatase activity of E-NPPs. Control assays were performed in the absence of nucleotide. For E-NTPDase inhibition experiments, 1 mM POM 1 was added to pre-incubation and enzymatic reaction buffers. For CD73 inhibition experiments, 1 mM α, β-meADP was added to pre-incubation and enzymatic reaction buffers. The reaction was revealed by incubation with 1% $(NH_4)_2S$ (*v/v*) for exactly 1 min. Nuclei were counterstained with haematoxylin. Samples were mounted with aqueous mounting medium (FluoromountTM, Sigma-Aldrich), observed under a light Nikon Eclipse E200 microscope, and photographed under a light Leica DMD 108 microscope.

4.5. Statistical Analysis

The predictive analytics software IBM SPSS Statistics v22 (IBM Corp., Armonk, NY, USA) was used for the creation of frequency tables with the distribution of ectonucleotidases in each endometrial component as well as the label intensity score in each case.

5. Conclusions

In the present study, we examined the presence of ectonucleotidases in eutopic and ectopic endometrial tissue in endometriosis. The main changes in expression and activity were found in the stromal compartment. We observed loss of the main route of ATP hydrolysis, the CD39-CD73 axis, in deep infiltrating endometriosis, the most severe endometriosis subtype. These findings point to ATP accumulation in the endometrial tissue microenvironment in endometriosis as possibly contributing to the two main symptoms of the disease: pain and infertility. Remarkably, we noted that immunodetection of NPP3 in endometrial stroma is exclusive to the endometriosis condition, and therefore it may well be a histological marker of the disease. Future studies on the role of purinergic signaling in endometriosis are needed to elucidate the underlying cellular and molecular mechanisms and to identify new diagnostic and therapeutic targets.

Supplementary Materials:
Figure S1. Immunolocalization of CD39 (A), NTPDase2 (B), NTPDase3 (C), NPP3 (D), CD73 (E), and CD26 (F) in atrophic endometria from women with endometriosis. Scale bars are 100 μm (A,C–F) and 200 μm (B). Figure S2. Immunolocalization of NTPDase2 in peritoneal (A), ovarian (B), and deep endometriosis lesions (C). There is NTPDase2 labelling in the connective tissue limiting the lesions (*arrows*). Scale bars are 100 μm (A,C) and 300 μm (B). Figure S3. Confocal fluorescence images of a proliferative endometrium (A–D) of a woman with endometriosis and an ovarian endometrioma (E–H) labeled with the antibodies against NTPDase2 (A,E) and the eMSC marker SUSD2 (B,F). Nuclei were labeled with DAPI (C,G). Merge images (D,H) show the co-localization of NTPDase2 and SUSD2 in perivascular cells in the eutopic and ectopic endometrial tissue. Scale bars are 50 μm (D,H).

Author Contributions: C.T. contributed to the design and execution of the experiments, and contributed to the writing of the paper. A.V., F.T., and X.M.-G. performed the histopathologic diagnostic. I.G.d.A. contributed to conducting the experiments. J.S. generated the antibodies against *ENTPD2* and *ENTPD3*. M.E.F.-M., P.B., B.C., and J.P. visited the women included in the study, made the clinical diagnoses, and performed the surgery to obtain the samples. M.M.-S. conceived the study and contributed to conducting the experiments and to the writing of the paper.

Acknowledgments: We dedicate this work to the memory of our beloved colleague and friend Lluís de Jover Armengol. We thank CERCA Programme (Generalitat de Catalunya) for institutional support, Tom Yohannan for language editing, and Serveis Científics i Tecnològics (Campus Bellvitge, Universitat de Barcelona) for technical support. We are grateful to the women who donated their samples for the study and to the endometriosis association Endo&Cat for supporting the project.

Abbreviations

ATP	Adenosine triphosphate
E-NPP	Ecto-nucleotide pyrophophotase/phosphodiesterase
E-NTPDase	Ecto-nucleoside triphosphate diphosphohydrolase
ADP	Adenosine diphosphate
AMP	Adenosine monophosphate
5'-NT	5'-nucleotidase
ADA	Adenosine deaminase
eMSC	Endometrial mesenchymal stem cell
SUSD2	Sushi domain containing 2
SMA	Smooth muscle actin
TPP	Thiamine pyrophosphate
α, β-meADP	α, β-methylene-ADP
ATP1B4	ATPase Na+/K+ Transporting Family Member Beta 4
DPPIV	Dipeptidyl peptidase IV
HRP	Horseradish peroxidase
DAB	3, 3'-diaminobenzidine substrate
AP	Alkaline phosphatase

Appendix A

Table A1. Summary of the number and proportion of tissues labeled with different antibodies.

Samples Stained	NTPDase1 (CD39)	NTPDase2	NTPDase3	NPP3	5'-NT (CD73)	CD26
	Positive Cases/Total of Samples (% of Tissues Stained)					
Eutopic endometrium						
Surface epithelium	1/14 (7.1%)	14/14 (100%)	7/13 (53.8%)	12/13 (92.3%)	9/12 (75%)	7/14 (50%)
Glandular epithelium	1/20 (5%)	20/20 (100%)	16/20 (80%)	18/19 (94.7%)	20/20 (100%)	15/20 (75%)
Endometrial stromal cells	7/20 (35%)	20/20 (100%)	0/20 (0%)	15/19 (78.9%)	12/20 (60%)	0/20 (0%)
Spiral arteries	19/20 (95%)	3/20 (15%)	5/20 (25%)	16/18 (88.9%)	3/20 (15%)	3/19 (15.8%)
Peritoneal endometriosis						
Endometrial epithelial cells	1/7 (14.3%)	7/7 (100%)	7/7 (100%)	7/7 (100%)	5/7 (71.4%)	4/7 (57.1%)
Endometrial stromal cells	6/7 (85.7%)	7/7 (100%)	0/7 (0%)	7/7 (100%)	5/7 (71.4%)	2/7 (28.6%)
Vessels of the lesion	5/7 (71.4%)	0/7 (0%)	0/7 (0%)	0/7 (0%)	1/7 (14.28%)	0/7 (0%)
Ovarian endometriosis						
Endometrial epithelial cells	8/28 (28.6%)	20/28 (71.4%)	16/28 (57.1%)	24/28 (85.7%)	24/28 (85.7%)	19/28 (67.9%)
Endometrial stromal cells	16/27 (59.3%)	10/27 (37%)	3/27 (11.1%)	16/27 (59.3%)	13/27 (48.1%)	2/27 (7.4%)
Vessels of the lesion	23/28 (82.1%)	1/28 (3.6%)	2/28 (7.1%)	8/28 (28.6%)	3/28 (10.7%)	3/28 (10.7%)
Deep endometriosis						
Endometrial epithelial cells	6/28 (21.4%)	23/26 (88.5%)	12/27 (44.4%)	24/28 (85.7%)	17/28 (60.7%)	15/28 (53.6%)
Endometrial stromal cells	9/25 (36%)	17/26 (65.4%)	1/27 (3.7%)	18/27 (66.7%)	6/27 (22.2%)	1/27 (3.7%)
Vessels of the lesion	11/24 (45.8%)	5/25 (20%)	1/27 (3.7%)	7/27 (25.9%)	7/27 (25.9%)	0/27 (0%)

References

1. Ponandai-Srinivasan, S.; Andersson, K.L.; Nister, M.; Saare, M.; Hassan, H.A.; Varghese, S.J.; Peters, M.; Salumets, A.; Gemzell-Danielsson, K.; Lalitkumar, P.G.L. Aberrant expression of genes associated with stemness and cancer in endometria and endometrioma in a subset of women with endometriosis. *Hum. Reprod.* **2018**, *33*, 1924–1938. [CrossRef] [PubMed]

2. Grandi, G.; Mueller, M.D.; Papadia, A.; Kocbek, V.; Bersinger, N.A.; Petraglia, F.; Cagnacci, A.; McKinnon, B. Inflammation influences steroid hormone receptors targeted by progestins in endometrial stromal cells from women with endometriosis. *J. Reprod. Immunol.* **2016**, *117*, 30–38. [CrossRef] [PubMed]

3.   Nothnick, W.; Alali, Z. Recent advances in the understanding of endometriosis: The role of inflammatory mediators in disease pathogenesis and treatment. *F1000Research* **2016**, *5*. [CrossRef] [PubMed]

4.   Ahn, S.H.; Khalaj, K.; Young, S.L.; Lessey, B.A.; Koti, M.; Tayade, C. Immune-inflammation gene signatures in endometriosis patients. *Fertil. Steril.* **2016**, *106*, 1420–1431. [CrossRef]

5.   Zhang, T.; De Carolis, C.; Man, G.C.W.; Wang, C.C. The link between immunity, autoimmunity and endometriosis: A literature update. *Autoimmun. Rev.* **2018**, *17*, 945–955. [CrossRef]

6.   Yegutkin, G.G. Enzymes involved in metabolism of extracellular nucleotides and nucleosides: Functional implications and measurement of activities. *Crit. Rev. Biochem. Mol. Biol.* **2014**, *49*, 473–497. [CrossRef]

7.   Ziganshin, A.U.; Zaitcev, A.P.; Khasanov, A.A.; Shamsutdinov, A.F.; Burnstock, G. Term-dependency of P2 receptor-mediated contractile responses of isolated human pregnant uterus. *Eur. J. Obstet. Gynecol. Reprod. Biol.* **2006**, *129*, 128–134. [CrossRef]

8.   Aliagas, E.; Vidal, A.; Torrejon-Escribano, B.; Taco Mdel, R.; Ponce, J.; de Aranda, I.G.; Sevigny, J.; Condom, E.; Martin-Satue, M. Ecto-nucleotidases distribution in human cyclic and postmenopausic endometrium. *Purinergic Signal.* **2013**, *9*, 227–237. [CrossRef]

9.   Burnstock, G. Purinergic signalling in the reproductive system in health and disease. *Purinergic Signal.* **2014**, *10*, 157–187. [CrossRef]

10.   Bellezza, I.; Minelli, A. Adenosine in sperm physiology. *Mol. Asp. Med.* **2017**, *55*, 102–109. [CrossRef]

11.   Villamonte, M.L.; Torrejon-Escribano, B.; Rodriguez-Martinez, A.; Trapero, C.; Vidal, A.; Gomez de Aranda, I.; Sevigny, J.; Matias-Guiu, X.; Martin-Satue, M. Characterization of ecto-nucleotidases in human oviducts with an improved approach simultaneously identifying protein expression and in situ enzyme activity. *Histochem. Cell Biol.* **2018**, *149*, 269–276. [CrossRef] [PubMed]

12.   Barrera, N.P.; Morales, B.; Villalon, M. Plasma and intracellular membrane inositol 1,4,5-trisphosphate receptors mediate the Ca(2+) increase associated with the ATP-induced increase in ciliary beat frequency. *Am. J. Physiol. Cell Physiol.* **2004**, *287*, C1114–C1124. [CrossRef] [PubMed]

13.   Yegutkin, G.G. Nucleotide- and nucleoside-converting ectoenzymes: Important modulators of purinergic signalling cascade. *Biochim. Biophys. Acta* **2008**, *1783*, 673–694. [CrossRef] [PubMed]

14.   Trapero, C.; Vidal, A.; Rodriguez-Martinez, A.; Sevigny, J.; Ponce, J.; Coroleu, B.; Matias-Guiu, X.; Martin-Satue, M. The ectonucleoside triphosphate diphosphohydrolase-2 (NTPDase2) in human endometrium: A novel marker of basal stroma and mesenchymal stem cells. *Purinergic Signal.* **2019**, *15*, 225–236. [CrossRef] [PubMed]

15.   Texido, L.; Romero, C.; Vidal, A.; Garcia-Valero, J.; Fernandez Montoli, M.E.; Baixeras, N.; Condom, E.; Ponce, J.; Garcia-Tejedor, A.; Martin-Satue, M. Ecto-nucleotidases activities in the contents of ovarian endometriomas: Potential biomarkers of endometriosis. *Mediat. Inflamm.* **2014**, *2014*, 120673. [CrossRef]

16.   Trapero, C.; Jover, L.; Fernandez-Montoli, M.E.; Garcia-Tejedor, A.; Vidal, A.; Gomez de Aranda, I.; Ponce, J.; Matias-Guiu, X.; Martin-Satue, M. Analysis of the ectoenzymes ADA, ALP, ENPP1, and ENPP3, in the contents of ovarian endometriomas as candidate biomarkers of endometriosis. *Am. J. Reprod. Immunol.* **2018**, *79*. [CrossRef] [PubMed]

17.   Bono, M.R.; Fernandez, D.; Flores-Santibanez, F.; Rosemblatt, M.; Sauma, D. CD73 and CD39 ectonucleotidases in T cell differentiation: Beyond immunosuppression. *FEBS Lett.* **2015**, *589*, 3454–3460. [CrossRef]

18.   Aliagas, E.; Torrejon-Escribano, B.; Lavoie, E.G.; de Aranda, I.G.; Sevigny, J.; Solsona, C.; Martin-Satue, M. Changes in expression and activity levels of ecto-5′-nucleotidase/CD73 along the mouse female estrous cycle. *Acta Physiol.* **2010**, *199*, 191–197. [CrossRef]

19.   Mate, G.; Bernstein, L.R.; Torok, A.L. Endometriosis is a cause of infertility. Does reactive oxygen damage to gametes and embryos play a key role in the pathogenesis of infertility caused by endometriosis? *Front. Endocrinol.* **2018**, *9*, 725. [CrossRef]

20.   Ahn, S.H.; Monsanto, S.P.; Miller, C.; Singh, S.S.; Thomas, R.; Tayade, C. Pathophysiology and immune dysfunction in endometriosis. *Biomed. Res. Int.* **2015**, *2015*, 795976. [CrossRef]

21.   Faas, M.M.; Saez, T.; de Vos, P. Extracellular ATP and adenosine: The yin and yang in immune responses? *Mol. Asp. Med.* **2017**, *55*, 9–19. [CrossRef] [PubMed]

22.   Zhang, C.; Gao, L.; Yi, Y.; Han, H.; Cheng, H.; Ye, X.; Ma, R.; Sun, K.; Cui, H.; Chang, X. Adenosine triphosphate regresses endometrial explants in a rat model of endometriosis. *Reprod. Sci.* **2016**, *23*, 924–930. [CrossRef] [PubMed]

23.   Zhang, H.; Niu, Y.; Feng, J.; Guo, H.; Ye, X.; Cui, H. Use of proteomic analysis of endometriosis to identify different protein expression in patients with endometriosis versus normal controls. *Fertil. Steril.* **2006**, *86*, 274–282. [CrossRef] [PubMed]

24.   Zhao, Y.; Liu, Y.N.; Li, Y.; Tian, L.; Ye, X.; Cui, H.; Chang, X.H. Identification of biomarkers for endometriosis using clinical proteomics. *Chin. Med. J.* **2015**, *128*, 520–527. [CrossRef] [PubMed]

25.   Ding, S.; Zhu, L.; Tian, Y.; Zhu, T.; Huang, X.; Zhang, X. P2X3 receptor involvement in endometriosis pain via ERK signaling pathway. *PLoS ONE* **2017**, *12*, e0184647. [CrossRef]

26.   Yuan, M.; Ding, S.; Meng, T.; Lu, B.; Shao, S.; Zhang, X.; Yuan, H.; Hu, F. Effect of A-317491 delivered by glycolipid-like polymer micelles on endometriosis pain. *Int. J. Nanomed.* **2017**, *12*, 8171–8183. [CrossRef]

27.   Alimi, Y.; Iwanaga, J.; Loukas, M.; Tubbs, R.S. The clinical anatomy of endometriosis: A review. *Cureus* **2018**, *10*, e3361. [CrossRef]

28.   Bowser, J.L.; Blackburn, M.R.; Shipley, G.L.; Molina, J.G.; Dunner, K., Jr.; Broaddus, R.R. Loss of CD73-mediated actin polymerization promotes endometrial tumor progression. *J. Clin. Investig.* **2016**, *126*, 220–238. [CrossRef]

29.   Sampson, J. Peritoneal endometriosis due to the menstrual dissemination of endometrial tissue into the peritoneal cavity. *Am. J. Obstet. Gynecol.* **1927**, *14*, 422–469. [CrossRef]

30.   Hood, B.L.; Liu, B.; Alkhas, A.; Shoji, Y.; Challa, R.; Wang, G.; Ferguson, S.; Oliver, J.; Mitchell, D.; Bateman, N.W.; et al. Proteomics of the human endometrial glandular epithelium and stroma from the proliferative and secretory phases of the menstrual cycle. *Biol. Reprod.* **2015**, *92*, 106. [CrossRef]

31.   Boggavarapu, N.R.; Lalitkumar, S.; Joshua, V.; Kasvandik, S.; Salumets, A.; Lalitkumar, P.G.; Gemzell-Danielsson, K. Compartmentalized gene expression profiling of receptive endometrium reveals progesterone regulated ENPP3 is differentially expressed and secreted in glycosylated form. *Sci. Rep.* **2016**, *6*, 33811. [CrossRef] [PubMed]

32.   Donate, F.; Raitano, A.; Morrison, K.; An, Z.; Capo, L.; Avina, H.; Karki, S.; Yang, P.; Ou, J.; Moriya, R.; et al. AGS16F is a novel antibody drug conjugate directed against ENPP3 for the treatment of renal cell carcinoma. *Clin. Cancer Res.* **2016**, *22*, 1989–1999. [CrossRef] [PubMed]

33.   Tsai, S.H.; Takeda, K. Regulation of allergic inflammation by the ectoenzyme E-NPP3 (CD203c) on basophils and mast cells. *Semin. Immunopathol.* **2016**, *38*, 571–579. [CrossRef] [PubMed]

34.   Chen, Q.; Xin, A.; Qu, R.; Zhang, W.; Li, L.; Chen, J.; Lu, X.; Gu, Y.; Li, J.; Sun, X. Expression of ENPP3 in human cyclic endometrium: A novel molecule involved in embryo implantation. *Reprod. Fertil. Dev.* **2018**, *30*, 1277–1285. [CrossRef]

35.   Deissler, H.; Blass-Kampmann, S.; Bruyneel, E.; Mareel, M.; Rajewsky, M.F. Neural cell surface differentiation antigen gp130(RB13-6) induces fibroblasts and glioma cells to express astroglial proteins and invasive properties. *FASEB J.* **1999**, *13*, 657–666. [CrossRef]

36.   Thompson, J.A.; Motzer, R.J.; Molina, A.M.; Choueiri, T.K.; Heath, E.I.; Redman, B.G.; Sangha, R.S.; Ernst, D.S.; Pili, R.; Kim, S.K.; et al. Phase I Trials of Anti-ENPP3 Antibody-drug conjugates in advanced refractory renal cell carcinomas. *Clin. Cancer Res.* **2018**, *24*, 4399–4406. [CrossRef]

37.   Rockenbach, L.; Braganhol, E.; Dietrich, F.; Figueiro, F.; Pugliese, M.; Edelweiss, M.I.; Morrone, F.B.; Sevigny, J.; Battastini, A.M. NTPDase3 and ecto-5'-nucleotidase/CD73 are differentially expressed during mouse bladder cancer progression. *Purinergic Signal.* **2014**, *10*, 421–430. [CrossRef]

38.   Yang, X.; Zhang, X.; Wu, R.; Huang, Q.; Jiang, Y.; Qin, J.; Yao, F.; Jin, G.; Zhang, Y. DPPIV promotes endometrial carcinoma cell proliferation, invasion and tumorigenesis. *Oncotarget* **2017**, *8*, 8679–8692. [CrossRef]

39.   Tan, C.W.; Lee, Y.H.; Tan, H.H.; Lau, M.S.; Choolani, M.; Griffith, L.; Chan, J.K. CD26/DPPIV down-regulation in endometrial stromal cell migration in endometriosis. *Fertil. Steril.* **2014**, *102*, 167–177. [CrossRef]

40.   Busacca, M.; Chiaffarino, F.; Candiani, M.; Vignali, M.; Bertulessi, C.; Oggioni, G.; Parazzini, F. Determinants of long-term clinically detected recurrence rates of deep, ovarian, and pelvic endometriosis. *Am. J. Obstet. Gynecol.* **2006**, *195*, 426–432. [CrossRef]

41.   Koninckx, P.R.; Meuleman, C.; Demeyere, S.; Lesaffre, E.; Cornillie, F.J. Suggestive evidence that pelvic endometriosis is a progressive disease, whereas deeply infiltrating endometriosis is associated with pelvic pain. *Fertil. Steril.* **1991**, *55*, 759–765. [CrossRef]

42.   Burnstock, G. Purinergic mechanisms and pain. *Adv. Pharmacol.* **2016**, *75*, 91–137. [CrossRef] [PubMed]

43.   Fung, C.Y.; Marcus, A.J.; Broekman, M.J.; Mahaut-Smith, M.P. P2X(1) receptor inhibition and soluble CD39 administration as novel approaches to widen the cardiovascular therapeutic window. *Trends Cardiovasc. Med.* **2009**, *19*, 1–5. [CrossRef] [PubMed]

Uncovering Potential Roles of Differentially Expressed Genes, Upstream Regulators and Canonical Pathways in Endometriosis Using an In Silico Genomics Approach

Zeenat Mirza [1,2,*] and Umama A. Abdel-dayem [1,2]

[1]   King Fahd Medical Research Center, King Abdulaziz University, Jeddah 21589, Saudi Arabia;
      uabdelsalam@kau.edu.sa
[2]   Department of Medical Lab Technology, Faculty of Applied Medical Sciences, King Abdulaziz University,
      Jeddah 21589, Saudi Arabia
*   Correspondence: zmirza1@kau.edu.sa

Abstract: Endometriosis is characterized by ectopic endometrial tissue implantation, mostly within the peritoneum, and affects women in their reproductive age. Studies have been done to clarify its etiology, but the precise molecular mechanisms and pathophysiology remain unclear. We downloaded genome-wide mRNA expression and clinicopathological data of endometriosis patients and controls from NCBI's Gene Expression Omnibus, after a systematic search of multiple independent studies comprising 156 endometriosis patients and 118 controls to identify causative genes, risk factors, and potential diagnostic/therapeutic biomarkers. Comprehensive gene expression meta-analysis, pathway analysis, and gene ontology analysis was done using a bioinformatics-based approach. We identified 1590 unique differentially expressed genes (129 upregulated and 1461 downregulated) mapped by IPA as biologically relevant. The top upregulated genes were *FOS, EGR1, ZFP36, JUNB, APOD, CST1, GPX3,* and *PER1,* and the top downregulated ones were *DIO2, CPM, OLFM4, PALLD, BAG5, TOP2A, PKP4, CDC20B,* and *SNTN.* The most perturbed canonical pathways were mitotic roles of Polo-like kinase, role of Checkpoint kinase proteins in cell cycle checkpoint control, and ATM signaling. Protein–protein interaction analysis showed a strong network association among FOS, EGR1, ZFP36, and JUNB. These findings provide a thorough understanding of the molecular mechanism of endometriosis, identified biomarkers, and represent a step towards the future development of novel diagnostic and therapeutic options.

Keywords: endometriosis; microarray; transcriptomics; biomarker; canonical pathways

1. Introduction

Endometriosis is a painful gynecological ailment marked by the presence of endometrial tissue outside the uterine cavity, commonly involving the uterus, ovaries, fallopian tubes, and pelvic tissues [1]. It is a complex and chronic estrogen-dependent disorder, wherein abnormal growth of uterine-lining (endometrium) tissue occurs outside the uterus, which can lead to serious complications like diabetes, obesity, mood disorders, dysmenorrhea, chronic pelvic pain, or even fatal endometrial cancer and cardiovascular disorders if left untreated for long. The most common site of endometriosis is the Douglas pouch (rectovaginal region) of the pelvic peritoneum [2]. Common symptoms include agonizing abdominal pain, period cramps (dysmenorrhea), heavy periods, pain with bowel movements or urination, dyspareunia, and infertility [3].

Pelvic exams and sonography are done to visualize abnormalities, and laparoscopy is required for diagnosis as well as treatment. Modes of treatment are primarily hormonal suppression and ultrasonographically guided surgical/laparoscopic management, which only provide symptomatic relief and the condition can recur with time [4]. Unfortunately, invasive surgery and the lack of a disease biomarker presently causes a mean latency of 7–11 years from symptom onset to definitive diagnosis. This substantial lag possibly has negative consequences in terms of disease progression.

An estimated 176 million women are affected by it worldwide, and studies suggest that 10% of females of reproductive age suffer from this inflammatory disorder. The prevalence of endometriosis is 11.1% among Saudi Arabian women [5]. However, the condition is often underdiagnosed and undertreated. Future higher risk for endometrial polyps [6] and rare progression to endometriosis-associated adenocarcinoma exists in endometriosis patients. They also have a lifetime predisposition to clear-cell and endometrioid types of ovarian cancer [7], which are endometriosis-derived, and which are possibly associated with retrograde menstruation [8]. The identification of a sufficiently specific and sensitive marker for the non-surgical detection of endometriosis would promise early diagnosis and prevention of detrimental effects, underscoring the need for comprehensive research. The most extensively studied potential biomarker for endometriosis is cancer antigen 125, but its use as a sole diagnostic marker is impractical due to its low sensitivity [9].

Recent innovations of high-throughput transcriptomics-based genome-wide approaches have had a major impact on medical research [10], thereby aiding in clinical classification and treatment predictions [10–12]. Understanding the genetic basis of the pathophysiology of endometriosis is important to explain the strong genetic association with heritability, estimated at around 50% [13]. Dysregulation of several genes has been implicated in the etiology of this ectopic condition.

In a menstrual cycle, endometrium undergoes transition from estrogen-dominant proliferative (follicular) phases (early-proliferative (EP), mid-proliferative (MP), and late-proliferative (LP)) to progesterone-dominant secretory (luteal) phases ((early-secretory (ES), mid-secretory (MS), and late-secretory (LS)), followed by the menstrual phase. A distinct differential transcriptional profile exists for each endometrial cycle phase [14,15]. As the uterine linings in endometriosis patients have altered transcriptomic profiles, molecular classification is needed for disease identification and staging [16]. Previous works have focused on expression profiling of different stages of the endometrial cycle in small groups. Herein, we integrated data to conduct comprehensive differential transcriptional profiling of a large cohort in order to identify differentially expressed genes, upstream regulators, and perturbed canonical pathways that could possibly be used in future to identify novel potential biomarkers and therapeutic targets for endometriosis.

Etiology

Decrease in age of menarche, fewer pregnancies, less breast feeding, and increase in maternal age at first birth all cause an overall increase in the number of ovulations and menstruations within a reproductive lifespan. These changes are associated strongly with the risk of endometriosis development and tend to be more pronounced during the decade of highest risk for endometriosis, i.e., 25–35 years of age [17]. Estrogen dependence, immune modulation, and certain environmental pollutants, mostly dioxins and polychlorinated biphenyls, perhaps contribute to the disease's pathobiology [18]. Immunological or hormonal dysfunction make some women predisposed to endometriosis. Higher macrophage activation and humoral immune responsiveness with reduced cell-mediated immunity, with weakened T-cell and NK-cell responses, are seen in women suffering from endometriosis. Humoral autoantibodies against endometrial and ovarian tissue have been detected in endometriosis patient sera [19].

The pathogenesis of endometriosis has been speculated to result from aberrant angiogenesis that occurs in the eutopic endometrium with retrograde menstruation—"Sampson's hypothesis" [2]. Factors that increase the rate of retrograde menstruation, such as congenital outflow tract obstructions, might also predispose to endometriosis. Detailed understanding on the basis of gene expression studies is lacking, and findings are often inconsistent or even contradictory.

2. Materials and Methods

2.1. Data Retrieval and Sample Description

Our approach was the integration of publicly available gene expression data generated by different microarray platforms. We first retrieved whole-transcript array datasets (.CEL files) along with provided clinical details of endometriosis patients dated up to 30 March 2020 from the Gene Expression Omnibus (GEO, NCBI) databank, a public domain hosting high-throughput genomic data. The present study included following expression data series with GEO accession numbers GSE7846, GSE7305, GSE6364, GSE4888, GSE51981, GSE31683, and GSE25628 and their sample information to compare the transcriptomic status of affected and control patients (Table 1). The GSE51981 dataset has a total of 148 endometrial samples from patients with ages ranging from 20–50 years. It includes samples from women in different menstrual cycle phases, including endometriosis with severe pelvic pain/infertility ($n = 77$) and normal without endometriosis ($n = 71$). Normal women with uterine fibroids, adenomyosis, or pelvic organ prolapse were further grouped as normal with uterine/pelvic pathology ($n = 37$), and others as normal without uterine pathology ($n = 34$). The GSE7846 dataset includes five arrays for human endometrial endothelial cells (HEECs) derived from eutopic endometria of patients with endometriosis, and five from patients without endometriosis (controls). GSE7305 includes expression profiles of 10 each of normal and diseased cases.

2.2. Gene Expression Analysis

To generate expression profiles of endometriosis samples, .CEL files were imported to Partek Genomics Suite, version 7.0 (Partek Inc., St. Louis, MO, USA) followed by log-transformation and normalization of the robust background-adjusted array dataset. Principal component analysis (PCA) was done on high-dimensional data to assess quality and overall variance in gene expression of individuals among sample groups. Analysis of variance (ANOVA) was employed to create a list of differentially expressed genes (DEGs) with a cut-off p-value of ≤ 0.05 and fold change of ± 2. Hierarchical clustering was done to reveal the pattern of most differentially expressed (up- and downregulated) genes across samples.

2.3. Gene Ontology, Pathway, and Upstream Regulators Analysis

The identified statistically significant DEGs with corresponding probe sets ID, p-value, fold-change values, and other relevant data were uploaded into the Ingenuity Pathways Analysis (IPA, QIAGEN's Ingenuity Systems, Redwood City, CA, USA) software for molecular network and canonical pathway analysis to define interaction amongst the differentially regulated genes using functional algorithms. The Benjamini–Hochberg method was used to adjust p-values for canonical pathways, and p-values below 0.01 and Altman z-scores of ± 2 were considered significant. Positive and negative values of z-score represent activation and inhibition of dysregulated canonical pathways. Gene ontology study was done to functionally categorize endometriosis-significant genes. All endometriosis-associated DEGs were imported to figuratively represent all identified connections and potential relationships among them, in order to identify significant pathways leading to endometriosis initiation and progression.

2.4. Protein–Protein Interaction Analysis

To check the interactions at the protein level, the STRING v11.0 database (http://string-db.org) was used to search for possible physical and functional associations among proteins encoded by the top DEGs (including both up- and downregulated) for a better understanding of disease pathobiology [20]. This prediction gives a visual idea about the possible interconnections between the proteins involved in a specific disease network.

3. Results

Differentially Expressed Genes from Meta-Analysis

Integration of the seven GEO data series included in present study comprised a total of 156 endometriosis patients and 118 controls. Data were merged before analysis as all had used the same GPL570 platform, except GSE25628 which used the GPL571 platform (Table 1).

Table 1. **Gene expression Omnibus** (GEO) data series, platform, and sample description of endometrium-based expression studies (total 156 endometriosis patients + 118 normal cases).

GEO Data Series	Total No. of Cases (Diseased + Normal)	Platform	Sample Description
GSE 7846	10 (5 + 5)	GPL570	Endometriosis ($n = 5$), Normal ($n = 5$)
GSE 7305	20 (10 +10)	GPL570	Endometriosis ($n = 10$), Normal ($n = 10$)
GSE 6364	37 (21 + 16)	GPL570	Proliferative ($n = 6$), Proliferative normal ($n = 5$); Early-secretory ($n = 6$), Early-secretory normal ($n = 3$); Mid-secretory ($n = 9$), Mid-secretory normal ($n = 8$)
GSE 4888	27 (21 + 6)	GPL570	Proliferative ($n = 4$), Early-secretory ($n = 3$), Mid-secretory ($n = 8$), Late-secretory ($n = 6$), Ambiguous histology ($n = 6$)
GSE 51981	148 (77 + 71)	GPL570	Severe endometriosis ($n = 48$), Mild endometriosis ($n = 29$), Normal without pelvic/uterine pathology ($n = 34$), Normal with pelvic/uterine pathology ($n = 37$)
GSE 31683	10 (6 + 4)	GPL570	*KLF9* silenced ($n = 2$), *PGR* silenced ($n = 2$), Both *KLF9* and *PGR* silenced ($n = 2$), Normal ($n = 4$)
GSE 25628	22 (16 + 6)	GPL571	Eutopic ($n = 9$), Ectopic ($n = 7$), Normal ($n = 6$)

Principal component analysis showed the grouping of the samples in three-dimensional space as per their whole-genome expression patterns, where each circle represents an individual (Figure 1). Comparing endometriosis with normal non-endometriosis tissue without any pelvic/uterine pathology resulted in the detection of 1590 differentially expressed genes (129 upregulated and 1461 downregulated). The top upregulated genes, including *FOS, EGR1, ZFP36, JUNB, APOD, CST1, GPX3,* and *PER1*, are shown in Table 2 and the top downregulated genes, including *DIO2, CPM, OLFM4, PALLD, BAG5, TOP2A, PKP4, CDC20B,* and *SNTN*, are shown in Table 3. Hierarchical clustering of DEGs showed a clear difference in expression pattern of genes between endometriosis cases and controls (Figure 2). Disease and functional annotation of DEGs broadly predicted endometrial adenocarcinoma. However, DEGs like *FOS, EGR1, ZFP36, JUNB, GPX3, PAEP, DUSP1, MT1M, COL6A1, NR4A1, TGFB1, CITED2, IL2RG, ACKR1, JUN, PTGER3, COL6A2, PGR, PLK2, PLA2G4A, FBN1, MPPED2, EZR, MMP11, GALNT4, PTEN, PIK3CA, CREB1, ERBIN, DNMT3A, REL, SDC2, ZNF25, ITGA6, GUCY1A2, PDGFD, OVGP1, ITGB1, APOBEC3B, OLFM1, NRIP1, MEF2A, CNTN1, BUB1B, MEST, KIF20A, RRM1, ANK3,* and *CCNA2* showed significant association with endometriosis (p-value = 0.0006).

Ingenuity pathway analysis for the DEGs of endometriosis revealed altered canonical pathways that were either activated or inhibited (Figure 3, Table 4). Mitotic roles of polo-like kinase (z-score −2.71), aldosterone signaling in epithelial cells (z-score −3.464), and role of CHK proteins in cell cycle checkpoint control (z-score −0.632) were found to be inhibited while ATM signaling (z-score + 1.698) and SUMOylation pathways (z-score + 2.668) were activated (Figure 4, Figure 5). IPA predicted the activation status of upstream regulators among identified DEGs of endometriosis. REL (transcription factor, z-score −4.13, Pval 0.0002), CTNNB1 (transcription factor, z-score −3.2, Pval 0.01), PGR (ligand-dependent nuclear receptor, z-score −2.2, Pval 0.0005), and VCAN (proteoglycan, z-score −2.6, Pval 0.02) were the top inhibited upstream regulators (Table 5). We also used a biological database, STRING, to predict functional associations and interaction between the proteins encoded by the identified significant DEGs (top up- and downregulated ones), and the results are shown in

Figure 6. The network indicated a strong interplay of various proteins and their specific involvement in endometriosis.

Figure 1. PCA showing two clear distinct clusters for severe endometriosis cases and normal healthy controls without uterine pathology.

Table 2. Top overexpressed/upregulated differentially expressed genes in endometriosis.

Gene Symbol	Gene Name	p-Value	Fold-Change
FOS	FBJ murine osteosarcoma viral oncogene homolog	3.02×10^{-13}	9.94558
EGR1	early growth response 1	7.67×10^{-17}	7.95823
FOSB	FBJ murine osteosarcoma viral oncogene homolog B	1.87×10^{-10}	7.14284
ZFP36	ZFP36 ring finger protein	5.23×10^{-14}	4.01565
JUNB	jun B proto-oncogene	8.28×10^{-15}	4.01404
APOD	apolipoprotein D	1.21×10^{-7}	3.7376
CST1	cystatin SN	2.52×10^{-5}	3.42216
GPX3	glutathione peroxidase 3	0.0057	3.34348
PER1	period circadian clock 1	6.14×10^{-13}	3.23599
CTSW	cathepsin W	8.08×10^{-7}	3.22223
SOCS3	suppressor of cytokine signaling 3	4.99×10^{-5}	3.11348
CFD	complement factor D (adipsin)	0.000993	2.99141
HSPB6	heat shock protein, alpha-crystallin-related, B6	9.31×10^{-8}	2.98362
LEFTY1	left-right determination factor 1	0.004712	2.89285
PAEP	progestagen-associated endometrial protein	0.029113	2.88223
DUSP1	dual specificity phosphatase 1	1.48×10^{-7}	2.88219
GNLY	Granulysin	1.52×10^{-5}	2.83639
EPHX1	epoxide hydrolase 1, microsomal (xenobiotic)	6.69×10^{-10}	2.78618
MT1M	metallothionein 1M	0.011648	2.76574
CLEC3B///EXOSC7	C-type lectin domain family 3, member B///exosome component 7	7.13×10^{-5}	2.74002
GNLY	Granulysin	1.61×10^{-5}	2.73433
TPSAB1///TPSB2	tryptase alpha/beta 1///tryptase beta 2 (gene/pseudogene)	1.20×10^{-6}	2.73381
IER2	immediate early response 2	4.65×10^{-14}	2.67138
PTPRO	protein tyrosine phosphatase, receptor type, O	2.70×10^{-14}	2.66719
ELN	Elastin	2.26×10^{-7}	2.6637
IER3	immediate early response 3	5.70×10^{-5}	2.61981
SOX13	SRY box 13	4.59×10^{-9}	2.60666
SOD3	superoxide dismutase 3, extracellular	2.00×10^{-9}	2.60457
SLC30A2	solute carrier family 30 (zinc transporter), member 2	0.002566	2.59508
AQP3	aquaporin 3 (Gill blood group)	0.000604	2.58706
HSPB6	heat shock protein, alpha-crystallin-related, B6	2.81×10^{-6}	2.57421
CD37	CD37 molecule	3.56×10^{-8}	2.48625
IRX3	iroquois homeobox 3	0.00585	2.48441
CREB3L1	cAMP responsive element binding protein 3-like 1	1.53×10^{-7}	2.48023

Table 3. The top downregulated differentially expressed genes in meta-analysis of endometriosis.

Gene Symbol	Gene Title	p-Value	Fold-Change
DIO2	deiodinase, iodothyronine, type II	6.84×10^{-12}	−5.38638
CPM	carboxypeptidase M	1.52×10^{-7}	−5.20763
OLFM4	olfactomedin 4	1.22×10^{-6}	−4.77761
PALLD	palladin, cytoskeletal associated protein	1.20×10^{-13}	−4.47775
BAG5	BCL2-associated athanogene 5	1.62×10^{-8}	−4.38993
TOP2A	topoisomerase (DNA) II alpha	4.50×10^{-8}	−4.22713
PKP4	plakophilin 4	5.35×10^{-19}	−3.97475
CDC20B	cell division cycle 20B	1.36×10^{-6}	−3.96043
SNTN	sentan, cilia apical structure protein	5.43×10^{-12}	−3.95899
SET	SET nuclear proto-oncogene	5.39×10^{-11}	−3.90488
CRISPLD1	cysteine-rich secretory protein LCCL domain containing 1	5.12×10^{-7}	−3.85982
NPAS3	neuronal PAS domain protein 3	1.57×10^{-6}	−3.83298
CADM1	cell adhesion molecule 1	4.63×10^{-15}	−3.78248
SMC3	structural maintenance of chromosomes 3	2.59×10^{-16}	−3.7407
SFRP4	secreted frizzled-related protein 4	0.000481	−3.72407
ANK2	ankyrin 2, neuronal	2.00×10^{-7}	−3.71876
ANLN	anillin actin binding protein	4.54×10^{-8}	−3.70838
WIF1	WNT inhibitory factor 1	1.73×10^{-6}	−3.65345
MMP26	matrix metallopeptidase 26	0.002107	−3.63998
PCSK5	proprotein convertase subtilisin/kexin type 5	7.33×10^{-8}	−3.63558
OXR1	oxidation resistance 1	1.62×10^{-13}	−3.61905
CTNNB1	catenin (cadherin-associated protein), beta 1	6.39×10^{-12}	−3.55057
PCSK5	proprotein convertase subtilisin/kexin type 5	1.69×10^{-8}	−3.53439
EIF5B	eukaryotic translation initiation factor 5B	1.60×10^{-8}	−3.52153
HSP90B1	heat shock protein 90kDa beta (Grp94), member 1	2.11×10^{-9}	−3.49988
PCYOX1	prenylcysteine oxidase 1	3.06×10^{-11}	−3.47374
MIB1	mindbomb E3 ubiquitin protein ligase 1	1.96×10^{-9}	−3.46544
OSBPL1A	oxysterol binding protein-like 1A	2.08×10^{-14}	−3.46429
CBX3	chromobox homolog 3	2.18×10^{-12}	−3.45307
TCAF1	TRPM8 channel-associated factor 1	1.87×10^{-13}	−3.42665
KMO	kynurenine 3-monooxygenase (kynurenine 3-hydroxylase)	2.06×10^{-5}	−3.42531
CTSZ	cathepsin Z	3.75×10^{-13}	−3.40201
KMO	kynurenine 3-monooxygenase (kynurenine 3-hydroxylase)	2.13×10^{-5}	−3.38857
PCSK5	proprotein convertase subtilisin/kexin type 5	5.06×10^{-8}	−3.38299
YWHAB	tyrosine 3-monooxygenase/tryptophan 5-monooxygenase activation protein, beta	2.64×10^{-13}	−3.35541
NMT2	N-myristoyltransferase 2	5.60×10^{-12}	-3.34186
CADM1	cell adhesion molecule 1	3.18×10^{-9}	−3.3281
CEP57	centrosomal protein 57kDa	3.21×10^{-15}	−3.28628

Hierarchical Clustering: DEGs of Endometriosis

Figure 2. Hierarchical clustering showing distribution of DEGs and cases. Downregulated and upregulated genes are shown in blue and red, respectively, showing a distinct pattern with a majority of genes found to be downregulated in endometriosis.

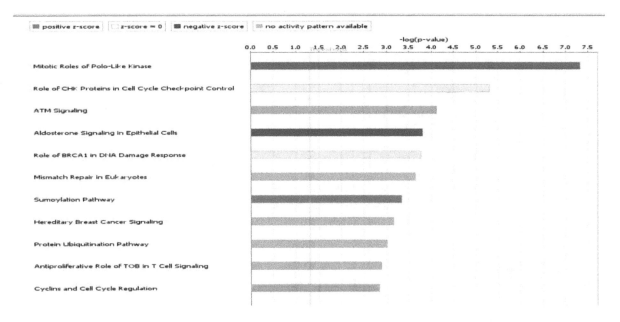

Figure 3. Significant pathways identified by IPA. The top 11 altered canonical pathways predicted from DEGs of endometriosis. Negative and positive z-scores, colored in shades of blue and red, represent inhibition and activation of pathways, respectively.

Table 4. Significant canonical pathways based on DEGs of endometriosis. Positive and negative z- scores indicate overall activation and inhibition status of pathways, respectively.

Ingenuity Canonical Pathways	−log (p-Value)	Ratio	Predicted z-Score	Molecules
Mitotic Roles of Polo-Like Kinase	7.34	0.333	−2.714 (Inhibited)	ANAPC4, CCNB1, CCNB2, CDC23, CDC27, CDK1, FBXO5, HSP90AA1, HSP90AB1, HSP90B1, KIF11, KIF23, PLK2, PPM1L, PPP2R2C, PPP2R5C, PPP2R5E, PRC1, RAD21, SMC3, TGFB1
ATM Signaling	4.11	0.219	1.698 (Activated)	ATF1, CBX1, CBX3, CBX5, CCNB1, CCNB2, CDK1, CHEK1, CREB1, FANCD2, JUN, PPM1L, PPP2R2C, PPP2R5C, PPP2R5E, RAD17, RAD50, SMC2, SMC3, TLK1, ZNF420
Aldosterone Signaling in Epithelial Cells	3.8	0.183	−3.464 (Inhibited)	DNAJA1, DNAJB14, DNAJC10, DNAJC27, DNAJC3, DNAJC9, DUSP1, HSP90AA1, HSP90AB1, HSP90B1, HSPA4, HSPA9, HSPB6, HSPD1, HSPH1, ITPR2, PDIA3, PDPK1, PIK3C2A, PIK3CA, PIK3R3, PIP5K1B, PLCB1, PRKCI, PRKD3, SACS, SCNN1G
Role of CHK Proteins in Cell Cycle Checkpoint Control	5.3	0.298	−0.632	ATMIN, CDK1, CHEK1, E2F7, E2F8, PCNA, PPM1L, PPP2R2C, PPP2R5C, PPP2R5E, RAD17, RAD50, RFC3, RFC4, RFC5, RPA1, TLK1
SUMOylation Pathway	3.34	0.198	2.668 (Activated)	DNMT3A, EP300, FOS, HDAC2, JUN, MYB, PCNA, PIAS1, RFC3, RFC4, RFC5, RHOB, RHOBTB1, RHOQ, RHOT1, RND3, RPA1, SERBP1, SMAD4, UBA2
Role of BRCA1 in DNA Damage Response	3.77	0.225	−0.707	ABRAXAS1, ATF1, BRCC3, BRD7, BRIP1, CHEK1, E2F7, E2F8, FANCD2, FANCL, MSH2, MSH6, RAD50, RFC3, RFC4, RFC5, RPA1, SMARCC1
Cyclins and Cell Cycle Regulation	2.83	0.2	−1.604	CCNA1, CCNA2, CCNB1, CCNB2, CCNE2, CDK1, CDK6, E2F7, E2F8, HDAC2, PPM1L, PPP2R2C, PPP2R5C, PPP2R5E, SKP2, TGFB1
PI3K/AKT Signaling	2.7	0.171	−1.091	CTNNB1, EIF4E, HSP90AA1, HSP90AB1, HSP90B1, INPP5F, ITGB1, JAK1, PDPK1, PIK3CA, PIK3R3, PPM1L, PPP2R2C, PPP2R5C, PPP2R5E, PTEN, RASD1, RHEB, RPS6KB1, SFN, SYNJ2, YWHAB

Figure 4. Significant inhibition of mitotic polo-like kinase pathway predicted by IPA. Pathway genes were overlaid to the DEGs; upregulated (*TGFB1, CDC25, FZR1*) genes are shown in red/pink, while downregulated genes (*PRC1, PLK, Cyclin B1, SMC3*) are shown in green.

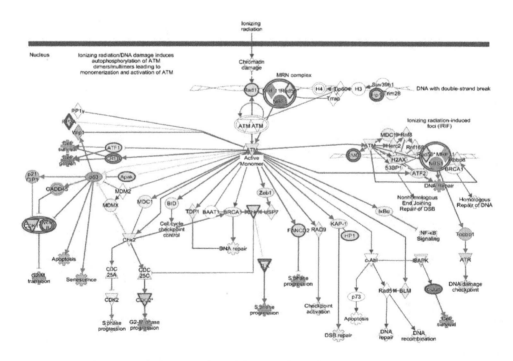

Figure 5. Activation of ATM signaling predicted by IPA-based pathway analysis. Pathway genes were overlaid to the DEGs, with upregulated ones shown in shades of red and downregulated ones shown in green.

Table 5. Most significant upstream regulators and target molecules in endometriosis dataset.

Upstream Regulator	Molecule Type	Predicted Activation z-score	p-Value of Overlap	Target Molecules in Dataset
REL	transcription regulator	−4.137 (Inhibited)	0.00021	AGA, AGPS, ANLN, APP, ARFGAP3, ATXN1, BCL3, CAMK2D, CCNY, CDC6
CTNNB1	transcription regulator	−3.208 (Inhibited)	0.0104	AKAP13, ALDH1A1, APOD, APP, ARFGAP3, ARMH4, AURKA, CADM1, CALM1, CCL3
PGR	ligand-dependent nuclear receptor	−2.237 (Inhibited)	0.00051	ABCG2, ACOX1, AHCYL1, AK3, AKAP13, ATP1B1, ATXN1, BUB1, CA12, CCNB1
VCAN	Proteoglycan	−2.625 (Inhibited)	0.024	COMP, CPE, ELN, IFI44L, IFIT1, ITGB1, MYH10, PCSK5, PENK, PLA2G2A
ACTL6A	Other	−2.236 (Inhibited)	0.093	CCNA2, CCNB1, CCNB2, CCNE2, SFN
DUSP1	phosphatase	−2.155 (Inhibited)	1	CMPK2, DUSP1, IER3, IFIT1, IFIT3, JUN, PTEN, ZFP36
HELLS	Enzyme	−2 (Inhibited)	0.0024	CCNA2, CCNB1, CDC6, HSPD1, PCNA, SLC44A1
RASSF8	Other	−2 (Inhibited)	0.0016	ENPP5, MRPL30, NEDD9, POSTN
TCF4	transcription regulator	−1.912	0.040	CCNA2, CCNB2, CDK1, CEP55, E2F8, FOS, HMGB2, HMMR, HSP90B1, IFI16
IGF2R	transmembrane receptor	−2 (Inhibited)	0.0080	ENPP5, MRPL30, NEDD9, POSTN
TGFB1	growth factor	−1.276	0.00087	ABCG2, ACKR1, ADAM12, ALDH5A1, APP, ARHGAP19, ASPM, ATG12, ATXN1, BCL3
HSF2	transcription regulator	−1.408	0.026	CCT2, HSBP1, HSPA4, HSPH1, JUN, PSMA5, TCP1
EDN3	other	0.816	0.0024	CDH2, CTNNB1, EGR1, FOS, ITGB1, LAMA1
FOS	transcription regulator	0.917	0.0020	ACOX1, ADAM12, AGPS, ANK3, AQP3, ATP2C1, CADM1, CALU, CAMK2D, CAT
RTN4	other	1.51	0.0041	APP, CFL1, IMPACT, JUN, JUND, LAP3, MAP2, RHOB, RTN4, YWHAB
ZFP36	transcription regulator	1.873	0.00015	CCNE2, CDC6, CENPA, CLCN3, CLMP, CTSS, E2F8, FOS, IER3, JUN
EPHB1	kinase	1.98	0.0052	EGR1, FOS, JUN, JUNB

Figure 6. STRING-based protein–protein interaction (PPI) network of selected differentially expressed genes, showing predicted interconnectivities.

4. Discussion

Endometriosis, a growth/deposition of endometrial tissue at extra-uterine sites, affects around 10% of reproductive women. In addition to abnormal reproductive physiological problems, cases are increasing drastically due to adverse consequences of treatment with oral contraceptives, GnRH agonists, synthetic progestins, and aromatase inhibitors (letrozole) to prevent the menstrual cycle and/or pregnancy [1,21]. Understanding the molecular etiology of origin and progression of endometriosis is necessary to explore therapeutic options and provide better treatment. We therefore conducted transcriptomic meta-analysis to identify endometriosis-associated significant DEGs and essential pathological pathways.

Combining multiple studies has always been challenging, as different studies use varied protocols, platforms, and analysis methods. We used raw data (.CEL) files to integrate multiple data series to get a bigger cohort and analyzed the data. We identified transcriptomic signatures of endometriosis and evaluated the roles of specific genes, upstream regulators, and dysregulated pathways. Our results provide some insight into the molecular mechanisms underlying endometriosis pathogenesis. Pathogenic genes and pathways may serve as novel targets for diagnostic and prognostic biomarkers and potential therapies for endometriosis. In the present study, we had a long list of genes and pathways, but have restricted our discussion to the most prominent genes and pathways.

4.1. Molecular Etiology of Endometriosis

Retrograde or "reverse" menstruation has been suggested as an initial cause of endometriosis, where menstrual blood is thrown back into pelvic cavity outside the uterus, instead of flowing out of the cervix. This endometrial tissue growth out of the uterus is the result of an estrogen-dependent hormonal local imbalance. Higher prevalence has been also seen in women with immune disorders (like rheumatoid arthritis, multiple sclerosis, systemic lupus erythematosus, and hypo- or hyperthyroidism) [17]. Recently, a small-molecule agonist G-1 (Tespria) against the G-protein-coupled estrogen receptor also showed reduction in endometrial growth [22].

Unusual transformation of certain abdominal wall cells into endometrial cells has been reported in some women [23] and, interestingly, it is believed that during embryonic development, the same cells are responsible for the growth of female reproductive organs. Researchers also think that pelvic inflammation, damage, or infection of cells that line the pelvis like a prior caesarean surgery can also trigger endometriosis [23–25]. The exact pathogenesis still remains uncertain. We therefore conducted a transcriptomics study in order to understand the genetic factors that allow cells to grow as endometrial tissue outside the uterus.

In our results, we found high expression of early and immediate early-response genes such as FBJ murine osteosarcoma viral oncogene homolog or *Fos proto-Oncogene (FOS)*, *FosB Proto-Oncogene (FOSB)*, *Early Growth Response 1 (EGR1)*, *ZFP36 Ring Finger Protein (ZFP36)*, *Immediate Early Response 2 (IER2)*, *Immediate Early Response 3 (IER3)*, *Jun B Proto-Oncogene (JUNB)*, and *Transcription Factor SOX-13 (SOX 13)*. The majority of these are DNA-binding proteins that act as transcriptional factors. Some others, like *Dual specificity protein phosphatase 1 (DUSP1)* and *Receptor-type tyrosine-protein phosphatase O (PTPRO)*, possess phosphatase activity.

c-Fos is the transcription factor of the Fos family, including *FosB*, *Fra-1*, and *Fra-2* [26]. It is an immediate early-response gene involved in cell proliferation and differentiation of normal tissue after extracellular stress stimuli. Its deregulation has been linked to oncogenic transformation and tumor progression. *FOS* plays a significant role in endometrial cells' proliferation and its overexpression is associated with a poor prognosis of endometrial carcinoma [27]. Fos and Jun family proteins form a heterodimer complex of AP-1 transcription factor, shown to be involved in endometrial carcinogenesis [28]. Upstream regulator analysis revealed genes such as *REL*, *CTNNB1*, *PGR*, and *VCAN* by analyzing linkage to DEGs that were experimentally shown to affect gene expression [29]. All upstream regulators were inhibited.

REL: *REL* (*V-Rel Avian Reticuloendotheliosis Viral Oncogene Homolog*) encodes for the proto-oncogene c-Rel protein, a transcription factor of the NF-κB family that regulates genes involved in B- and T-cell differentiation, immune response, survival, apoptosis, proliferation, and oncogenic processes, including endometrial carcinogenesis [30,31].

CTNNB1: *CTNNB1* (*Catenin β1*) codes for a protein that regulates and coordinates cell–cell adhesion, embryonic development, epithelial–mesenchymal transition, and gene transcription. It is an integral part of the canonical Wnt pathway. Aberrant Wnt/β-catenin signaling pathway function is allied with loose cytoskeleton organization and cell-to-cell contacts of epithelial cells, along with a high motility of mesenchymal cells to promote invasiveness and fibrosis. This might lead to multiple cancers, including endometrial cancer [32–36]. Targeting the Wnt/β-catenin signaling was shown to avert fibrogenesis in a xenograft endometriosis mice model [35].

VCAN: *VCAN* (*Versican*) codes for four extracellular matrix isoforms like large chondroitin sulfate proteoglycan in different tissues and organs that regulate cell adhesion, proliferation, migration, and survival [2]. Higher expression of *VCAN* has been reported in angiogenesis, tumor growth, cancer relapse, and inflammatory lung disorders [37–39]. Significantly high expression of *VCAN* was also reported in the mid-secretory phase of endometrial epithelial cells after combination estrogen/progesterone treatment. The V1 isoform of *VCAN* was recently reported to the facilitate development of endometrial receptivity and human embryo implantation [40]. Higher expression of *VCAN* is connected with pathogenesis of peritoneal endometriosis and seems to be an indicator of poor prognosis endometrial cancer [2,41].

Alteration in expression of *HOXB4* [42], apelin peptide [43], interleukin 18 [44], estrogen and progesterone receptors [45], integrin β3 and osteopontin (*OPN*) [46], microRNA-29c, and FKBP4 [47] have been reported. Varied expression levels of metastasis-inducing proteins (*S100P*, *S100A4*, *OPN*, and anterior gradient homologue 2 (*AGR2*)) have been shown to enhance pathogenesis by increasing endometrial cell invasiveness and establishing endometriotic ectopic deposits after retrograde menstruation [48].

Aromatase activates estrogen biosynthesis locally from androgens, thereby sequentially stimulating a positive feedback cycle of prostaglandin E2 production by upregulating cyclooxygenase-2 (*COX-2*). Because of lack of aromatase (estrogen synthase) in the normal endometrium, androgens cannot be converted into estrogen [49]. In contrast, numerous studies have described aberrantly high expression of aromatase in eutopic and ectopic endometrium [17]. Increased *COX-2* expression in the stromal cells and aberrant aromatase overexpression in eutopic endometrium have both been indicated as potential therapeutic biomarkers, and therefore, their specific inhibitors are being increasingly employed for therapeutic management [50]. A probable connection of Krüppel-like Factor 9 (*KLF9*) dysregulation has been suggested in both pregnancy failure and endometrial pathogenesis [51]. The progesterone resistance and subsequent infertility seen in endometriosis seems to have an association with *KLF9*, a progesterone-receptor-interacting protein, as mice null for Klf9 are sub-fertile. It is implicated that deficiency of *KLF9* contributes to progesterone resistance of eutopic endometrium in patients [52] and exhibits simultaneous abrogation of Hedgehog-, Notch-, and steroid-receptor-regulated networks [53].

Based on serum proteomic differential expression, a possible biomarker panel comprising zinc-alpha-2-glycoprotein, albumin, and complement C3 has been proposed for effective and non-invasive diagnosis of endometriosis [54]. Importantly, the three markers were independent from the endometriosis stage and cycle phase. Brain Derived Neurotrophic Factor (*BDNF*) has been identified as a potential peripheral early diagnostic marker, as its mean plasma concentrations were twice as high in endometriosis cases in contrast to asymptomatic or healthy controls [9]. Based on this, a nano-chip-based electrochemical detection technique was developed. The only limitation to this is its non-specificity, as the variations in *BDNF* expression have been reported in numerous unconnected pathologies [55].

4.2. Canonical Pathways Involved in Endometriosis

Molecular pathway analysis revealed a couple of significantly altered canonical pathways for DEGs of endometriosis. Herein, we discuss the role of key pathways like Mitotic roles of polo-like kinase, Role of CHK proteins in cell cycle checkpoint control, Aldosterone signaling in epithelial cells, and ATM Signaling in endometriosis progression.

Mitotic Roles of Polo-Like Kinase Pathway: The Polo-like kinase (Plks) is a member of the serine/threonine protein kinase (*PLK1-5*) family that regulates the mitotic checkpoint during M phase of cell division. Plks can act either as oncogene or tumor suppressor, and has been found to be overexpressed in different cancer types including endometrial [56] and ovarian [57] cancers. Because of its direct association with increased cellular proliferation and poor prognosis, it is considered a bona fide cancer biomarker [58,59]. Direct association of Plks expression with serum estrogen (ovarian hormone) levels and abnormal regulation of ectopic endometrial cell proliferation strongly suggest its role in the pathogenesis of endometriosis [60]. Plks inhibitors such as volasertib and rigosertib are in advanced stage of clinical trials and might be used for endometriosis treatment [61].

Role of CHK Proteins in Cell Cycle Checkpoint Control Pathway: Activation of cell cycle checkpoint kinases including Chk1 and Chk2 are an instant response to repair any type of DNA damage [62]. In response to DNA damage, this signaling pathway temporarily delays cell cycle progression, allowing time for DNA repair, or triggers programmed cell death. Activated ATM kinase phosphorylates Chk2 which phosphorylates *CDC25C* to block the progression from G2 to M phase. Chk2 also phosphorylates p53, attenuating p53 binding to *MDM2* and activating p21/WAF1 to arrest the G1 phase of the cell cycle. *Rad3*-dependent activation of Chk1 phosphorylates *CDC25A* and *CDC2* to inhibit their activity to block G2–M transition. Overall, CHK protein signaling depends on the type of stress and extent of DNA damage and is involved in endometrial cancer [63].

Cisplatin exerts an anticancer effect by activating DNA-damage-response genes Chk1/2, which generates both survival (repair) and apoptotic signals that lead to cell death. Cisplatin-resistant cells have dominant repair signaling that allows cells to survive. Chk1/2 inhibitor AZD7762 has been shown to overcome cisplatin resistance in endometriosis-associated ovarian cancer by reducing repair signaling [64].

ATM Signaling Pathway: Ataxia telangiectasia mutated (*ATM*) gene codes for serine/threonine protein kinase and participates in cell division and DNA repair. DNA damage induces autophosphorylation of ATM which activates DNA repair enzymes by phosphorylating Chk1/2 to fix the broken strands [65]. Efficient cross-talk between ATR-Chk1 and ATM-Chk2 leads to repair of damaged DNA strands which helps to maintain the cell's genomic stability and integrity [66]. The ATM signaling pathway, because of its central role in cell division and DNA repair, has been a focus of cancer research, especially endometrial cancer, for exploring novel molecular therapies targeting ATM pathways [67].

Aldosterone Signaling in Epithelial Cells Pathway: Aldosterone is a mineralocorticoid steroid hormone produced by the adrenal cortex. Aldosterone signaling primarily controls blood pressure and inflammation by regulating its target genes (*FKBP5, IGF1, KRAS, PKCε, NCOA1, NCOR1, NEDD4L, SGK,* and *MR/NR3C2* as per RGD, https://rgd.mcw.edu [68] and IPA). Recent studies have shown the possible involvement of aldosterone in multiple gynecological problems and inflammatory disorders [69]. There is a well-established association of endometriosis with intraperitoneal inflammation diseases like atherosclerosis and hypertension, and also with autoimmune diseases like diabetes, hypothyroidism, and cancer [9]. A metabolomics-based study revealed high aldosterone levels in endometriosis patients with infertility [70].

4.3. Future Directions

The strength of present work lies in the inclusion of multiple endometriosis-related expression datasets in order to understand endometriosis at the molecular level. However, the absence of a validation study was its limitation. In future, we plan to conduct RT-PCR-based validation studies for differentially expressed genes on endometriosis samples collected from the Jeddah region. Further cell cultures and animal models could be used to assess the effect of activated/suppressed genes on molecular pathways and disease phenotypes for potential clinical translation. Virtual screening of potential lead compounds against identified therapeutic biomarkers for rational drug design will be done. This could facilitate imminent tailor-made personalized therapies.

5. Conclusions

Endometriosis is an estrogen-dependent, progesterone-resistant, inflammatory multifactorial gynecological disorder. Identification of distinct molecular signatures and potential therapeutic molecules corresponding to endometriosis is needed for better diagnosis. The present microarray-based genomics and molecular pathway analysis method helped to establish a better understanding of endometriosis at the molecular level, as multiple expression datasets were integrated to determine differentially expressed genes and identify canonical molecular pathways related to endometriosis in a broad way. The study identified alterations of gene expression and molecular signaling, including aldosterone signaling, that result in the hormonal imbalances and pathogenesis of endometriosis. An anti-inflammatory diet and increased levels of antioxidants and phytonutrients can be recommended to patients to reverse inflammation and oxidative damage, while also supporting healthy hormone balance.

Author Contributions: Z.M. and U.A.A.-D. Study design, U.A.A.-D. Acquisition of data, Z.M. Analysis and interpretation of data, Z.M. Manuscript writing, U.A.A.-D. Critical review of manuscript. All authors have read and agreed to the published version of the manuscript.

References

1.   Cho, Y.J.; Lee, S.H.; Park, J.W.; Han, M.; Park, M.J.; Han, S.J. Dysfunctional signaling underlying endometriosis: Current state of knowledge. *J. Mol. Endocrinol.* **2018**, *60*, R97–R113. [CrossRef]

2.   Tani, H.; Sato, Y.; Ueda, M.; Miyazaki, Y.; Suginami, K.; Horie, A.; Konishi, I.; Shinomura, T. Role of Versican in the Pathogenesis of Peritoneal Endometriosis. *J. Clin. Endocrinol. Metab.* **2016**, *101*, 4349–4356. [CrossRef] [PubMed]

3.   Alimi, Y.; Iwanaga, J.; Loukas, M.; Tubbs, R.S. The Clinical Anatomy of Endometriosis: A Review. *Cureus* **2018**, *10*, e3361. [CrossRef] [PubMed]

4.   Yeung, P., Jr. The laparoscopic management of endometriosis in patients with pelvic pain. *Obstet. Gynecol. Clin. N. Am.* **2014**, *41*, 371–383. [CrossRef] [PubMed]

5.   Rouzi, A.A.; Sahly, N.; Kafy, S.; Sawan, D.; Abduljabbar, H. Prevalence of endometriosis at a university hospital in Jeddah, Saudi Arabia. *Clin. Exp. Obstet. Gynecol.* **2015**, *42*, 785–786.

6.   Zheng, Q.M.; Mao, H.I.; Zhao, Y.J.; Zhao, J.; Wei, X.; Liu, P.S. Risk of endometrial polyps in women with endometriosis: A meta-analysis. *Reprod. Biol. Endocrinol.* **2015**, *13*, 103. [CrossRef]

7.   Kim, H.S.; Kim, T.H.; Chung, H.H.; Song, Y.S. Risk and prognosis of ovarian cancer in women with endometriosis: A meta-analysis. *Br. J. Cancer* **2014**, *110*, 1878–1890. [CrossRef]

8.   Vaughan, S.; Coward, J.I.; Bast, R.C.; Berchuck, A.; Berek, J.S.; Brenton, J.D.; Coukos, G.; Crum, C.C.; Drapkin, R.; Etemadmoghadam, D.; et al. Rethinking ovarian cancer: Recommendations for improving outcomes. *Nat. Rev. Cancer* **2011**, *11*, 719–725. [CrossRef]

9.   Hughes, C.; Foster, W.; Agarwal, S. The impact of endometriosis across the lifespan of women: Foreseeable research and therapeutic prospects. *Biomed. Res. Int.* **2015**, *2015*, 158490. [CrossRef]

10.   Sorlie, T.; Tibshirani, R.; Parker, J.; Hastie, T.; Marron, J.S.; Nobel, A.; Deng, S.; Johnsen, H.; Pesich, R.; Geisler, S.; et al. Repeated observation of breast tumor subtypes in independent gene expression data sets. *Proc. Natl. Acad. Sci. USA* **2003**, *100*, 8418–8423. [CrossRef]

11. Hedenfalk, I.; Duggan, D.; Chen, Y.; Radmacher, M.; Bittner, M.; Simon, R.; Meltzer, P.; Gusterson, B.; Esteller, M.; Kallioniemi, O.P.; et al. Gene-expression profiles in hereditary breast cancer. *N. Engl. J. Med.* **2001**, *344*, 539–548. [CrossRef] [PubMed]

12. Chang, J.C.; Wooten, E.C.; Tsimelzon, A.; Hilsenbeck, S.G.; Gutierrez, M.C.; Elledge, R.; Mohsin, S.; Osborne, C.K.; Chamness, G.C.; Allred, D.C.; et al. Gene expression profiling for the prediction of therapeutic response to docetaxel in patients with breast cancer. *Lancet* **2003**, *362*, 362–369. [CrossRef]

13. Borghese, B.; Zondervan, K.T.; Abrao, M.S.; Chapron, C.; Vaiman, D. Recent insights on the genetics and epigenetics of endometriosis. *Clin. Genet.* **2017**, *91*, 254–264. [CrossRef] [PubMed]

14. Ponnampalam, A.P.; Weston, G.C.; Trajstman, A.C.; Susil, B.; Rogers, P.A.W. Molecular classification of human endometrial cycle stages by transcriptional profiling. *Mol. Hum. Reprod.* **2004**, *10*, 879–893. [CrossRef] [PubMed]

15. Sherwin, R.; Catalano, R.; Sharkey, A. Large-scale gene expression studies of the endometrium: What have we learnt? *Reproduction* **2006**, *132*, 1–10. [CrossRef]

16. Miller, L.M.; Johnson, N.P. EPHect—The Endometriosis Phenome (and Biobanking) Harmonisation Project—May be very helpful for clinicians and the women they are treating. *F1000Res* **2017**, *6*, 14. [CrossRef]

17. Parazzini, F.; Vercellini, P.; Pelucchi, C. Endometriosis: Epidemiology, and Etiological Factors. In *Endometriosis*; Linda, C.G., Johannes, L.H.E., David, L.H., Eds.; Wiley-Blackwell: Oxford, UK, 2012; pp. 19–26. [CrossRef]

18. Porpora, M.G.; Resta, S.; Fuggetta, E.; Storelli, P.; Megiorni, F.; Manganaro, L.; De Felip, E. Role of environmental organochlorinated pollutants in the development of endometriosis. *Clin. Exp. Obstet. Gynecol.* **2013**, *40*, 565–567.

19. Mathur, S.; Peress, M.R.; Williamson, H.O.; Youmans, C.D.; Maney, S.A.; Garvin, A.J.; Rust, P.F.; Fudenberg, H.H. Autoimmunity to endometrium and ovary in endometriosis. *Clin. Exp. Immunol.* **1982**, *50*, 259–266. [CrossRef]

20. Szklarczyk, D.; Gable, A.L.; Lyon, D.; Junge, A.; Wyder, S.; Huerta-Cepas, J.; Simonovic, M.; Doncheva, N.T.; Morris, J.H.; Bork, P.; et al. STRING v11: Protein-protein association networks with increased coverage, supporting functional discovery in genome-wide experimental datasets. *Nucleic Acids Res.* **2019**, *47*, D607–D613. [CrossRef]

21. Attar, E.; Bulun, S.E. Aromatase inhibitors: The next generation of therapeutics for endometriosis? *Fertil. Steril.* **2006**, *85*, 1307–1318. [CrossRef]

22. Sharma, G.; Hu, C.; Staquicini, D.I.; Brigman, J.L.; Liu, M.; Mauvais-Jarvis, F.; Pasqualini, R.; Arap, W.; Arterburn, J.B.; Hathaway, H.J. Preclinical efficacy of the GPER-selective agonist G-1 in mouse models of obesity and diabetes. *Sci. Transl. Med.* **2020**, *12*. [CrossRef] [PubMed]

23. Marques, C.; Silva, T.S.; Dias, M.F. Clear cell carcinoma arising from abdominal wall endometriosis - Brief report and review of the literature. *Gynecol. Oncol. Rep.* **2017**, *20*, 78–80. [CrossRef] [PubMed]

24. Yıldırım, D.; Tatar, C.; Doğan, O.; Hut, A.; Dönmez, T.; Akıncı, M.; Toptaş, M.; Bayık, R.N. Post-cesarean scar endometriosis. *Turk. J. Obstet. Gynecol.* **2018**, *15*, 33–38. [CrossRef] [PubMed]

25. Sosa-Durán, E.E.; Aboharp-Hasan, Z.; Mendoza-Morales, R.C.; García-Rodríguez, F.M.; Jiménez-Villanueva, X.; Peñavera-Hernández, J.R. Clear cell adenocarcinoma arising from abdominal wall endometriosis. *Cirugía Cir.* **2016**, *84*, 245–249. [CrossRef] [PubMed]

26. Milde-Langosch, K. The Fos family of transcription factors and their role in tumourigenesis. *Eur. J. Cancer* **2005**, *41*, 2449–2461. [CrossRef] [PubMed]

27. Nemos, C.; Delage-Mourroux, R.; Jouvenot, M.; Adami, P. Onset of direct 17-beta estradiol effects on proliferation and c-fos expression during oncogenesis of endometrial glandular epithelial cells. *Exp. Cell Res.* **2004**, *296*, 109–122. [CrossRef]

28. Mahner, S.; Baasch, C.; Schwarz, J.; Hein, S.; Wölber, L.; Jänicke, F.; Milde-Langosch, K. C-Fos expression is a molecular predictor of progression and survival in epithelial ovarian carcinoma. *Br. J. Cancer* **2008**, *99*, 1269–1275. [CrossRef]

29. Krämer, A.; Green, J.; Pollard, J., Jr.; Tugendreich, S. Causal analysis approaches in ingenuity pathway analysis. *Bioinformatics* **2014**, *30*, 523–530. [CrossRef]

30. Gilmore, T.D.; Gerondakis, S. The c-Rel Transcription Factor in Development and Disease. *Genes Cancer* **2011**, *2*, 695–711. [CrossRef]

31. Pallares, J.; Martínez-Guitarte, J.L.; Dolcet, X.; Llobet, D.; Rue, M.; Palacios, J.; Prat, J.; Matias-Guiu, X. Abnormalities in the NF-κB family and related proteins in endometrial carcinoma. *J. Pathol.* **2004**, *204*, 569–577. [CrossRef]

32. Lecarpentier, Y.; Schussler, O.; Hébert, J.-L.; Vallée, A. Multiple Targets of the Canonical WNT/β-Catenin Signaling in Cancers. *Front. Oncol.* **2019**, *9*. [CrossRef] [PubMed]

33. Morin, P.J. beta-catenin signaling and cancer. *Bioessays News Rev. Mol. Cell. Dev. Biol.* **1999**, *21*, 1021–1030. [CrossRef]

34. Chen, Y.; Song, W. Wnt/catenin β1/microRNA 183 predicts recurrence and prognosis of patients with colorectal cancer. *Oncol Lett.* **2018**, *15*, 4451–4456. [CrossRef] [PubMed]

35. Matsuzaki, S.; Darcha, C. Involvement of the Wnt/beta-Catenin Signaling Pathway in the Cellular and Molecular Mechanisms of Fibrosis in Endometriosis. *PLoS ONE* **2013**, *8*, e76808. [CrossRef] [PubMed]

36. Yang, Y.-M.; Yang, W.-X. Epithelial-to-mesenchymal transition in the development of endometriosis. *Oncotarget* **2017**, *8*, 41679–41689. [CrossRef]

37. Kischel, P.; Waltregny, D.; Dumont, B.; Turtoi, A.; Greffe, Y.; Kirsch, S.; De Pauw, E.; Castronovo, V. Versican overexpression in human breast cancer lesions: Known and new isoforms for stromal tumor targeting. *Int. J. Cancer* **2010**, *126*, 640–650. [CrossRef]

38. Du, W.W.; Yang, W.; Yee, A.J. Roles of versican in cancer biology—Tumorigenesis, progression and metastasis. *Histol. Histopathol.* **2013**, *28*, 701–713. [CrossRef]

39. Andersson-Sjöland, A.; Hallgren, O.; Rolandsson, S.; Weitoft, M.; Tykesson, E.; Larsson-Callerfelt, A.K.; Rydell-Törmänen, K.; Bjermer, L.; Malmström, A.; Karlsson, J.C.; et al. Versican in inflammation and tissue remodeling: The impact on lung disorders. *Glycobiology* **2015**, *25*, 243–251. [CrossRef]

40. Miyazaki, Y.; Horie, A.; Tani, H.; Ueda, M.; Okunomiya, A.; Suginami, K.; Kondoh, E.; Baba, T.; Konishi, I.; Shinomura, T.; et al. Versican V1 in human endometrial epithelial cells promotes BeWo spheroid adhesion in vitro. *Reproduction* **2019**, *157*, 53. [CrossRef]

41. Kodama, J.; Kusumoto, T.; Seki, N.; Matsuo, T.; Ojima, Y.; Nakamura, K.; Hongo, A.; Hiramatsu, Y. Prognostic significance of stromal versican expression in human endometrial cancer. *Ann. Oncol.* **2007**, *18*, 269–274. [CrossRef]

42. AlKusayer, G.M.; Pon, J.R.; Peng, B.; Klausen, C.; Lisonkova, S.; Kinloch, M.; Yong, P.; Muhammad, E.M.S.; Leung, P.C.K.; Bedaiwy, M.A. HOXB4 Immunoreactivity in Endometrial Tissues From Women With or Without Endometriosis. *Reprod. Sci.* **2017**. [CrossRef]

43. Ozkan, Z.S.; Cilgin, H.; Simsek, M.; Cobanoglu, B.; Ilhan, N. Investigation of apelin expression in endometriosis. *J. Reprod. Infertil.* **2013**, *14*, 50–55.

44. Luo, Q.; Ning, W.; Wu, Y.; Zhu, X.; Jin, F.; Sheng, J.; Huang, H. Altered expression of interleukin-18 in the ectopic and eutopic endometrium of women with endometriosis. *J. Reprod. Immunol.* **2006**, *72*, 108–117. [CrossRef] [PubMed]

45. Jones, R.K.; Bulmer, J.N.; Searle, R.F. Immunohistochemical characterization of proliferation, oestrogen receptor and progesterone receptor expression in endometriosis: Comparison of eutopic and ectopic endometrium with normal cycling endometrium. *Hum. Reprod.* **1995**, *10*, 3272–3279. [CrossRef] [PubMed]

46. Xiao, Y.; Yang, X.L.; Sun, X.; Peng, C.; Li, X.; Wang, M.; Zhou, Y.F. [Expression of integrin beta3 and osteopontin in endometrium of patients with adenomyosis]. *Zhonghua Fu Chan Ke Za Zhi* **2009**, *44*, 354–358. [PubMed]

47. Joshi, N.R.; Miyadahira, E.H.; Afshar, Y.; Jeong, J.W.; Young, S.L.; Lessey, B.A.; Serafini, P.C.; Fazleabas, A.T. Progesterone Resistance in Endometriosis Is Modulated by the Altered Expression of MicroRNA-29c and FKBP4. *J. Clin. Endocrinol. Metab.* **2017**, *102*, 141–149. [CrossRef] [PubMed]

48. Hapangama, D.K.; Raju, R.S.; Valentijn, A.J.; Barraclough, D.; Hart, A.; Turner, M.A.; Platt-Higgins, A.; Barraclough, R.; Rudland, P.S. Aberrant expression of metastasis-inducing proteins in ectopic and matched eutopic endometrium of women with endometriosis: Implications for the pathogenesis of endometriosis. *Hum. Reprod.* **2012**, *27*, 394–407. [CrossRef] [PubMed]

49. Bulun, S.E.; Yang, S.; Fang, Z.; Gurates, B.; Tamura, M.; Zhou, J.; Sebastian, S. Role of aromatase in endometrial disease. *J. Steroid Biochem. Mol. Biol.* **2001**, *79*, 19–25. [CrossRef]

50. Ebert, A.D.; Bartley, J.; David, M. Aromatase inhibitors and cyclooxygenase-2 (COX-2) inhibitors in endometriosis: New questions—Old answers? *Eur. J. Obstet. Gynecol. Reprod. Biol.* **2005**, *122*, 144–150. [CrossRef]

51. Simmen, F.A.; Su, Y.; Xiao, R.; Zeng, Z.; Simmen, R.C.M. The Krüppel-like factor 9 (KLF9) network in HEC-1-A endometrial carcinoma cells suggests the carcinogenic potential of dys-regulated KLF9 expression. *Reprod. Biol. Endocrinol.* **2008**, *6*, 41. [CrossRef]

52. Pabona, J.M.; Simmen, F.A.; Nikiforov, M.A.; Zhuang, D.; Shankar, K.; Velarde, M.C.; Zelenko, Z.; Giudice, L.C.; Simmen, R.C. Kruppel-like factor 9 and progesterone receptor coregulation of decidualizing endometrial stromal cells: Implications for the pathogenesis of endometriosis. *J. Clin. Endocrinol. Metab.* **2012**, *97*, E376–E392. [CrossRef] [PubMed]

53. Heard, M.E.; Simmons, C.D.; Simmen, F.A.; Simmen, R.C. Kruppel-like factor 9 deficiency in uterine endometrial cells promotes ectopic lesion establishment associated with activated notch and hedgehog signaling in a mouse model of endometriosis. *Endocrinology* **2014**, *155*, 1532–1546. [CrossRef] [PubMed]

54. Signorile, P.G.; Baldi, A. Looking for an effective and non-invasive diagnostic test for endometriosis: Where are we? *Ann. Transl. Med.* **2018**, *17*, S106. [CrossRef] [PubMed]

55. Bockaj, M.; Fung, B.; Tsoulis, M.; Foster, W.G.; Soleymani, L. Method for Electrochemical Detection of Brain Derived Neurotrophic Factor (BDNF) in Plasma. *Anal. Chem.* **2018**, *90*, 8561–8566. [CrossRef] [PubMed]

56. Takai, N.; Miyazaki, T.; Fujisawa, K.; Nasu, K.; Hamanaka, R.; Miyakawa, I. Polo-like kinase (PLK) expression in endometrial carcinoma. *Cancer Lett.* **2001**, *169*, 41–49. [CrossRef]

57. Takai, N.; Miyazaki, T.; Fujisawa, K.; Nasu, K.; Hamanaka, R.; Miyakawa, I. Expression of polo-like kinase in ovarian cancer is associated with histological grade and clinical stage. *Cancer Lett.* **2001**, *164*, 41–49. [CrossRef]

58. de Cárcer, G. The Mitotic Cancer Target Polo-Like Kinase 1: Oncogene or Tumor Suppressor? *Genes* **2019**, *10*, 208. [CrossRef]

59. Fu, Z.; Wen, D. The Emerging Role of Polo-Like Kinase 1 in Epithelial-Mesenchymal Transition and Tumor Metastasis. *Cancers (Basel)* **2017**, *9*, 131. [CrossRef]

60. Tang, L.; Wang, T.-T.; Wu, Y.-T.; Zhou, C.-Y.; Huang, H.-F. High expression levels of cyclin B1 and Polo-like kinase 1 in ectopic endometrial cells associated with abnormal cell cycle regulation of endometriosis. *Fertil. Steril.* **2009**, *91*, 979–987. [CrossRef]

61. Gutteridge, R.E.A.; Ndiaye, M.A.; Liu, X.; Ahmad, N. Plk1 Inhibitors in Cancer Therapy: From Laboratory to Clinics. *Mol. Cancer Ther.* **2016**, *15*, 1427–1435. [CrossRef]

62. Zhou, B.-B.S.; Elledge, S.J. The DNA damage response: Putting checkpoints in perspective. *Nature* **2000**, *408*, 433–439. [CrossRef] [PubMed]

63. Vassileva, V.; Millar, A.; Briollais, L.; Chapman, W.; Bapat, B. Genes involved in DNA repair are mutational targets in endometrial cancers with microsatellite instability. *Cancer Res.* **2002**, *62*, 4095–4099. [PubMed]

64. Itamochi, H.; Nishimura, M.; Oumi, N.; Kato, M.; Oishi, T.; Shimada, M.; Sato, S.; Naniwa, J.; Sato, S.; Kudoh, A.; et al. Checkpoint Kinase Inhibitor AZD7762 Overcomes Cisplatin Resistance in Clear Cell Carcinoma of the Ovary. *Int. J. Gynecol. Cancer* **2014**, *24*, 61–69. [CrossRef] [PubMed]

65. Daniel, J.A.; Pellegrini, M.; Lee, J.-H.; Paull, T.T.; Feigenbaum, L.; Nussenzweig, A. Multiple autophosphorylation sites are dispensable for murine ATM activation in vivo. *J. Cell. Biol.* **2008**, *183*, 777–783. [CrossRef] [PubMed]

66. Smith, J.; Mun Tho, L.; Xu, N.; A. Gillespie, D. Chapter 3—The ATM–Chk2 and ATR–Chk1 Pathways in DNA Damage Signaling and Cancer. In *Advances in Cancer Research*; Vande Woude, G.F., Klein, G., Eds.; Academic Press: Cambridge, MA, USA, 2010; Volume 108, pp. 73–112.

67. Takeuchi, M.; Tanikawa, M.; Nagasaka, K.; Oda, K.; Kawata, Y.; Oki, S.; Agapiti, C.; Sone, K.; Miyagawa, Y.; Hiraike, H.; et al. Anti-Tumor Effect of Inhibition of DNA Damage Response Proteins, ATM and ATR, in Endometrial Cancer Cells. *Cancers (Basel)* **2019**, *11*, 1913. [CrossRef] [PubMed]

68. Smith, J.R.; Hayman, G.T.; Wang, S.J.; Laulederkind, S.J.F.; Hoffman, M.J.; Kaldunski, M.L.; Tutaj, M.; Thota, J.; Nalabolu, H.S.; Ellanki, S.L.R.; et al. The Year of the Rat: The Rat Genome Database at 20: A multi-species knowledgebase and analysis platform. *Nucleic Acids Res.* **2020**, *48*, D731–D742. [CrossRef]

69. Sabbadin, C.; Andrisani, A.; Ambrosini, G.; Bordin, L.; Donà, G.; Manso, J.; Ceccato, F.; Scaroni, C.; Armanini, D. Aldosterone in Gynecology and Its Involvement on the Risk of Hypertension in Pregnancy. *Front. Endocrinol.* **2019**, *10*, 575. [CrossRef]

70. Letsiou, S.; Peterse, D.P.; Fassbender, A.; Hendriks, M.M.; van den Broek, N.J.; Berger, R.; Dorien, F.O.; Vanhie, A.; Vodolazkaia, A.; Van Langendonckt, A.; et al. Endometriosis is associated with aberrant metabolite profiles in plasma. *Fertil. Steril.* **2017**, *107*, 699–706.e696. [CrossRef]

Assessment of Coagulation Parameters in Women Affected by Endometriosis: Validation Study and Systematic Review of the Literature

Jessica Ottolina [1], Ludovica Bartiromo [1], Carolina Dolci [1], Noemi Salmeri [1],
Matteo Schimberni [1], Roberta Villanacci [1], Paola Viganò [2,*] and Massimo Candiani [1]

[1] Gynecology/Obstetrics Unit, IRCCS San Raffaele Scientific Institute, 20132 Milan, Italy;
ottolina.jessica@hsr.it (J.O.); bartiromo.ludovica@hsr.it (L.B.); dolci.carolina@hsr.it (C.D.);
salmeri.noemi@hsr.it (N.S.); schimberni.matteo@hsr.it (M.S.); villanacci.roberta@hsr.it (R.V.);
candiani.massimo@hsr.it (M.C.)
[2] Reproductive Sciences Lab, Division of Genetics and Cell Biology, IRCCS San Raffaele Scientific Institute,
20132 Milan, Italy
* Correspondence: vigano.paola@hsr.it

Abstract: The presence of endometriosis determines an inflammatory response locally. The objective of this validation study and systematic review was to assess systemic levels of coagulation and inflammatory parameters in women with or without the disease. We conducted a retrospective analysis of a database prospectively collected from January 2017 to February 2020 including $n = 572$ women who underwent laparoscopic surgery for endometriosis (cases, $n = 324$) or other benign gynecologic diseases (controls, $n = 248$). Inflammatory markers and coagulation parameters were determined. An advanced systematic search of the literature on the same parameters was conducted up to April 2020. A significantly higher neutrophil count was found in endometriosis patients. Patients with endometriomas and stage III–IV disease had a significantly lower absolute lymphocyte count and shortened activated partial thromboplastin time (aPTT) values. In the final regression model, aPTT retained significant predictive value for stage III–IV endometriosis (odds ratio (OR) = 0.002, 95% confidence interval (CI) = 0.00–0.445; $p = 0.024$). Results from the $n = 14$ included studies in the systematic review are characterized by a high variability, but some consistency has been found for alterations in thrombin time, platelet-to-lymphocyte ratio, and neutrophil count associated with endometriosis. Modest systemic changes of some inflammatory and coagulation parameters are associated with endometriosis. Indeed, all the modifications detected are still within the normal reference intervals, explaining the high heterogeneity among studies.

Keywords: endometriosis; coagulation; thrombin time; activated partial thromboplastin time; platelet-to-lymphocyte ratio; neutrophil-to-lymphocyte ratio

1. Introduction

Endometriosis, defined as the presence of endometrial tissue and fibrosis located outside the uterine cavity, is a common chronic disease that affects around 10% of women of reproductive age and is associated with infertility and pelvic pain [1–4]. Traditionally defined as a hormonal disease with an increased local production of estrogens due to aberrant steroidogenesis, it is also characterized by features of a pelvic chronic inflammatory condition. The presence of ectopic tissue in the peritoneal cavity is associated with overproduction of pro-inflammatory and pro-fibrotic cytokines and chemokines (i.e., interleukin (IL)-1β, IL-6, tumor necrosis factor (TNF)-α, and transforming growth factor-β (TGF-β)) detected in endometriotic lesions, endometriotic cyst fluid, and peritoneal fluid [5–8].

Macrophages infiltrating the ectopic lesions express typical markers of alternative activation, favoring the growth of the lesions and promoting their angiogenesis. Some inflammatory parameters, such as the neutrophil-to-lymphocyte ratio (NLR), have also been found elevated in the peripheral blood in patients with some forms of the disease [9,10]. The close association of inflammatory conditions and coagulatory processes has been known for a long time [11]. Platelets are the first immunomodulatory cells at the site of injury and inflammation, providing a functional link between host response and coagulation. Monocytes and neutrophils contribute to coagulation by the expression of tissue factor [7,8], which is upregulated upon inflammation. Other cells of the circulation and vasculature are altered by inflammatory conditions toward a pro-thrombotic state, as well. Moreover, in their activated state, neutrophils are capable of expelling neutrophil extracellular traps, which exert antibacterial functions, but also induce a strong coagulatory response. In line with the presence of a cross-talk between these two systems, platelet count (PLC) has been found to be increased in patients affected by endometriosis [12,13], while activated partial thromboplastin time (aPTT) and thrombin time (TT) were shown to be shortened [12,14]. In 2018, our group specifically demonstrated that endometriosis patients had a significantly shorter aPTT than women not affected by the disease and, in the subgroup analysis, women with ovarian disease had significantly shortened aPTT values in comparison to women without this form. Furthermore, both platelet-to-lymphocyte ratio (PLR) and aPTT were shown to be altered in the less severe forms. Since endometriotic cells express tissue factor (TF), these alterations were suggested to represent the subtle manifestation of the activation of this factor in the lesions and were portrayed in the context of angiogenesis and, thus, the development and progression of the disease [15]. Based on this evidence, coagulation and inflammatory parameters have also been proposed as systemic biomarkers for the presence of endometriosis. However, although their values seem to be significantly different from controls, they still remain in the normal range. In light of these data, other evidence is needed in order to confirm the presence of subtle alterations of coagulation parameters in endometriosis before setting up investigations on the pathogenetic and clinical significance of these findings. We have herein analyzed systemic levels of coagulation and inflammatory parameters in a validation study including women with or without endometriosis undergoing gynecologic pelvic surgery. In addition, to offer a general view of available data, we systematically reviewed and compared our findings with results from the current literature focused on this topic.

2. Materials and Methods

2.1. Retrospective Case–Control Study

This study was based on a retrospective analysis of a surgical database prospectively collected from January 2017 to February 2020 at San Raffaele Scientific Institute in Milan, Italy. All patients had a surgical indication for gynecologic diseases and underwent laparoscopic surgery. All participants met the following inclusion criteria: non-pregnant, reproductive-age women; normal hepatic and renal function tests; and a surgical indication for endometriosis or other benign gynecologic diseases. Women with coagulation disorders, autoimmune diseases, diagnosis of uterine or ovarian malignancy, or concomitant use of antiplatelet or anticoagulant therapy at the time of surgery were excluded. Women whose data on coagulation status were not available were also excluded. Information about age, body mass index (BMI), smoking status, medical history, previous history of gynecological surgery, intraoperative findings, histopathological diagnosis, and routine blood tests were collected. The routine preoperative tests included complete blood count parameters, NLR, PLR, PT (prothrombin time) ratio, aPTT ratio, and international normalized ratio (INR). A peripheral blood sample (2 mL) was obtained from the median cubital vein of each patient and mixed with 3.2% citric acid for anticoagulation purposes. All blood analyses were obtained at a maximum of 1 month before surgery. The NLR was obtained by dividing the absolute neutrophil count by the absolute lymphocyte count, while the PLR was obtained by dividing the absolute platelet count by the absolute lymphocyte count. All blood analyses were done during either the follicular or the luteal phase of the cycle before surgery. The case group included patients with a diagnosis of endometriosis. The stage of endometriosis was established according to the revised American Fertility Society (r-AFS) classification [16]. Endometriotic lesions were classified according to their phenotype as ovarian endometrioma (OMA), deep infiltrating endometriosis (DIE), and superficial peritoneal endometriosis (SPE) [17]. Since these phenotypes are frequently combined, patients were assigned to the group corresponding to the most severe lesion detected, with the severity scale going from the least to the most severe as follows: SPE, OMA, DIE. The control group consisted of women with a surgical diagnosis of tubal pathology and ovarian benign cysts. Both the surgical and the histopathological examinations confirmed no evidence of endometriosis in the control population. According to the abovementioned selection criteria, $n = 572$ women were included: $n = 324$ had a diagnosis of endometriosis, and $n = 248$ had a diagnosis of other gynecologic diseases. All the women signed a written informed consent to record their data for scientific purposes. The Institutional Review Board of our Institution approved the study (Comitato Etico Ospedale San Raffaele; No. 01END, approved 12 April 2012).

2.2. Systematic Review of the Literature

The study was registered and accepted for inclusion in the database PROSPERO (ID CRD42020171524). The systematic review was carried out in accordance with the methods proposed by Preferred Reporting Item for Systematic Reviews and Meta-analysis (PRISMA) guidelines [18]. We performed an advanced, systematic search of online medical databases PubMed and Medline using the following keywords: "endometriosis" in combination with "thrombin", "thrombin time", "thromboplastin", "partial thromboplastin time", "activated partial thromboplastin time", "INR", "international normalized ratio", "coagulation/blood coagulation", "platelets/blood platelets", "lymphocyte", "platelets-to-lymphocyte ratio/platelets-lymphocyte ratio", or "neutrophil-to-lymphocyte ratio/ neutrophil-lymphocyte ratio". To optimize search output, we used specific tools available in each database, such as Medical Subject Headings (MeSH) terms (PubMed/Medline). The EndNote software (available online: https://endnote.com, accessed on 31 May 2020) was used to remove duplicate articles. Only full-length manuscripts written in English up to April 2020 were considered. We checked all citations found by title and abstract to establish the eligibility of the source and obtained the full text of eligible articles. We also performed a manual scan of the references list of the review articles to identify any additional relevant citations. Three review authors (J.O., M.S., and L.B.) independently assessed the risk of bias for each study using the risk-of-bias tool for case–control studies developed by clarity group [19]. We assessed the risk of bias according to the following domains: i) Can we be confident in the assessment of exposure?; ii) Can we be confident that cases had developed the outcome of interest and controls had not?; iii) Were the cases properly selected?; iv) Were the controls properly selected?; v) Were cases and controls matched according to important prognostic variables or was statistical adjustment carried out for those variables?. We graded each potential source of bias as Definitely yes (low risk of bias), Probably yes (Moderate risk of bias), Probably no (Serious risk of bias), or Definitely no (Critical, high risk of bias). We summarized the risk of bias judgments across different studies for each of the domains listed.

2.3. Statistical Analysis

Statistical analysis was performed using IBM SPSS Statistics, Version Chicago 24.0 (IBM Corp. Realesd 2016. Version 24.0. Armonk, NY, USA). Differences in systemic inflammatory response markers between cases and controls were investigated. Coagulation parameters were analyzed including only patients who were not taking any hormonal therapy at the time of surgery. Categorical variables were expressed as absolute value and percentages, and between-groups comparisons were evaluated using the Pearson's chi square test with a Monte Carlo approximation at 95% confidence interval (CI). Continuous and normally distributed variables were presented as mean, range, and standard deviation (SD), and between-groups differences were investigated using the independent Student's t-test. Subgroup analyses according to the stage and type of endometriosis were performed using the one-way analysis of variance (ANOVA) test. Before conducting means comparisons, the assumption of homogeneity of variances was tested and satisfied based on Levene's F tests. In order to evaluate the nature of the differences between the means further, each statistically significant ANOVA test was followed-up with a Bonferroni's post hoc test. A binary logistic regression was conducted in order to evaluate coagulation and inflammatory parameters as independent predictor factors of endometriosis. Adjusted odds ratios with 95% CI were evaluated when a statistically significant correlation was found. p-values < 0.05 were considered statistically significant.

3. Results

3.1. Results of the Retrospective Analysis

Of the $n = 324$ women affected by endometriosis, $n = 85$ were stage I or II (26.2%) disease, whereas the remaining $n = 239$ patients (73.76%) were stages III or IV. According to the type of disease, $n = 214$ patients (66%) were classified as having OMA, $n = 69$ patients (21.3%) as having DIE, and $n = 41$ patients (12.7%) as having SPE. Endometriosis could not be detected in $n = 248$ women. These cases were used as controls. The main diagnosis of this group was as follows: ovarian dermoids ($n = 110$), serous or seromucinous ovarian cysts ($n = 77$), tubal pathology ($n = 43$), and normal pelvis ($n = 18$). The baseline characteristics of patients with and without endometriosis are shown in Table 1.

Table 1. Baseline characteristics of the endometriosis and control groups.

Baseline Characteristics	Endometriosis Group ($n = 324$)	Control Group ($n = 248$)	p-Value
Age (years)	33.53 ± 5.51	31.15 ± 7.9	**0.001**
BMI (kg/m^2)	21.37 ± 3.9	22.29 ± 4.0	**0.028**
Smoking habit	28 (14.7%)	35 (18.3%)	0.09
Indication for surgery			
Symptoms	174 (55.4%)	69 (29%)	
Offspring desire	113 (36%)	56 (23.5%)	**0.001**
Occasional findings	12 (3.8%)	104 (43.7%)	
Symptoms and offspring desire	15 (4.8%)	8 (3.4%)	
Prophylactic surgery		1 (0.4%)	
HT before surgery	128 (39.5%)	64 (25.8%)	0.43
Previous pelvic surgery	82 (25.9%)	85 (34.6%)	**0.027**

Note: values are mean ± SD or absolute value (%). Abbreviations: BMI, body mass index; HT, hormonal therapy. p-values < 0.05 were considered statistically significant (bold values).

In line with previous observations [20], patients with endometriosis had a significantly lower BMI compared with controls; moreover, patients with endometriosis were older than non-endometriosis patients. Results from comparisons of systemic inflammatory parameters between cases and controls are reported in Table 2. A significantly higher neutrophil count was found in patients with endometriosis when compared to controls. No difference in lymphocytes count and NLR was detected between the two groups. When we considered the various manifestations of endometriosis separately, we found that women with ovarian disease had a borderline significant lower absolute lymphocyte count in comparison with controls, SPE group, and DIE group. In addition, women with stage III to IV disease had a slightly lower lymphocyte count than those with stage I to II disease, and the difference reached statistical significance. In order to evaluate the real effect of endometriosis on the coagulation status, we decided to include in the comparisons only cases ($n = 163$) and controls ($n = 96$) who were not taking any hormonal therapy at the time of surgery because of the well-known impact of the treatment on the coagulation parameters [21,22]. Intergroups differences of coagulation parameters and inflammatory response markers in patients without hormonal therapy are shown in Table 3.

Table 2. Systemic inflammatory response parameters according to the different stage and type of endometriosis versus controls.

Diagnosis	L (10^9/L)	N (10^9/L)	NLR
Endometriosis ($n = 324$)	2.05 ± 0.53	4.30 ± 1.51	2.21 ± 0.95
Controls ($n = 248$)	2.12 ± 0.55	4.03 ± 1.57	2.05 ± 1.50
	$p = 0.13$	$p = \mathbf{0.038}$	$p = 0.13$
OMA ($n = 214$)	2.01 ± 0.52	4.32 ± 1.51	2.27 ± 0.97
DIE ($n = 69$)	2.19 ± 0.64	4.36 ± 1.51	2.12 ± 0.95
SPE ($n = 41$)	2.04 ± 0.56	4.08 ± 1.55	2.04 ± 0.78
Controls ($n = 248$)	2.12 ± 0.55	4.03 ± 1.57	2.05 ± 1.50
	$p = \mathbf{0.049}$	$p = 0.15$	$p = 0.27$
Stage I–II ($n = 85$)	2.16 ± 0.56	4.29 ± 1.49	2.06 ± 0.81
Stage III–IV ($n = 239$)	2.01 ± 0.52	4.30 ± 1.52	2.25 ± 0.99
Controls ($n = 248$)	2.12 ± 0.55	4.03 ± 1.57	2.05 ± 1.50
	$p = \mathbf{0.032}$	$p = 0.11$	$p = 0.15$

Note: values are mean ± SD or absolute value (%). Abbreviations: OMA, ovarian endometrioma; DIE, deep infiltrating endometriosis; SPE, superficial peritoneal endometriosis; N, neutrophil count; L, lymphocyte count; NLR, neutrophil-to-lymphocyte ratio. p-values < 0.05 were considered statistically significant (bold values).

For inflammatory parameters, in line with the above reported results, patients with OMAs had significantly lower absolute lymphocytes count if compared to both controls and DIE group. No difference in neutrophils count and NLR was detected among the endometriosis phenotypes. Focusing on the coagulation parameters, a significant between-group difference emerged in aPTT values, as women with OMA disease had shortened aPTT values if compared to patients with SPE, DIE, and controls. Moreover, women with stage III–IV disease had slightly, but significantly, shorter aPTT values than those with stage I–II endometriosis or than controls. No difference was found for platelet count or PLR among the various groups. Boxplots of levels of coagulation parameters and systemic inflammatory response markers according to the different stages of endometriosis are presented in Figure 1. A logistic regression was conducted in order to evaluate whether a certain coagulation or inflammatory status could be a predictor of the disease. The binary logistic regression was able to correctly classify 78.5% of cases ($R^2 = 0.05$, $\chi^2(1) = 5.29$, $p = 0.021$). In the final regression model, aPTT retained significant predictive value for stages III–IV endometriosis ($b = -6.091$, standard error (SE) = 2.695; OR = 0.002, 95% CI = 0.00–0.445; $p = 0.024$) (Table 4).

Table 3. Coagulation parameters and systemic inflammatory response markers according to the different stage and type of endometriosis versus controls, excluding patients taking hormonal drugs.

Diagnosis	PT Ratio	aPTT Ratio	INR	PLC (10⁹/L)	L (10⁹/L)	N (10⁹/L)	NLR	PLR
OMA (n = 118)	1.05 ± 0.06	1.01 ± 0.07	1.06 ± 0.07	253.5 ± 62.0	1.93 ± 0.49	3.99 ± 1.48	2.18 ± 1.03	69.81 ± 25.6
DIE (n = 28)	1.05 ± 0.06	1.05 ± 0.08	1.05 ± 0.07	268.7 ± 73.0	2.29 ± 0.64	3.96 ± 1.27	1.79 ± 0.60	72.43 ± 22.7
SPE (n = 17)	1.07 ± 0.09	1.04 ± 0.07	1.07 ± 0.12	254.5 ± 53.1	1.97 ± 0.33	3.51 ± 1.26	1.80 ± 0.63	81.43 ± 33.0
Controls (n = 96)	1.05 ± 0.06	1.03 ± 0.06	1.06 ± 0.06	249.4 ± 50.2	2.11 ± 0.49	3.99 ± 1.57	1.99 ± 0.96	72.93 ± 37.6
	$p = 0.61$	$p = \mathbf{0.049}$	$p = 0.59$	$p = 0.50$	$p = \mathbf{0.003}$ [b]	$p = 0.64$	$p = 0.117$	$p = 0.52$
Stage I–II (n = 35)	1.06 ± 0.08	1.05 ± 0.08	1.06 ± 0.09	262.3 ± 64.7	2.12 ± 0.59	3.77 ± 1.36	1.83 ± 0.62	76.55 ± 27.4
Stage III–IV (n = 128)	1.02 ± 0.07	1.01 ± 0.07	1.06 ± 0.06	254.6 ± 62.8	1.97 ± 0.49	3.98 ± 1.45	2.14 ± 1.01	70.09 ± 25.6
Controls (n = 96)	1.05 ± 0.06	1.03 ± 0.06	1.06 ± 0.06	249.4 ± 50.2	2.11 ± 0.49	3.99 ± 1.57	1.99 ± 0.96	72.93 ± 37.6
	$p = 0.78$	$p = \mathbf{0.040}$ [b]	$p = 0.82$	$p = 0.53$	$p = 0.07$	$p = 0.73$	$p = 0.18$	$p = 0.51$

Note: values are mean ± SD or absolute value (%). Abbreviations: OMA, ovarian endometrioma; DIE, deep infiltrating endometriosis; SPE, superficial peritoneal endometriosis; PT, prothrombin time; aPTT, activated partial thromboplastin time; INR, international normalized ratio; PLC, platelet count; N, neutrophil count; L, lymphocyte count; NLR, neutrophil-to-lymphocyte ratio; PLR, platelet-to-lymphocyte ratio. [b] When $p < 0.05$, a Bonferroni's post hoc test was performed for within-groups differences. p-values < 0.05 were considered statistically significant (bold values).

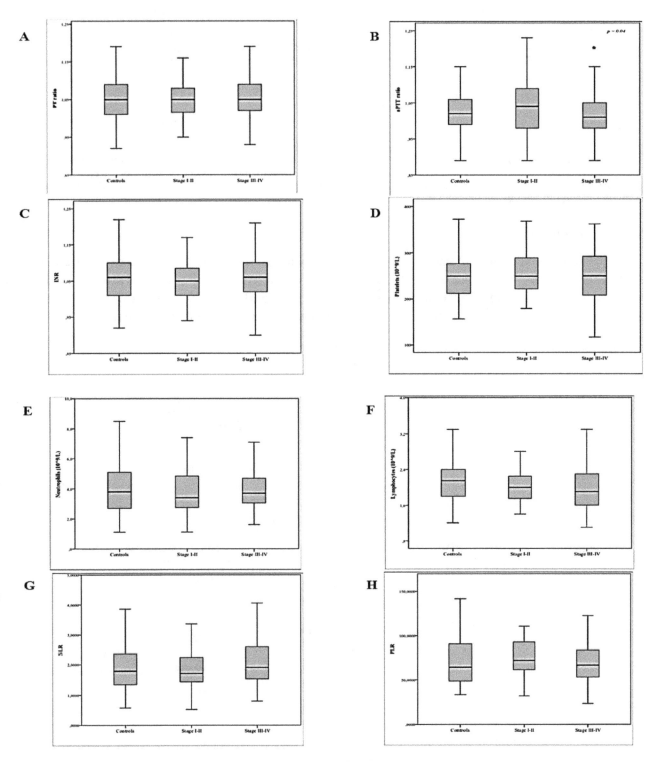

Figure 1. Boxplots of levels of coagulation parameters and systemic inflammatory response parameters according to different stages of endometriosis (n = 259). (**A**) PT, prothrombin time; (**B**) aPTT, activated partial thromboplastin time; (**C**) INR, international normalized ratio; (**D**) PLC, platelet count; (**E**) N, neutrophil count; (**F**) L, lymphocyte count; (**G**) NLR, neutrophil-to-lymphocyte ratio; (**H**) PLR, platelet-to-lymphocyte ratio. * p = 0.04.

Table 4. Logistic regression of coagulation and inflammatory parameters predicting the stage of endometriosis.

Variable	B Coefficient	SE	OR	p-Value
PT ratio	−4.084	12.301		0.74
aPTT ratio	−6.091	2.695	**0.002**	**0.024**
INR	3.611	11.279		0.75
PLC (10^9/L)	0.000	0.006		0.95
L (10^9/L)	−0.587	0.728		0.42
N (10^9/L)	0.645	1.355		0.63
NLR	1.342	1.402		0.34
PLR	−0.007	0.018		0.71

Abbreviations: SE, standard error; OR, odds ratio; PT, prothrombin time; aPTT, activated partial thromboplastin time; INR, international normalized ratio; PLC, platelet count; N, neutrophil count; L, lymphocyte count; NLR, neutrophil-to-lymphocyte ratio; PLR, platelet-to-lymphocyte ratio. p-values < 0.05 were considered statistically significant (bold values).

3.2. Results of the Systematic Review

The search revealed $n = 17$ studies eligible for inclusion in this systematic review. Of these, $n = 14$ were finally included [9,12–14,23–32]. A flow diagram of the systematic review is shown in Figure 2 (PRISMA template). The main characteristics of the included studies are summarized in Table 5. The risks of bias of the included studies are summarized in Supplementary Figure S1.

Figure 2. Flow diagram of the search strategy, screening, eligibility, and inclusion criteria.

Table 5. Main characteristics of considered studies.

Author, Years	Country	Study Design	Study Period	Cases/Controls Sample Size (n)	Age (Years)	Parameters Assessed (When)	Confounding Factors
Cho et al., 2008 [23]	South Korea	Retrospective case–control study	01/2004 12/2007	Endometriosis [1] (231)/ Benign ovarian cysts [1] (231) Healthy women [2] (384)	33.3 ± 7.3 * (Overall) 32.6 ± 7.35 * (endometriosis) 34.2 ± 8.9 * (benign ovarian cyst) 33.9 ± 5.7 * (healthy women)	Complete blood cell count, NLR, and CA125 (before surgery or as part of routine health examination [3])	Unclear
Yavuzcan et al., 2013 [25]	Turkey	Retrospective case–control study	11/2009 02/2013	Endometriosis [1] stage III/IV (61) - 33 with OMA - 28 non-OMA/Tubal ligation [1] (33)	36.21 ± 8.37 * (Overall)	Complete blood cell count, NLR, PLR, and CA125 (before surgery [3])	No
Avcioğlu et al., 2014 [26]	Turkey	Retrospective study	01/2001 06/2013	Endometriosi [1] stage III/IV (124)/Endometriosis [1] stage I/II (40)	33.7 ± 7.7 * (Overall)	Complete blood cell count, MPV, PDW, and PCT (before surgery [3])	No
Kim et al., 2014 [27]	South Korea	Retrospective study	04/2005 03/2013	Endometriosis [1] stage III (189)/Endometriosis [1] stage IV (230)	15–51 (Overall) 19-49 - 33.8 ± 6.8 * (stage III) 15-51 - 34.7 ± 7.0 * (stage IV)	Complete blood cell count, NLR, CRP, AMH, CEA, CA125, CA 19-9 (<1 month before surgery)	No
Chmaj-Wierzchowska et al., 2015 [13]	Poland	Hospital-based case-control	09/2009 11/2012	OMA [1] without coexisting foci of peritoneal endometriosis (48)/Mature teratomas [1] (38)	18–38 (Overall) 30.00 ± 4.6 * (OMA) 27.03 ± 4.52 * (teratomas)	Complete blood cell count, fibrinogen, urocortin, ghrelin, and leptin (<1 day before surgery)	No
Yang et al., 2015 [24]	China	Retrospective case–control study	01/2009 06/2012 [4]	Endometriosis [1] - 119 Stage III - 78 Stage IV/ Benign ovarian cysts [1] (102) Healthy women [2] (112)	32.58 ± 6.37 * (Overall) 32.17 ± 6.50 * (endometriosis) 32.03 ± 6.83 * (benign ovarian cyst) 33.81 ± 5.52 * (healthy women)	Complete blood cell count, PLR, and CA125 (before surgery or as part of routine health examination [3])	Unclear
Wu et al., 2015 [12]	China	Hospital-based case-control	06-12/2012	OMA [1] (50) -35 stage III -15 stage IV/Age-matched healthy women [2] (50)	23-44 - 32.9 ± 6.1 * (OMA) 20-48 - 31.4 ± 6.4 * (controls)	Complete blood cell count, aPTT, PT, TT, INR, fibrinogen, D-dimer, fasting serum glucose, and serum cortisol (before surgery [3])	Yes

Table 5. *Cont.*

Author, Years	Country	Study Design	Study Period	Cases/Controls Sample Size (n)	Age (Years)	Parameters Assessed (When)	Confounding Factors
Tokmak et al., 2016 [9]	Turkey	Retrospective case-control study	01/2008 01/2013	OMA [1](467)/Age- and BMI-matched benign ovarian cysts [1] (340)	16–50 (Overall) 18–49 – 33.7 ± 8.4 * (OMA) 16–50 - 33.9 ± 11.6 * (Controls)	Complete blood cell count, NLR, PLR, CA125, AFP, CA 19-9, CA-15.3 (<1 month before surgery)	Unclear
Ding et al., 2018 [14]	China	Cross-sectional study	04/2015 03/2016	OMA [1](100)/ Women without endometriosis (100); - 60 Healthy women [2] - 40 CINIII or ovarian teratoma [1]	21–49 (Overall) 32.0 ± 7.1 * (OMA) 33.0 ± 7.1 * (controls)	PLC, platelet activation rate, maximum platelet aggregation rate, D-dimer, fibrinogen, FDPs, sP-sel, F1 + 2, PT; TT; aPTT, INR (before surgery [3] and 3 months later only in OMA)	Unclear
Seckin et al., 2018 [28]	Turkey	Retrospective case-control study	01/2013 12/2016	OMA [1] (267)/ Benign ovarian cysts [1] (235)	15–49 – 27.1 ± 7.2 * (overall) 28.3 ± 6.6 * (cases) 25.8 ± 7.6 * (controls)	Complete blood cell count, NLR, PCT, PDW, PLR, and CA125 (before surgery [3])	Yes (only age </> 25 years)
Viganò et al., 2018 [14]	Italy	Retrospective case-control study	01/2013 12/2015	Endometriosis [1] (169) - 45 Stage I–II - 124 Stage III–IV/ Benign gynecologic pathology [1] (145)	35.8 ± 5.9 * (endometriosis) 36.9 ± 6.5 * (controls)	Complete blood cell count, NLR, PLR, TT ratio, aPTT, and INR (<1 month before surgery)	Yes
Coskun et al., 2019 [32]	Turkey	Retrospective case-control study	01/2013 01/2015	Adenomyosis [1] (84) Endometriosis [1] (102)/ Tubal ligation [1] (88)	52.9 ±7.4 * (adenomyosis) 35.3 ± 8.7 * (OMA) 37.9 ± 4.2 * (Controls)	Complete blood cell count, MPV, and CA125 (<1 week before the surgery)	Unclear
Ding et al., 2019 [30]	China	Retrospective case-control study	06/2015 06/2017	OMA [1] (226)/ Cyst group [1] (210) Tubal reanastomosis [1] (112)	35.7 ± 0.4 * (OMA) 35.9 ± 0.4 * (Cyst group) 35.8 ± 0.5 * (Controls)	Complete blood cell count, TT, PT, fibrinogen, CRP, PLR, NLR, aPTT, and CA125 (<1 month before surgery)	Yes
Turgut et al., 2019 [31]	Turkey	Retrospective case-control study	01/2012 02/2017	Endometriosis [1] (121) - 17 Stage I–II - 104 Stage III–IV/ Healthy women [2] (136)	22–53 (endometriosis) 17–51 (controls)	Complete blood cell count, MPV, and CA125 (before surgery [3])	Yes (age)

Note: * Mean ± SD. [1] Women with surgical and pathological diagnosis of endometriosis or other benign diseases/conditions with exclusion of endometriosis; [2] no surgery performed; [3] not specified when; [4] healthy women recruited only between 1/2012 and 06/2012; OMA, ovarian endometriosis; NLR, neutrophil–lymphocyte ratio; CA125, cancer antigen 125; PLR, platelet–lymphocyte ratio; MPV, mean platelet volume; PDW, platelet distribution width; PCT, plateletcrit; CPR, C-reactive protein; AMH, anti-Müllerian hormone; CEA, carcinoembryonic antigen; CA19-9, cancer antigen 19-9; aPTT, activated partial thromboplastin time; PT, prothrombin time; TT, thrombin time; INR, international normalized ratio; AFP, a- fetoprotein; CA15-3, cancer antigen 15-3; PLC, platelets; FDPs, fibrin degradation products; sP-sel, plasma-soluble P-selectin; F1 + 2, prothrombin fragment F1 + 2.

3.2.1. Coagulation Parameters in Endometriosis Patients

Table 6 shows the results of the studies that have investigated coagulation parameters in relation to the presence of endometriosis. The first studies that evaluated PLC did not find significant differences between endometriosis patients and the control groups [24,25]. The same results were obtained in other studies addressing PLC as a secondary outcome in the investigations of other coagulation parameters useful for the diagnosis of endometriosis [9,12–14,31]. In a retrospective case–control study that included women with adenomyosis, endometriosis, and a control group, Coskun et al. found a statistically higher PLC in endometriosis patients versus controls [32]. Similar results were obtained by Seckin and coworkers that, considering women with OMAs or other benign adnexal cysts, reported a significantly higher PLC in the OMA group compared to controls, and this difference remained even when considering the younger (<25 years old) and older (>25 years old) subgroups [28]. Avcioğlu et al. found that in patients with advanced endometriosis (stages III–IV), PLC was significantly higher when compared to minimal–mild endometriosis (stages I–II) and showed a significant positive correlation between PLC ($r = 0.8$; $p = 0.001$) and white blood cell (WBC) [26]. This finding was later supported by Ding et al., who reported a significantly higher PLC in women with endometriosis compared to controls and, within the OMA group, a significantly higher PLC mean value in case of severe endometriosis [30]. Opposite results were obtained by Kim and coworkers, since PLC was not significantly different in severe endometriosis [27]. Three studies have evaluated PT [12,29,30], and only Ding and coworkers showed a significantly shorter time in the OMA group compared to a benign cyst group and a control group [30]. Conversely, for TT, three studies [12,29,30] out of four showed significantly shorter values in patients affected by OMAs compared to control groups [12,14,29,30]. Three studies have evaluated differences in INR between patients with and without endometriosis finding no difference [12,14,29]. Four studies have addressed aPTT [12,14,29,30], and two of them have reported shortened aPTT in cases when compared to controls [12,14]. In particular, in our previous study, considering the various manifestations of endometriosis separately, we found that women with ovarian disease had shortened aPTT values in comparison to controls and women with SPE and DIE. In addition, women with stage I to II endometriosis had slightly shorter, but significant, aPTT values than those with stage III to IV disease [14]. In a multivariate logistic regression analysis, after controlling for potential confounders (age, parity, BMI, and smoking), aPTT retained significant predictive value for endometriosis [14]. Interestingly, in a cross-sectional study considering 100 women with OMA before and three months after surgery, Ding and colleagues found that, after the surgical removal of all visible lesions by laparoscopy, the coagulation measurements (PLC, INR, PT, aPTT, and TT) were all significantly changed suggesting a possible role for active endometriotic lesions in this modification [29].

Table 6. Systematic review: coagulation parameters of women with and without endometriosis in the included studies.

Author	Year	Study Population (n)	PT	TT	aPTT	PLC (10⁹/L)	INR
Yavuzcan et al. [25]	2013	Cases (OMA): 33				269.8 ± 65.2	
		Cases (non-OMA): 28				298.9 ± 107.8	
		Controls: 33				286.4 ± 67.6	
Avcıoğlu et al. [26]	2014	Stage I–II: 40				187 ± 36.18 *	
		Stage III–IV: 124				309.15 ± 54.43 *	
Kim et al. [27]	2014	Stage III (OMA): 189				NR	
		Stage IV (OMA): 230				NR	
Wu et al. [12]	2015	Cases (OMA): 50	NR	NR *	NR *	NR	NR
		Controls: 50	NR	NR *	NR *	NR	NR
Chmaj-Wierzchowska et al. [13]	2015	Cases (OMA): 48				267.80	
		Controls: 38				258.90	
		Cases: 197				253.25 ± 59.98	
Yang et al. [24]	2015	Benign tumor: 102				248.83 ± 61.69	
		Controls: 112				246.47 ± 52.55	
Tokmak et al. [9]	2016	Cases (OMA): 467				275.9 ± 72.1	
		Controls: 340				276.2 ± 71.3	
Seckin et al. [28]	2018	Cases (OMA): 267				292.9 ± 67.6 *	
		Controls: 235				269.7 ± 61.3 *	
Viganò et al. [14]	2018	Cases: 169		1.00 ± 0.9	1.12 ± 0.19 *	250.00 ± 55.8	0.99 ± 056
		Controls: 145		0.970 ± 0.10	1.13 ± 0.15 *	262.20 ± 63.4	0.98 ± 0.16
		Cases (OMA): 98		0.99 ± 0.06	1.08 ± 0.07 *	254.5 ± 61.47	0.99 ± 0.71
		Controls: 145		0.99 ± 0.09	1.14 ± 0.07 *	254.7 ± 58.62	0.99 ± 0.11
Ding et al. [29]	2018	Cases (OMA): 100	NR	NR *	NR	NR	NR
		Controls: 100	NR	NR *	NR	NR	NR
		Post-surgery (OMA): 100	NR *	NR *	NR *	NR *	NR *
Turgut et al. [31]	2019	Cases: 121				265 ± 86	
		Controls: 136				258 ± 70.5	
Ding et al. [30]	2019	Cases (OMA): 226	12.69 ± 0.04 *	15.42 ± 0.04 *	NR	239.8 ± 3.6 *	
		Controls: 112	12.99 ± 0.06 *	15.78 ± 0.06 *	NR	220.0 ± 5.4 *	
		Benign cyst: 210	13.00 ± 0.04 *	15.68 ± 0.05 *	NR	228.4 ± 4.0 *	
		Stage III (OMA): 91	12.64 ± 0.06	15.38 ± 0.06	35.68 ± 0.30	243.8 ± 5.4 *	
		Stage IV (OMA): 135	12.72 ± 0.05	15.44 ± 0.05	35.44 ± 0.26	237.1 ± 4.7 *	
Coskun et al. [32]	2019	Cases: 102				292.9 ± 73.9 *	
		Adenomyosis: 84				295.1 ± 77.5	
		Controls: 88				269.9 ± 59 *	

Note: * statistically significant; PT: prothrombin time; TT: thrombin time; aPTT: activated partial thromboplastin time; PLC: platelet count; INR: international normalized ratio; OMA: ovarian endometrioma; NR: not reported.

3.2.2. Systemic Inflammatory Markers in Endometriosis Patients

Results for the inflammatory markers, including neutrophils, lymphocytes, PLR, and NLR, from the systematic review are presented in Table 7. Three studies showed that neutrophil count was higher in patients with endometriosis than in women without the disease [9,23,31]. On the other hand, three studies showed no significant difference among groups, either when considering OMAs or in non-OMA patients [14,25,28]. Importantly, our present study confirmed a significantly higher neutrophil count in patients with endometriosis. Among eight studies investigating the lymphocyte count [9,14,23–25,27,28,31], only three of them reported a significantly lower mean cell count in endometriosis compared to controls [9,23,31], and no correlation between the stage of endometriosis and the lymphocyte count was observed by Kim et al. [27]. Two studies found no difference between cases and controls in terms of NLR [25,28]. In our previous study, we found no difference in NLR between women with endometriosis and controls, although, when considering the various manifestations of endometriosis separately, a significant difference among groups emerged, as women with peritoneal lesions had lower NLR compared to patients without this form [14]. On the contrary, NLR was found to be significantly increased in the endometriosis group by Cho et al., who evaluated the usefulness of NLR in diagnosing endometriosis compared to benign ovarian tumors and healthy controls [23]. The same result was subsequently confirmed by three other studies [9,30,31]. Kim and coworkers, comparing stage I–II to stage III–IV endometriosis cases who underwent laparoscopic conservative surgery for OMAs, did not find any difference in NLR [27]. Among six studies investigating PLR [9,14,24,25,28,30], results obtained were more consistent. Four groups reported a significantly higher PLR in women with endometriosis [9,24,28,30]. In our previous case–control study [14], considering the various manifestations of endometriosis separately, we found that women with stage I to II endometriosis had significantly higher PLR than those with stage III to IV disease. A higher PLR in stage III–IV of endometriosis has been reported by Yang et al., compared to benign adnexal tumors and controls [24]. Only the study by Yavuzcan et al. reported no statistically significant difference in terms of PLR between endometriosis patients and controls and among the various endometriosis subgroups [25].

Table 7. Systematic review: inflammatory parameters of women with or without endometriosis in the included studies.

Author	Year	Study Population (n)	Neutrophils 10^9/L	Lymphocytes 10^9/L	NLR	PLR
Cho et al. [23]	2008	Cases: 231	4.41 *	1.82 *	2.66 *	
		Benign tumor: 145	4.17 *	1.96 *	2.31 *	
		Controls: 384	3.6 *	1.95 *	1.99 *	
Yavuzcan et al. [25]	2013	Cases (OMA): 33	4.14 ± 1.73	2.12 ± 0.87	2.40 ± 2.04	162.84 ± 141.28
		Cases (non-OMA): 28	4.68 ± 2.18	2.02 ± 0.68	2.51 ± 1.37	159.14 ± 61.20
		Controls:33	4.50 ± 1.57	2.25 ± 0.66	2.11 ± 0.86	132.45 ± 35.74
Kim et al. [27]	2014	Stage III (OMA): 189		NR	NR	
		Stage IV (OMA):230		NR	NR	
Yang et al. [24]	2015	Cases: 197		1.91 ± 0.52		141.79 ± 51.78 *
		Benign tumor:102		2.02 ± 0.52		129.28 ± 39.20 *
		Controls: 112		2.05 ± 0.49		126.68 ± 39.67 *
Tokmak et al. [9]	2016	Cases (OMA): 467	4.8 ± 1.8 *	1.98 ± 5.92 *	2.8 ± 2.0 *	153.3 ± 71.3 *
		Controls: 340	3.8 ± 1.2 *	2.41 ± 7.17 *	1.7 ± 0.5 *	122.4 ± 42.7 *
Viganò et al. [14]	2018	Cases: 169	3.76 ± 1.34	2.04 ± 0.56	NR	NR
		Cases (OMA): 98	3.9 ± 1.62	2.02 ± 0.66	2.08 ± 1.01	135.18 ± 68.69
		Controls:145	3.99 ± 1.6	1.97 ± 0.55	2.16 ± 1.25	130.65 ± 52.8
Seckin et al. [28]	2018	Cases: 267	4.6 ± 1.8	2.2 ± 0.6	2.3 ± 1.3	142.3 ± 48.4 *
		Controls:235	4.5 ± 2.1	2.2 ± 0.7	2.1 ± 1.2	129.3 ± 40.4 *
Turgut et al. [31]	2019	Cases: 121	4.4 ± 1.9 *	2 ± 0.8 *	2.18 ± 0.86 *	
		Controls:136	3.55 ± 1.53 *	2.15 ± 0.8 *	1.70 ± 0.8 *	
Ding et al. [30]	2019	Cases: 226 (OMA)			2.56 ± 0.07 *	146.4 ± 2.8 *
		Benign cyst: 210			2.34 ± 0.07 *	137.7 ± 3.4 *

Note: * p-value statistically significant; OMA: ovarian endometrioma; NLR: neutrophil-to-lymphocyte ratio; PLR: platelet-to-lymphocyte ratio; NR: not reported.

4. Discussion

We have herein confirmed our previous results documenting the present of subtle alterations of the peripheral coagulation system in patients with endometriosis. More specifically, in the validation study, the sub-analysis according to the various forms of the disease showed a shortened aPTT to be associated with the presence of moderate–severe endometriosis and with the presence of OMAs. This result is in line with previous evidence demonstrating a shortened aPTT in women with endometriosis, in particular with the ovarian form [12,14].

Results from the systematic reviews are characterized by a high variability, but a certain rate of consistency has been found also for alterations in TT and PLR in association with endometriosis.

In relation to the inflammatory parameters, we found a significantly higher neutrophil count in patients with endometriosis and a significantly lower absolute lymphocyte count in women affected by OMAs. We failed to detect similar results in our previous study thus supporting again the high variability of the observations. On the other hand, in line with our present findings, some groups had already reported that neutrophil count and NLR were significantly increased in the endometriosis group [9,23,30,31].

Variability of the results among the different studies may have different explanations. First, numbers of cases enrolled in the various studies are limited and, given the small changes observed among groups, the possibility of detecting significant differences is reduced. This is the reason for our choice to proceed with a systematic review. Second, the control groups are quite different among the studies, from only surgical patients as controls, or comparing women with other benign ovarian disease to endometriosis. A benign ovarian cyst may be responsible of an inflammatory pelvic environment as well, with a consequential alteration in inflammatory markers. Third, endometriosis is characterized by a plethora of manifestations and forms that are differently represented in the selected studies; some authors considered both minimal–mild and moderate–severe endometriosis, while other studies included only women with an advanced disease (stages III–IV) [27,30]. Similarly, some studies included only women without an ovarian disease while others considered only OMA patients [9,27,30] and others a combination of the two forms [25].

Overall, these results tend to confirm the idea that women with endometriosis are characterized by systemic changes of some inflammatory parameters [1,20,33,34] as well as by a modest change of the coagulation function. Indeed, all the modifications of the coagulation process detected are still within the normal reference intervals. Interestingly, Ding and coworkers have shown that three months after surgery for the removal of endometriotic lesions, the coagulation measurements were all significantly changed, suggesting a possible role for active endometriosis in the alterations of coagulation parameters, either locally or systemically [29].

The subtle variations observed in affected patients may be due to the TF pathway activation at the level of endometriotic lesions. Immunohistochemical studies revealed a marked elevation of TF expression pattern in eutopic and ectopic endometrium from women with endometriosis [35]. Moreover, the protease-activated receptor 2 (PAR-2), which is activated by TF/FVIIa, was as well demonstrated to be highly upregulated in the glandular epithelium of eutopic endometrium. Hence, both TF and the PAR-2 receptor are strategically poised for angiogenic and inflammatory signaling in endometriotic lesions [36,37]. Once TF is exposed to blood, it starts a reaction cascade that culminates in the increased production of thrombin. A shortened aPTT is correlated with elevated levels of coagulation factors (except factor VII) and of all markers for increased thrombin generation in plasma (prothrombin fragment 1,2, thrombin–antithrombin complexes, D-dimers, and factor VIII coagulant activity), thus determining a change in hemostatic balance in favor of a prothrombotic state [38,39]. In our multivariate logistic regression analysis, aPTT retained significant predictive value for stage III–IV endometriosis, but given the small difference detected, this diagnostic parameter is unlikely to be useful to fully differentiate women with and without disease. Endometriosis would not more frequently develop in women with shorter aPTT; however, we cannot exclude that these perturbations of the coagulation system may occur at some time during the pathogenetic process starting from repeated tissue repair lesions. Indeed, cyclic bleeding of endometriotic lesions determines the local release of factors such as those activating platelets (PAFs), thrombin and thromboxane A2 (TXA2), resulting in increased angiogenesis, increased vascular permeability and in the induction of platelet activation and aggregation [4,40–42]. The activated platelets would further release von Willebrand factor (vWF), adenosine diphosphate (ADP), serotonin, PAF, TXA2, and Chemokine (C-X-C motif) ligand 4 (CXCL4), causing further platelet aggregation and perpetuating the coagulation activation [43]. Importantly, the consequent extravasation and aggregation of platelets can finally induce fibrosis in endometriosis lesions through TGF-β1 release and induction of the TGF-β1/Smad3 signaling pathway, which is a potent inducer of epithelial–mesenchymal transition and fibroblast-to-myofibroblast transition in endometriotic cells [40,43,44].

Controversial data have been reported in relation to the platelet count among the various studies, while a quite consistent significantly higher PLR was observed in women in endometriosis. A possible explanation for this inconsistency is that platelets exert their role as "activated platelets", without necessarily increasing their absolute mean value in peripheral blood. The elevated percentage of activated platelets in the peripheral blood of women with endometriosis is consistent with the observed shortened TT and aPTT. The release of TXA2, a potent platelet activation inducer, can generate a vicious cycle in maintaining platelet activation, the activation of the coagulation cascade, higher plasma fibrinogen levels, and short aPTTs in endometriosis [44,45].

Recently, increased cardiovascular and thrombotic morbidity in terms of myocardial infarction, angina, and coronary bypass graft intervention has been recognized in women with endometriosis. The relative risk of combined coronary heart disease events was 1.62 (95% confidence interval: 1.39–1.89) after adjustment for confounders [46,47]. Moreover, endometriosis has been interestingly identified as a novel predicting factor for venous thromboembolism during pregnancy and postpartum in a Japanese birth cohort study [48]. Factors contributing to this increased risk have not been deeply investigated. Possible causes could be the hormonal treatment or previous hysterectomy/oophorectomy in affected women. On the other hand, another hypothesis could attribute these events to these subtle alterations in coagulation and fibrinolysis parameters recently identified in affected patients causing a hypercoagulable status [12].

Our validation study has some limitations: (1) the retrospective design of the study that could have influenced the interpretation of the data; (2) patients on hormonal treatment have been included, but, in order to evaluate the unique effect of the endometriosis on the coagulation status, we did include only cases and controls with a negative history of hormonal therapy before surgery in the comparisons of coagulation parameters; (3) age was different between cases and controls; nevertheless, since a limited age range was set as a case selection criteria, a selection bias may be excluded.

5. Conclusions

In conclusion, our findings suggest that women with OMAs and moderate–severe forms of endometriosis show a modest strength of the coagulation function potentially attributable to the inflammatory nature of the lesions. Endometriosis also seems to be associated with systemic changes of some inflammatory parameters, for instance, a modest increase of neutrophil count. All the alterations detected are still within the normal reference intervals, explaining the high heterogeneity among studies. We cannot, however, rule out that these systemic perturbations may contribute to the pathogenetic process of the disease or to the increased cardiovascular and thrombotic morbidity observed in patients affected.

Author Contributions: Conceptualization, P.V. and J.O.; methodology, P.V.; software, N.S.; validation, P.V., M.C., and J.O.; formal analysis, N.S.; investigation, M.S., L.B., and R.V.; resources, M.S., L.B., R.V., N.S., and C.D.; data curation, N.S. and J.O.; writing—original draft preparation, M.S., L.B., N.S., R.V., C.D., and P.V.; writing—review and editing, J.O. and P.V.; visualization, J.O., P.V., and M.C.; supervision, J.O., P.V., and M.C.; project administration, M.C. and P.V. All authors have read and agreed to the published version of the manuscript.

References

1. Vercellini, P.P.; Vigano, P.; Somigliana, E.; Fedele, L. Endometriosis: Pathogenesis and treatment. *Nat. Rev. Endocrinol.* **2013**, *10*, 261–275. [CrossRef]

2. Zondervan, K.; Becker, C.M.; Koga, K.; Missmer, S.A.; Taylor, R.N.; Vigano, P. Endometriosis. *Nat. Rev. Dis. Prim.* **2018**, *4*, 9. [CrossRef]

3. Vigano, P.; Candiani, M.; Monno, A.; Giacomini, E.; Vercellini, P.P.; Somigliana, E. Time to redefine endometriosis including its pro-fibrotic nature. *Hum. Reprod.* **2018**, *33*, 347–352. [CrossRef]

4. Vigano, P.; Ottolina, J.; Bartiromo, L.; Bonavina, G.; Schimberni, M.; Villanacci, R.; Candiani, M. Cellular Components Contributing to Fibrosis in Endometriosis: A Literature Review. *J. Minim. Invasive Gynecol.* **2020**, *27*, 287–295. [CrossRef]

5. Sikora, J.; Mielczarek-Palacz, A.; Kondera-Anasz, Z. Imbalance in Cytokines from Interleukin-1 Family - Role in Pathogenesis of Endometriosis. *Am. J. Reprod. Immunol.* **2012**, *68*, 138–145. [CrossRef]

6. Wickiewicz, D.; Chrobak, A.; Gmyrek, G.B.; Halbersztadt, A.; Gabryś, M.; Goluda, M.; Chełmońska-Soyta, A. Diagnostic accuracy of interleukin-6 levels in peritoneal fluid for detection of endometriosis. *Arch. Gynecol. Obstet.* **2013**, *288*, 805–814. [CrossRef]

7. Birt, J.A.; Nabli, H.; Stilley, J.A.; Windham, E.A.; Frazier, S.R.; Sharpe-Timms, K.L. Elevated Peritoneal Fluid TNF-α Incites Ovarian Early Growth Response Factor 1 Expression and Downstream Protease Mediators. *Reprod. Sci.* **2013**, *20*, 514–523. [CrossRef] [PubMed]

8. Velasco, I.; Acién, P.; Campos, A.; Acién, M.I.; Ruiz-Maciá, E. Interleukin-6 and other soluble factors in peritoneal fluid and endometriomas and their relation to pain and aromatase expression. *J. Reprod. Immunol.* **2010**, *84*, 199–205. [CrossRef] [PubMed]

9. Tokmak, A.; Yildirim, G.; Öztaş, E.; Akar, S.; Erkenekli, K.; Gülşen, P.; Yilmaz, N.; Uğur, M. Use of Neutrophil-to-Lymphocyte Ratio Combined With CA-125 to Distinguish Endometriomas From Other Benign Ovarian Cysts. *Reprod. Sci.* **2015**, *23*, 795–802. [CrossRef] [PubMed]

10. Boss, E.A.; Massuger, L.F.A.G.; Thomas, C.M.; Geurts-Moespot, A.; Van Schaik, J.H.M.; Boonstra, H.; Sweep, F.C.G.J. Clinical value of components of the plasminogen activation system in ovarian cyst fluid. *Anticancer. Res.* **2002**, *22*, 275–282.

11. Esmon, C.T. The interactions between inflammation and coagulation. *Br. J. Haematol.* **2005**, *131*, 417–430. [CrossRef] [PubMed]

12. Wu, Q.; Ding, D.; Liu, X.; Guo, S.-W. Evidence for a Hypercoagulable State in Women With Ovarian Endometriomas. *Reprod. Sci.* **2015**, *22*, 1107–1114. [CrossRef] [PubMed]

13. Chmaj-Wierzchowska, K.; Kampioni, M.; Wilczak, M.; Sajdak, S.; Opala, T. Novel markers in the diagnostics of endometriomas: Urocortin, ghrelin, and leptin or leukocytes, fibrinogen, and CA-125? *Taiwan. J. Obstet. Gynecol.* **2015**, *54*, 126–130. [CrossRef] [PubMed]

14. Also, P.; Ottolina, J.; Sarais, V.; Rebonato, G.; Somigliana, E.; Candiani, M. Coagulation Status in Women With Endometriosis. *Reprod. Sci.* **2017**, *25*, 559–565. [CrossRef]

15. Sanchez, A.M.; Vigano, P.; Somigliana, E.; Panina-Bordignon, P.; Vercellini, P.P.; Candiani, M. The distinguishing cellular and molecular features of the endometriotic ovarian cyst: From pathophysiology to the potential endometrioma-mediated damage to the ovary. *Hum. Reprod. Updat.* **2013**, *20*, 217–230. [CrossRef]

16. Reproductive, A.S.F. Revised American Society for Reproductive Medicine classification of endometriosis: 1996. *Fertil. Steril.* **1997**, *67*, 817–821. [CrossRef]

17. Nisolle, M.; Donnez, J. Peritoneal endometriosis, ovarian endometriosis, and adenomyotic nodules of the rectovaginal septum are three different entities. *Fertil. Steril.* **1997**, *68*, 585–596. [CrossRef]

18. Moher, D.; Liberati, A.; Tetzlaff, J.; Altman, D.G. Preferred Reporting Items for Systematic Reviews and Meta-Analyses: The PRISMA Statement. *Ann. Intern. Med.* **2009**, *151*, 264–269. [CrossRef]

19. EFSA Scientific Committee; Benford, D.; Halldorsson, T.; Jeger, M.J.; Knutsen, H.K.; More, S.; Naegeli, H.; Noteborn, H.; Ockleford, C.; Ricci, A.; et al. The principles and methods behind EFSA's Guidance on Uncertainty Analysis in Scientific Assessment. *EFSA J.* **2018**, *16*, 5122. [CrossRef]

20. Vigano, P.; Somigliana, E.; Panina, P.; Rabellotti, E.; Vercellini, P.P.; Candiani, M. Principles of phenomics in endometriosis. *Hum. Reprod. Updat.* **2012**, *18*, 248–259. [CrossRef]

21. World Health Organization Collaborative Study of Cardiovascular Disease and Steroid Hormone Contarception Venous thromboembolic disease and combined oral contraceptives: Results of international multicentre case-control study. *Lancet* **1995**, *346*, 1575–1582. [CrossRef]

22. Farmer, R.; Lawrenson, R.; Thompson, C.; Kennedy, J.; Hambleton, I.R. Population-based study of risk of venous thromboembolism associated with various oral contraceptives. *Lancet* **1997**, *349*, 83–88. [CrossRef]

23. Cho, S.; Cho, H.; Nam, A.; Kim, H.Y.; Choi, Y.S.; Park, K.H.; Cho, D.J.; Lee, B.S. Neutrophil-to-lymphocyte ratio as an adjunct to CA-125 for the diagnosis of endometriosis. *Fertil. Steril.* **2008**, *90*, 2073–2079. [CrossRef]

24. Yang, H.; Zhu, L.; Wang, S.; Lang, J.; Xu, T. Noninvasive Diagnosis of Moderate to Severe Endometriosis: The Platelet-Lymphocyte Ratio Cannot Be a Neoadjuvant Biomarker for Serum Cancer Antigen 125. *J. Minim. Invasive Gynecol.* **2015**, *22*, 373–377. [CrossRef] [PubMed]

25. Yavuzcan, A.; Caglar, M.; Ustun, Y.; Dilbaz, S.; Ozdemir, I.; Yıldız, E.; Ozkara, A.; Kumru, S. Evaluation of mean platelet volume, neutrophil/lymphocyte ratio and platelet/lymphocyte ratio in advanced stage endometrioma with endometrioma. *J. Turk. Gynecol. Assoc.* **2013**, *14*, 210–215. [CrossRef]

26. Avcioğlu, S.N.; Altinkaya, S.Ö.; Küçük, M.; Demircan-Sezer, S.; Yüksel, H. Can Platelet Indices Be New Biomarkers for Severe Endometriosis? *ISRN Obstet. Gynecol.* **2014**, *2014*, 1–6. [CrossRef]

27. Kim, S.K.; Park, J.Y.; Jee, B.C.; Suh, C.S.; Kim, S.H. Association of the neutrophil-to-lymphocyte ratio and CA 125 with the endometriosis score. *Clin. Exp. Reprod. Med.* **2014**, *41*, 151–157. [CrossRef]

28. Seckin, B.; Ates, M.C.; Kirbas, A.; Yesilyurt, H. Usefulness of hematological parameters for differential diagnosis of endometriomas in adolescents/young adults and older women. *Int. J. Adolesc. Med. Health* **2018**. [CrossRef]

29. Ding, D.; Liu, X.; Guo, S.-W. Further Evidence for Hypercoagulability in Women With Ovarian Endometriomas. *Reprod. Sci.* **2018**, *25*, 1540–1548. [CrossRef]

30. Ding, S.; Lin, Q.; Zhu, T.; Li, T.; Zhu, L.; Wang, J.; Zhang, X. Is there a correlation between inflammatory markers and coagulation parameters in women with advanced ovarian endometriosis? *BMC Women's Health* **2019**, *19*, 1–8. [CrossRef]

31. Turgut, A.; Hocaoglu, M.; Ozdamar, O.; Usta, A.; Gunay, T.; Akdeniz, E. Could hematologic parameters be useful biomarkers for the diagnosis of endometriosis? *Bratisl. Med. J.* **2019**, *120*, 912–918. [CrossRef] [PubMed]

32. Çoşkun, B.; Ince, O.; Erkilinc, S.; Elmas, B.; Saridogan, E.; Çoşkun, B.; Doğanay, M.; Erkılınç, S.; Saridogan, E. The feasibility of the platelet count and mean platelet volume as markers of endometriosis and adenomyosis: A case control study. *J. Gynecol. Obstet. Hum. Reprod.* **2019**, 101626. [CrossRef]

33. Cassarino, M.F.; Ambrogio, A.G.; Cassarino, A.; Terreni, M.R.; Gentilini, D.; Sesta, A.; Cavagnini, F.; Losa, M.; Giraldi, F.P. Gene expression profiling in human corticotroph tumours reveals distinct, neuroendocrine profiles. *J. Neuroendocr.* **2018**, *30*, e12628. [CrossRef] [PubMed]

34. Sanchez, A.M.; Somigliana, E.; Vercellini, P.; Pagliardini, L.; Candiani, M.; Viganò, P. Endometriosis as a detrimental condition for granulosa cell steroidogenesis and development: From molecular alterations to clinical impact. *J. Steroid Biochem. Mol. Biol.* **2016**, *155*, 35–46. [CrossRef] [PubMed]

35. Krikun, G.; Lockwood, C.J.; Paidas, M.J. Tissue factor and the endometrium: From physiology to pathology. *Thromb. Res.* **2009**, *124*, 393–396. [CrossRef] [PubMed]

36. Lin, M.; Weng, H.; Wang, X.; Zhou, B.; Yu, P.; Wang, Y. The role of tissue factor and protease-activated receptor 2 in endometriosis. *Am. J. Reprod. Immunol.* **2012**, *68*, 251–257. [CrossRef]

37. Osuga, Y. Proteinase-activated receptors in the endometrium and endometriosis. *Front. Biosci.* **2012**, *4*, 1201–1212. [CrossRef]

38. Senthil, M.; Chaudhary, P.; Smith, D.; Ventura, P.E.; Frankel, P.H.; Pullarkat, V.; Trisal, V. A shortened activated partial thromboplastin time predicts the risk of catheter-associated venous thrombosis in cancer patients. *Thromb. Res.* **2014**, *134*, 165–168. [CrossRef]

39. Mina, A.; Favaloro, E.J.; Koutts, J. Relationship between short activated partial thromboplastin times, thrombin generation, procoagulant factors and procoagulant phospholipid activity. *Blood Coagul. Fibrinolysis* **2012**, *23*, 203–207. [CrossRef]

40. Guo, S.-W.; Ding, D.; Geng, J.-G.; Wang, L.; Liu, X. P-selectin as a potential therapeutic target for endometriosis. *Fertil. Steril.* **2015**, *103*, 990–1000.e8. [CrossRef]

41. Zhang, Q.; Duan, J.; Olson, M.; Fazleabas, A.T.; Guo, S.-W. Cellular Changes Consistent With Epithelial–Mesenchymal Transition and Fibroblast-to-Myofibroblast Transdifferentiation in the Progression of Experimental Endometriosis in Baboons. *Reprod. Sci.* **2016**, *23*, 1409–1421. [CrossRef] [PubMed]

42. Zhang, Q.; Duan, J.; Liu, X.; Guo, S.-W. Platelets drive smooth muscle metaplasia and fibrogenesis in endometriosis through epithelial–mesenchymal transition and fibroblast-to-myofibroblast transdifferentiation. *Mol. Cell. Endocrinol.* **2016**, *428*, 1–16. [CrossRef] [PubMed]

43. Guo, S.-W.; Du, Y.; Liu, X. Endometriosis-Derived Stromal Cells Secrete Thrombin and Thromboxane A2, Inducing Platelet Activation. *Reprod. Sci.* **2016**, *23*, 1044–1052. [CrossRef] [PubMed]

44. Ding, D.; Liu, X.; Duan, J.; Guo, S.-W. Platelets are an unindicted culprit in the development of endometriosis: Clinical and experimental evidence. *Hum. Reprod.* **2015**, *30*, 812–832. [CrossRef] [PubMed]

45. Mikhailidis, D.P.; Barradas, M.A.; Maris, A.; Jeremy, J.Y.; Dandona, P. Fibrinogen mediated activation of platelet aggregation and thromboxane A2 release: Pathological implications in vascular disease. *J. Clin. Pathol.* **1985**, *38*, 1166–1171. [CrossRef]

46. Kvaskoff, M.; Mu, F.; Terry, K.L.; Harris, H.R.; Poole, E.M.; Farland, L.V.; Missmer, S.A. Endometriosis: A high-risk population for major chronic diseases? *Hum. Reprod. Updat.* **2015**, *21*, 500–516. [CrossRef]

47. Zuin, M.; Rigatelli, G.; Stellin, G.; Faggian, G.; Roncon, L. Should women with endometriosis be screened for coronary artery disease? *Eur. J. Intern. Med.* **2016**, *35*, e19–e20. [CrossRef]

48. Sugiura-Ogasawara, M.; Ebara, T.; Matsuki, T.; Yamada, Y.; Omori, T.; Matsumoto, Y.; Kato, S.; Kano, H.; Kurihara, T.; Saitoh, S.; et al. Endometriosis and Recurrent Pregnancy Loss as New Risk Factors for Venous Thromboembolism during Pregnancy and Post-Partum: The JECS Birth Cohort. *Thromb. Haemost.* **2019**, *119*, 606–617. [CrossRef]

Role of B-Cell Translocation Gene 1 in the Pathogenesis of Endometriosis

Jeong Sook Kim [1], Young Sik Choi [2,3], Ji Hyun Park [4], Jisun Yun [2], Soohyun Kim [4], Jae Hoon Lee [2], Bo Hyon Yun [2,3], Joo Hyun Park [3,4], Seok Kyo Seo [2,3], SiHyun Cho [3,4,*], Hyun-Soo Kim [5,*] and Byung Seok Lee [2,3]

[1] Department of Obstetrics and Gynecology, University of Ulsan College of Medicine, Ulsan University Hospital, Ulsan 44033, Korea
[2] Department of Obstetrics and Gynecology, Severance Hospital, Yonsei University College of Medicine, Seoul 03722, Korea
[3] Institute of Women's Life Medical Science, Yonsei University College of Medicine, Seoul 03722, Korea
[4] Department of Obstetrics and Gynecology, Gangnam Severance Hospital, Yonsei University College of Medicine, Seoul 06273, Korea
[5] Department of Pathology and Translational Genomics, Samsung Medical Center, Sungkyunkwan University School of Medicine, Seoul 06351, Korea
* Correspondence: sihyuncho@yuhs.ac (S.C.); hyun-soo.kim@samsung.com (H.-S.K.)

Abstract: Estrogen affects endometrial cellular proliferation by regulating the expression of the *c-myc* gene. B-cell translocation gene 1 (BTG1), a translocation partner of the *c-myc*, is a tumor suppressor gene that promotes apoptosis and negatively regulates cellular proliferation and cell-to-cell adhesion. The aim of this study was to determine the role of BTG1 in the pathogenesis of endometriosis. *BTG1* mRNA and protein expression was evaluated in eutopic and ectopic endometrium of 30 patients with endometriosis (endometriosis group), and in eutopic endometrium of 22 patients without endometriosis (control group). The effect of BTG1 downregulation on cellular migration, proliferation, and apoptosis was evaluated using transfection of primarily cultured human endometrial stromal cells (HESCs) with *BTG1* siRNA. *BTG1* mRNA expression level of eutopic and ectopic endometrium of endometriosis group were significantly lower than that of the eutopic endometrium of the control group. Migration and wound healing assays revealed that BTG1 downregulation resulted in a significant increase in migration potential of HESCs, characterized by increased expression of matrix metalloproteinase 2 (MMP2) and MMP9. Downregulation of BTG1 in HESCs significantly reduced Caspase 3 expression, indicating a decrease in apoptotic potential. In conclusion, our data suggest that downregulation of BTG1 plays an important role in the pathogenesis of endometriosis.

Keywords: BTG1; endometriosis; human endometrial stromal cells

1. Introduction

Endometriosis is a commonly occurring gynecological disorder that may cause pelvic pain and infertility [1]. The diagnosis of endometriosis is pathologically confirmed by the ectopic presence of endometrial-like epithelium and stroma. Endometriosis is prevalent in approximately 10% of all reproductive women, 20–30% of women with infertility, and 40–80% of women with chronic pelvic pain, or both [2]. Although several pathogenic theories have been suggested, the exact underlying mechanisms of endometriosis still remains unclear. The long-term management of endometriosis-related symptoms and recurrence after surgery also remains a challenge. Understanding endometrial cellular expression of certain genes and proteins may result in improved diagnosis and treatment of endometriosis.

Cellular proliferation, differentiation, and apoptosis are cell cycle-dependent processes [3]. Disruption of cell cycle regulation results in tumor formation and progression [4]. Estrogen regulates endometrial cellular proliferation by binding to an atypical *cis*-element in *c-myc* promoter [5]. Serum estrogen levels are 5–8 times higher than normal in women with endometriosis [6]. Estrogen receptor-α and *c-myc* are highly expressed in deeply infiltrating endometriotic tissue [7]. Therefore, the *c-myc* gene may play a crucial role in endometriosis.

B-cell translocation gene 1 (*BTG1*) was identified as a translocation partner of the *c-myc* gene in B-cell chronic lymphocytic leukemia [8]. BTG1 belongs to the BTG/TOB family of anti-proliferative proteins that include BTG2, BTG3, TOB1, and TOB2, which regulates cell growth and differentiation [9–11]. BTG1 is primarily expressed in quiescent cells at G_0/G_1 phase of cell cycle, and its level declines as cells enter S phase [12]. Exogenous overexpression of BTG1 reduces proliferation of murine fibroblasts by inducing G1 arrest and/or apoptosis [12]. BTG1 also negatively regulate proliferation of murine microglial cells [13].

BTG1 is also a known tumor suppressor gene that negatively regulates cellular proliferation, cell-to-cell adhesion, migration, and invasion in carcinomas of esophagus, nasopharynx, liver, breast, kidneys and lungs [14–18]. We recently demonstrated that BTG1 expression is significantly reduced in ovarian carcinoma tissues, and that BTG1 silencing in ovarian carcinoma occurs through epigenetic repression [19].

The role of BTG1 in endometrial cellular proliferation and the precise molecular mechanisms of BTG1 function in the pathogenesis of endometriosis remain unclear. In this study, we investigated BTG1 expression in eutopic and ectopic endometrial tissue samples obtained from patients with or without endometriosis. We also analyzed the expression levels of *BTG1* mRNA and protein and several cell cycle-related genes in primarily culture human endometrial stromal cells (HESCs), and examined whether downregulation of BTG1 affects cellular migration, proliferation, and/or apoptosis of HESCs.

2. Results

2.1. Clinical Characteristics

The clinical characteristics of the participants are shown in Table 1. The endometriosis group showed significantly decreased gravidity ($p = 0.034$) and parity ($p = 0.006$) compared to the control group. Patients with endometriosis exhibited lower body mass index than those without endometriosis, even though the difference between the groups was not statistically significant ($p = 0.092$). Serum levels of cancer antigen 125 were significantly higher in the endometriosis group than in the control group ($p = 0.002$). The differences in visual analogue scale (VAS) for pain between the groups were statistically significant. Mean VAS were significantly higher in the endometriosis group (6.57 ± 8.43) than in the control group (1.55 ± 9.88; $p < 0.001$).

Table 1. Patient characteristics.

Characteristic	Endometriosis Group	Control Group	*p*-Value
Number of patients	30	22	
Age (years)	34.93 ± 1.33	37.41 ± 1.78	0.349
Gravidity (frequency)	0.90 ± 0.24	1.91 ± 0.38	0.034 *
Parity (frequency)	0.47 ± 0.16	1.23 ± 0.22	0.006 *
Body mass index (kg/m^2)	20.67 ± 0.34	21.76 ± 0.53	0.092
Cancer antigen 125 (U/mL)	84.06 ± 25.83	18.60 ± 3.17	0.002 *
Visual analogue scale	6.57 ± 0.84	1.55 ± 0.98	<0.001 *

* Statistically significant. Data are expressed as mean ± standard error of mean.

2.2. Expression of BTG1 mRNA and Protein in Eutopic and Ectopic Endometrium of Patients with and without Endometriosis

Eutopic endometrium of the control group (1.95 ± 0.35) displayed significantly higher *BTG1* mRNA expression than both eutopic (1.12 ± 0.14; $p = 0.048$) and ectopic (0.81 ± 0.22; $p = 0.004$) endometrium of the endometriosis group (Figure 1A). In both groups, differences in *BTG1* mRNA expression between proliferative and secretory phases were not statistically significant, although the endometriosis groups exhibited lower expression levels than the control group in both the proliferative and secretory endometrial tissue samples (Table 2).

Figure 1. *BTG1* mRNA expression in eutopic and ectopic endometrial tissue samples obtained from patients with or without endometriosis. (**A**) Differences in *BTG1* mRNA expression levels among 3 groups: eutopic endometrium of the control group (Ctrl-Eut) and the endometriosis group (EM-Eut) and ectopic endometrium (EM-Ect). The expression levels of *BTG1* mRNA are normalized to that of *GAPDH* mRNA. (**B**) BTG1 protein expression in eutopic and ectopic endometrial tissue samples. (a) Eutopic endometrial tissue shows uniform and strong BTG1 immunoreactivity in the glandular and stromal cells (×100). (b) High-power view of image a. The cells in the endometrial glands and stroma exhibit strong BTG1 expression both in the nucleus and cytoplasm (×400). (c) Eutopic endometrial tissue of a patient with endometriosis displays patchy BTG1 expression with variable staining intensity (×100). (d) High-power view of image c. About half of the endometrial glandular epithelium and stromal cells show weak-to-moderate nuclear and cytoplasmic BTG1 immunoreactivity (×400). (e) Ectopic endometrial tissue in a patient with endometriosis (×100). (f) High-power view of image e. BTG1 expression is absent in the ectopic endometrial tissue. A faint nonspecific cytoplasmic staining is observed in the glandular epithelium (×400). (**C**) Differences in BTG1 staining intensity among 3 groups. * $p < 0.05$, ** $p < 0.01$. Error bars represent standard error of mean.

Table 2. *BTG1* mRNA expression in endometrium according to the phase of endometrium.

Phase of Endometrium	Group		p-Value
	Endometriosis	Control	
Proliferative phase	1.23 ± 0.21 ($n = 14$)	1.75 ± 0.50 ($n = 8$)	0.570
Secretory phase	1.03 ± 0.20 ($n = 15$)	1.88 ± 0.60 ($n = 10$)	0.091

Data are expressed as mean ± standard error of mean.

Using immunohistochemistry, we investigated BTG1 protein expression in eutopic and ectopic endometrial tissue samples in patients with and without endometriosis. Representative photomicrographs showing BTG1 immunoreactivity are shown in Figure 1B. Eutopic endometrial tissue of the control group showed strong BTG1 immunoreactivity in the endometrial glands and stroma. BTG1 was localized in both the nucleus and the cytoplasm of glandular epithelial and stromal cells. In contrast, BTG1 immunostaining was patchy and markedly reduced in the eutopic endometrium of the endometriosis group. About half of the glandular epithelial and stromal cells showed mild-to-moderate staining intensity. BTG1 staining intensity in eutopic and ectopic endometrium of the endometriosis group was markedly decreased compared with that in the eutopic endometrial tissue samples of the control group (Figure 1C). BTG1 was almost absent in the endometrial-type glands and stroma, although a faint nonspecific cytoplasmic staining was observed in the glandular epithelium. The BTG1 immunostaining results were in agreement with the mRNA expression data.

2.3. Effect of BTG1 Downregulation on Migration Potential of HESCs

We observed that the expression levels of BTG1 was reduced in endometriosis. Therefore, we speculated that downregulation of BTG1 may have effects on the migration of HESCs. We confirmed a reduction in BTG1 expression after *BTG1* siRNA transfection of HESCs (Figure 2A), and then examined the mRNA expression levels of *MMP2* and *MMP9*, which encode matrix metalloproteinase 2 (MMP2) and MMP9, respectively. They are well-known indicators for cell migration [20–23], and previous studies have shown that expression of MMP2 and/or MMP9 were elevated in endometriosis [24–26]. RT-PCR revealed that *BTG1* siRNA-transfected cells exhibited 1.18- and 1,94-fold increases in *MMP2* and *MMP9* mRNA expression levels compared to vehicle-treated control cells, with marginal significance ($p = 0.059$ and $p = 0.089$, respectively; Figure 2B). In line with this finding, the expression levels of MMP2 and MMP9 proteins were significantly increased in the transfected cells compared with the control cells (Figure 2C), indicating that BTG1 downregulation in HESCs induces an increase in their migration potential.

We further performed migration (Figure 2D) and wound healing (Figure 2E) assays. Compared to the control cells (4.40 ± 0.49), a significantly higher number of migrating cells was observed in the transfected cells (41.80 ± 1.07; $p < 0.001$). Wound healing assay revealed that scratched areas filled up with more HESCs in the transfected cells compared with the control cells ($p = 0.005$). Taken together, our observations suggest that BTG1 suppresses migration potential of in HESC.

Figure 2. Effect of BTG1 downregulation on migration potential in HESCs. (**A**) Marked reduction in BTG1 protein expression after *BTG1* siRNA transfection. (**B**) The increases in the expression levels of *MMP2* and *MMP9* mRNA after BTG1 downregulation. (**C,D**) The significant increases in (C) the expression levels of MMP2 and MMP9 protein and (D) the number of migrated HESCs after BTG1 downregulation (×100). (**E**) Significantly higher rate of wound closure in the *BTG1* siRNA-transfected cells (×100). ** $p < 0.01$. Error bars represent standard error of mean.

2.4. Effect of BTG1 Downregulation on Apoptotic Potential and Proliferative Activity of HESCs

To investigate the role of BTG1 in apoptosis of HESCs, the mRNA expression levels of *Caspase 3*, *Caspase 8*, *Fas*, and *FasL* were measured in HESCs transfected with *BTG1* siRNA or treated with vehicle control (Figure 3A). Among them, *Caspase 3* mRNA expression was significantly affected by BTG1 downregulation. The transfected cells showed a 0.78-fold decrease in the expression level of *Caspase 3* mRNA compared to the control cells ($p = 0.029$). To validate this finding, we evaluated the expression levels of pro- and anti-apoptotic proteins including Caspase 3, cleaved Caspase 3, Bax, and Bcl-2 (Figure 3B). BTG1 downregulation reduced the expression levels of pro-apoptotic factors (cleaved Caspase 3 and Bcl-2) and elevated the expression level of anti-apoptotic factor (Bax). *Fas* mRNA and protein expression appeared to be increased in the transfected cells, the alterations were not statistically significant. Flow cytometry analysis (Figure 4A) revealed that the percentage of Annexin V-positive cells decreased significantly after transfection (6.34 ± 0.34 versus $4.69 \pm 0.07\%$; $p = 0.008$). In addition, MTT assay (Figure 4B) revealed that relative cell proliferation of HESCs was increased significantly after BTG1 downregulation. These findings indicate that downregulation of BTG1 in HESCs induced a decrease in apoptotic potential and an increase in cellular proliferation.

Figure 3. Effect of BTG1 downregulation on the expression of apoptosis-related proteins in HESCs. (**A**) mRNA expression levels of *Caspase 3, Caspase 8, Fas,* and *FasL* after *BTG1* siRNA transfection. (**B**) Protein expression levels of Caspase 3, cleaved Caspase 3, Bax, Bcl-2, and Fas. * $p < 0.05$. Error bars represent standard error of mean.

Figure 4. Effect of BTG1 downregulation on apoptotic potential and proliferative activity of HESCs. (**A**) Flow cytometry analysis showing decreased apoptotic potential of HESCs after BTG1 downregulation. A significant decrease in the percentage of apoptosis cells is observed in the *BTG1* siRNA-transfected cells. (**B**) MTT assay showing a significant increase in the percentage of relative cell proliferation after BTG1 downregulation. * $p < 0.05$. Error bars represent standard error of mean.

3. Discussion

Although *BTG1* is a known anti-proliferative gene, the role of BTG1 in the pathophysiology of endometriosis has remained unclear. In this study, we observed that BTG1 expression was significantly reduced in ectopic and eutopic endometrial tissues of patients with endometriosis. Downregulation of BTG1 increased proliferative activity and migration potential of HESCs, and decreased their apoptotic potential. Our observations suggest that reduced expression of BTG1 facilitates proliferation and migration of HESCs and suppresses their apoptosis, resulting in the progression of endometriosis.

MMPs are enzymes that degrade extracellular matrix proteins and are important for the tissue remodeling process [27]. MMP2 (gelatinase A) and MMP9 (gelatinase B) degrade type IV collagen and fibronectin [20]. Previous studies reported that MMP2 expression is increased along with other proteases in the late secretory endometrium [23], and that the expression level of MMP9 is elevated in patients with endometriosis, suggesting that their endometrial tissue is inherently more invasive [22]. In this study, we demonstrated that downregulation of BTG1 in HESCs resulted in elevated MMP2 and MMP9 expression levels, suggesting that BTG1 negatively regulates endometrial cell migration.

The apoptotic signaling is classified into two major pathways: extrinsic or cytoplasmic and intrinsic pathways. The extrinsic pathway is regulated by the Fas death receptor, and the intrinsic pathway is regulated by the Bcl-2 family of proteins [28,29]. The ratio of anti-apoptotic Bcl-2 to pro-apoptotic Bax is a critical factor for the intrinsic pathway. Hetero-dimerization of Bcl-2 with Bax, which inhibits apoptosis, is controlled by a family of cysteinyl proteases called caspases [30–32]. In this study, we showed that cellular apoptosis was reduced after downregulation of BTG1 in HESCs. The expression levels of *Caspase 3* mRNA were significantly reduced after BTG1 downregulation, whereas there were no significant alterations in mRNA expression levels of *Caspase 8*, *Fas*, or *FasL*. The *BTG1* siRNA-transfected HESCs also displayed decreased Bax expression and increased Bcl-2 expression. A previous study documented that overexpression of BTG1 induces apoptosis of breast carcinoma cells, accompanied by a decline in the Bcl-2 level and an increase in the Bax and Caspase 3 levels [18]. Our data suggest that BTG1 regulates cellular apoptosis via the intrinsic pathway in HESCs, thus affecting the pathogenesis of endometriosis.

There are a few limitations in this study. First, we conducted a pilot study using a relatively small number of the endometriosis subjects. Nevertheless, a significant reduction in BTG1 expression was observed in ectopic and eutopic endometrium of patients with endometriosis. Second, the control group did not include disease-free subjects. Since surgical resection of nonpathological ovarian or endometrial tissues from healthy patients raises ethical implications, we inevitably used tissue samples obtained from patients with ovarian mature teratoma, ovarian serous cystadenoma, or paratubal cyst. These benign ovarian lesions are not associated with ovarian endometriosis or endometrial pathology. Third, the majority of patients had moderate-to-severe endometriosis; therefore, we failed to investigate the association between BTG1 expression status and the severity of endometriosis. Fourth, we did not observe any expression of BTG1 in the Ishikawa cell line before and after BTG1 downregulation. We additionally measured MMP2 and MMP9 expression levels in Ishikawa cell line, but there was no difference in the expression levels (Figure 5). Since BTG1 is a tumor suppressor and the Ishikawa cell line is derived from endometrial carcinoma, lack of BTG1 expression was an expected finding.

Figure 5. Effect of BTG1 downregulation on the protein expression levels of BTG1, MMP2 and MMP9 in Ishikawa cell line.

In conclusion, we demonstrated that downregulation of BTG1 could play an important role in the progression of endometriosis. We observed that BTG1 expression was significantly reduced in ectopic and eutopic endometrial tissues of patients with endometriosis. BTG1 downregulation via siRNA transfection increased migration potential and proliferative activity of HESCs, and decreased their apoptotic potential.

4. Materials and Methods

4.1. Patients and Tissue Samples

This study (3-2015-0250, 23 November 2015) was reviewed and approved by the Institutional Review Board of Gangnam Severance Hospital (Seoul, Korea). Between 1 June 2015 and 31 July 2015, 54 women who underwent laparoscopy for various gynecological conditions (pelvic mass, pelvic pain, endometriosis, and infertility) were enrolled after obtaining their written informed consent. Thirty-two and 22 patients participated in the endometriosis and control groups, respectively. Their ages ranged from 19 to 45 years. Patients with postmenopausal symptoms, previous hormone or gonadotropin-releasing hormone agonist use, uterine adenomyosis, endometrial lesion (polyp, hyperplasia, or malignancy), infectious disease, acute or chronic inflammatory disease, autoimmune disease, and cardiovascular disease were excluded.

All probable endometriotic lesions were surgically resected and sent to the pathology department for histopathological examination. Patients were assigned to the endometriosis group only after pathological confirmation of endometriosis. The extent of endometriosis was determined according to the revised American Society for Reproductive Medicine Classification of endometriosis [33]. Among 32 patients with peritoneal and/or ovarian endometriosis, 30 patients exhibited a moderate-to-severe form of endometriosis, while the remaining 2 patients had a mild form of the disease. The presence and intensity of endometriosis-related pain, including dysmenorrhea, deep dyspareunia, and/or non-menstrual pelvic pain, were assessed using VAS [34].

Fifteen of the 22 patients who participated in the control group were diagnosed as having mature cystic teratoma, and the remaining 7 patients had serous cystadenoma (5 patients) or paratubal cyst (2 patients). These benign ovarian lesions were not associated with ovarian endometriosis or endometrial pathology. Since surgical resection of nonpathological ovarian or endometrial tissues from healthy patients raises ethical implications, the control group did not include disease-free subjects. Endometrial tissue samples were obtained using a Pipelle catheter.

4.2. Culture of Primary Endometrial Stromal Cells and Ishikawa Cell Line

We cultured primary endothelial stromal cells as previously described [35]. Endometrial tissue was finely minced and the cells were dispersed by incubation in Hanks Balanced Salt Solution containing 4-(2-hydroxyethyl)-1-piperazineethanesulfonic acid (2 mmol/mL), 1% penicillin/streptomycin, and collagenase (1 mg/mL, 15 U/mg) for 60 min at 37 °C with agitation and pipetting. The cells were centrifuged and cell pellets were washed, suspended in Dulbecco's modified Eagle's medium:Ham F12 (1:Z1) solution containing 10% fetal bovine serum and 1% penicillin/streptomycin, passed through a 40-µm cell strainer (Corning Inc., Corning, NY, USA), and plated on commercially available 75 cm^2 tissue culture Falcon flasks (BD Biosciences, San Jose, CA, USA). We used cultured HESCs at 3–5 passages for analysis. We cultured the Ishikawa cell line in Minimum Essential Media (Invitrogen, Carlsbad, CA, USA) containing 2.0 mmol/L 1-glutamine and Earl salts, supplemented with 10% fetal bovine serum, 1% sodium pyruvate, and 1% penicillin/streptomycin.

4.3. Cell Transfection

Cells were seeded in 6-well plates, cultured to 70–80% confluence, and transfected with *BTG1* siRNA or control siRNA-A (Santa Cruz, Dallas, TX, USA) using Lipofectamine 3000 (Invitrogen) according to the manufacturer's recommendations at a final concentration of 50 nM. The transfected cells were harvested after 48 h.

4.4. RNA Isolation and Quantitative Real-Time Polymerase Chain Reaction (qRT-PCR)

To measure *BTG1* mRNA levels, total RNAs were isolated from cultured cells using the RNeasy Mini Kit (Qiagen Inc., Valencia, CA, USA). RNA sample concentrations were analyzed using a Nanodrop 2000 spectrophotometer (Thermo Fisher Scientific, Waltham, MA, USA). The Superscript III kit (Invitrogen) was used to synthesize cDNA using 1 μg of total RNA primed with oligo(dT). PCR was performed in a C1000 Thermal Cycler (Bio-Rad Laboratories, Hercules, CA, USA). The synthesized cDNA products were stored at −20 °C. qPCR was performed with 2 μL of synthesized cDNA as template using a 7300 Real-Time PCR System (Applied Biosystems, Foster City, CA, USA). Real-time PCR was performed using the Power SYBR Green PCR master mix (Applied Biosystems). The reaction mixture included the cDNA template, forward and reverse primers, ribonuclease-free water, and the SYBR Green PCR master mix at a final reaction volume of 20 μL. Reactions were performed at 95 °C for 5 min, followed by 40 cycles of 95 °C for 30 s, 60 °C for 30 s, 72 °C for 1 min, and a final extension at 72 °C for 5 min. Threshold cycle (Ct) values and melting curves were calculated using the 7300 Real-time PCR system software (Applied Biosystems). Each reaction was performed in triplicates. If not specified, the mRNA levels in each sample were normalized to those of *GAPDH*. Primer sequences for *BTG1*, *Caspase 3*, *Caspase 8*, *Fas*, *FasL*, *MMP2*, *MMP9* and *GAPDH* are shown in Table 3. The product amount was calibrated to the internal control reference using the ΔΔCt analysis [36].

Table 3. Primer sequences used.

Gene		Sequence
BTG1	Forward	CAA GGG ATC GGG TTA CCG TTG T
	Reverse	AGC CAT CCT CTC CAA TTC TGT AGG
Caspase 3	Forward	GGA AGC GAA TCA ATG GAC TCT GG
	Reverse	GCA TCG ACA TCT GTA CCA GAC C
Caspase 8	Forward	CCA GAG ACT CCA GGA AAA GAG A
	Reverse	GAT AGA GCA TGA CCC TGT AGG C
Fas	Forward	AGC TTG GTC TAG AGT GAA AA
	Reverse	GAG GCA GAA TCA TGA GAT AT
FasL	Forward	CAG CTC TTC CAC CTG CAG AAG G
	Reverse	AGA TTC CTC AAA ATT GAT CAG AGA GAG
MMP2	Forward	ACC GCG ACA AGA AGT ATG GC
	Reverse	CCA CTT GCG GTC ATC ATC GT
MMP9	Forward	CGA TGA CGA GTT GTG GTC CC
	Reverse	TCG TAG TTG GCC GTG GTA CT
GAPDH	Forward	ACC ACA GTC CAT GCC ATC AC
	Reverse	TCC ACC ACC CTG TTG CTG TA

4.5. Immunohistochemistry

BTG1 protein expression was assessed by immunohistochemistry using the Bond Polymer Intense Detection System (Leica Biosystems, Newcastle upon Tyne, UK) according to the manufacturer's recommendations. Surgically resected tissues were fixed in 10% neutral buffered formalin for 12–24 h. The tissues were then sectioned, processed with an automatic tissue processor, and embedded in paraffin blocks. A rotary microtome was used to cut 4-μm thick sections from each formalin-fixed, paraffin-embedded tissue block. Deparaffinization was performed using Bond Dewax Solution (Leica Biosystems). Antigen retrieval was performed using Bond Epitope Retrieval Solution (Leica Biosystems) for 30 min at 100 °C. Endogenous peroxidases were quenched with hydrogen peroxide for 5 min. Sections were incubated with anti-rabbit antibody against BTG1 (1:100, polyclonal, Abcam, Cambridge, MA, USA) for 15 min at ambient temperature. Biotin-free polymeric horseradish peroxidase-linker antibody conjugate system and Bond-maX automatic slide stainer (Leica Biosystems) were used. Visualization was performed using 1 mM 3,3'-diaminobenzidine, 50 mM Tris-hydrogen chloride buffer (pH 7.6), and 0.006% hydrogen peroxide. The sections were counterstained with hematoxylin. Positive and negative control samples were included with each reaction to minimize inter-assay variation. Normal colonic tissue was used as positive control. The negative control was prepared by replacing the primary antibody with non-immune serum; no detectable staining was evident. The staining intensity of BTG1 was assessed on a scale of 0–3, with 0 indicating negative staining; 1, weak; 2, moderate; and 3, strong.

4.6. Protein Extraction and Western Blot Analysis

We prepared protein extracts using a radio-immunoprecipitation assay buffer containing protease and a phosphatase inhibitor cocktail (Thermo Fisher Scientific). We determined the concentrations of total cell lysates using Pierce BCA protein assay kit (Thermo Fisher Scientific). We mixed 20 µg of total protein with 5× sample buffer, and then heated at 95 °C for 5 min. Samples were loaded on 12% sodium dodecyl sulfate-polyacrylamide gels and transferred to a polyvinylidene fluoride membrane (EMD Millipore, Burlington, MA, USA) with use of a Transblot apparatus (Bio-Rad Laboratories). Membranes (EMD Millipore) were blocked with 5% non-fat skim milk in Tris-buffered saline solution (10 mmol/L Tris-hydrogen chloride (pH 7.4) and 0.5 mol/L sodium chloride) with 0.1% v/v of Tween-20 (TBS-T). The blots were probed with primary antibodies against BTG1 (1:200, Abcam), MMP9 (1:250, Santa Cruz) with TBS-T; MMP2 (1:250, Santa Cruz) with TBS-T, Caspase 3 (1:1,000, Cell Signaling Technology, Danvers, MA, USA) with TBS plus 5% skim milk, Bax (1:500, Santa Cruz) with TBS plus 5% skim milk, Bcl-2 (1:1000, Cell Signaling Technology) with TBS plus 5% skim milk, and GAPDH (1:1000, Santa Cruz) with TBS plus 5% skim milk. They were then incubated in horseradish peroxidase-conjugated secondary antibodies (1:2000, Thermo Fisher Scientific). Proteins were detected using enhanced chemiluminescence (Santa Cruz). The experiment was repeated three times and the data shown are representative.

4.7. Migration and Wound Healing Assay

We performed migration assay for BTG1-transfected cells using 8-mm-pore polycarbonate membranes (EMD Millipore) within 24-well plates. Freshly treated by trypsin and washed cells were suspended in 200 mL of serum-free medium and positioned in the top chamber of each insert (5×10^4 cells/well); 600 mL of medium containing 10% fetal bovine serum was added into the lower chambers. Cells were fixed and stained with hematoxylin after incubation for 24 h at 37 °C in a 5% carbon dioxide humidified incubator. Cells in the inner chamber were removed using a cotton swab and the cells that were attached to the bottom side of the membrane were counted and imaged using an inverted microscope (Olympus, Tokyo, Japan) at 200× magnification over ten random fields in each well. For the wound healing assay, HESCs were transfected with control or *BTG1* siRNA for 48 h. The transfected cells were seeded using Dulbecco's modified Eagle's medium/F12 (1:1) with 10% fetal bovine serum and antibiotics and cultured in 24-well plates incubated at 37 °C with 5% carbon dioxide for 24 h. A linear wound (scratch) was generated using a sterile 100 µL pipette tip and debris was washed twice with phosphate-buffered saline. Cells were grown in culture for 18–24 h at 37 °C with 5% carbon dioxide. The scratched areas in each well were imaged using the EVOS inverted microscope (Advanced Microscopy Group, Mill Creek, WA, USA) to calculate the migration ability of *BTG1*-knockdown cells using ImageJ Version 1.51, a Java-based image processing program developed at the National Institutes of Health (Bethesda, MD, USA) [37]. The experiments were repeated four times.

4.8. Flow Cytometry

Cells were seeded in 6-well plates, incubated with indicated concentrations of chemical for 24 or 48 h, and transfected for 48 h. Cells were washed twice with phosphate-buffered saline; and suspended in 400 mL of binding buffer. Cells were stained with 5 mL Annexin V-fluorescein isothiocyanate (FITC) and 4 mL propidium iodide and incubated at room temperature for 10 min using Annexin V-FITC Apoptosis Detection Kit (BD Biosciences). The stained cells were quantified by flow cytometry using the FACS Canto II system (BD Biosciences) and the data were analyzed using DIVA software (version 8.0; BD Biosciences).

4.9. MTT Assay

Cytotoxicity was performed using the CellTiter 96 Non-Radioactive Cell Proliferation Assay (MTT) kit as manufacturer's recommendations (Promega, Madison, WI, USA). Briefly, 1×10^4 HESCs/well were seeded onto 96 well plates and incubated for 24 hr. After removal of supernatant, the plates were incubated with mixed solution (new media 100 μL and MTT solution 10 μL) for 4 h at 37 °C in a carbon dioxide incubator. Solubilization and stop solution mixture was added. The dark blue formazan product was quantified using a microplate reader at 570 nm (with a 690 nm reference filter; Molecular Device, Sunnyvale, CA, USA).

4.10. Statistical Analysis

All data were assessed for normal distribution using the Kolmogorov-Smirnov test or the Shapiro-Wilk test. The Student t-test or the Mann-Whitney U test was used for comparisons. One-way analysis of variance was performed in conjunction with the Tukey's post-hoc test to evaluate differences among groups. Statistical analyses were performed using SPSS for Windows, Version 16.0 (SPSS Inc., Chicago, IL, USA).

Author Contributions: All authors (J.S.K., Y.S.C., J.H.P. (Ji Hyun Park), J.Y., S.K., J.H.L., B.H.Y., J.H.P. (Joo Hyun Park), S.K.S., S.C., H.-S.K. and B.S.L.) were responsible for: acquisition of data, or analysis and interpretation of data, final approval of the version to be published. Additionally, J.S.K., Y.S.C., S.C. and H.-S.K. were responsible for substantial contributions to conception and design and drafting the manuscript. Especially, S.C. and H.-S.K. were responsible for revising the manuscript critically for important intellectual content.

Acknowledgments: We thank all other members, who were not listed here, in the department for their contribution of active discussions.

References

1. Zegers-Hochschild, F.; Adamson, G.D.; Dyer, S.; Racowsky, C.; de Mouzon, J.; Sokol, R.; Rienzi, L.; Sunde, A.; Schmidt, L.; Cooke, I.D.; et al. The International Glossary on Infertility and Fertility Care, 2017. *Hum. Reprod.* **2017**, *32*, 1786–1801. [CrossRef] [PubMed]
2. Giudice, L.C.; Kao, L.C. Endometriosis. *Lancet* **2004**, *364*, 1789–1799. [CrossRef]
3. Agathocleous, M.; Harris, W.A. Metabolism in physiological cell proliferation and differentiation. *Trends Cell Biol.* **2013**, *23*, 484–492. [CrossRef] [PubMed]
4. Shibata, D.; Aaltonen, L.A. Genetic predisposition and somatic diversification in tumor development and progression. *Adv. Cancer Res.* **2001**, *80*, 83–114. [PubMed]
5. Bulun, S.E. Endometriosis. *N. Engl. J. Med.* **2009**, *360*, 268–279. [CrossRef] [PubMed]
6. Huhtinen, K.; Desai, R.; Stahle, M.; Salminen, A.; Handelsman, D.J.; Perheentupa, A.; Poutanen, M. Endometrial and endometriotic concentrations of estrone and estradiol are determined by local metabolism rather than circulating levels. *J. Clin. Endocrinol. Metab.* **2012**, *97*, 4228–4235. [CrossRef] [PubMed]
7. Vinci, G.; Arkwright, S.; Audebourg, A.; Radenen, B.; Chapron, C.; Borghese, B.; Dousset, B.; Mehats, C.; Vaiman, D.; Vacher-Lavenu, M.C.; et al. Correlation Between the Clinical Parameters and Tissue Phenotype in Patients Affected by Deep-Infiltrating Endometriosis. *Reprod. Sci.* **2016**, *23*, 1258–1268. [CrossRef] [PubMed]
8. Waanders, E.; Scheijen, B.; van der Meer, L.T.; van Reijmersdal, S.V.; van Emst, L.; Kroeze, Y.; Sonneveld, E.; Hoogerbrugge, P.M.; van Kessel, A.G.; van Leeuwen, F.N.; et al. The origin and nature of tightly clustered BTG1 deletions in precursor B-cell acute lymphoblastic leukemia support a model of multiclonal evolution. *PLoS Genet.* **2012**, *8*, e1002533. [CrossRef] [PubMed]
9. Berthet, C.; Guehenneux, F.; Revol, V.; Samarut, C.; Lukaszewicz, A.; Dehay, C.; Dumontet, C.; Magaud, J.P.; Rouault, J.P. Interaction of PRMT1 with BTG/TOB proteins in cell signalling: Molecular analysis and functional aspects. *Genes Cells Devoted Mol. Cell. Mech.* **2002**, *7*, 29–39. [CrossRef]

10. Doidge, R.; Mittal, S.; Aslam, A.; Winkler, G.S. The anti-proliferative activity of BTG/TOB proteins is mediated via the Caf1a (CNOT7) and Caf1b (CNOT8) deadenylase subunits of the Ccr4-not complex. *PLoS ONE* **2012**, *7*, e51331. [CrossRef]

11. Rouault, J.P.; Rimokh, R.; Tessa, C.; Paranhos, G.; Ffrench, M.; Duret, L.; Garoccio, M.; Germain, D.; Samarut, J.; Magaud, J.P. BTG1, a member of a new family of antiproliferative genes. *Embo J.* **1992**, *11*, 1663–1670. [CrossRef] [PubMed]

12. Corjay, M.H.; Kearney, M.A.; Munzer, D.A.; Diamond, S.M.; Stoltenborg, J.K. Antiproliferative gene BTG1 is highly expressed in apoptotic cells in macrophage-rich areas of advanced lesions in Watanabe heritable hyperlipidemic rabbit and human. *Lab. Investig. A J. Tech. Methods Pathol.* **1998**, *78*, 847–858.

13. Lee, H.; Cha, S.; Lee, M.S.; Cho, G.J.; Choi, W.S.; Suk, K. Role of antiproliferative B cell translocation gene-1 as an apoptotic sensitizer in activation-induced cell death of brain microglia. *J. Immunol.* **2003**, *171*, 5802–5811. [CrossRef] [PubMed]

14. Sun, G.G.; Wang, Y.D.; Cheng, Y.J.; Hu, W.N. BTG1 underexpression is an independent prognostic marker in esophageal squamous cell carcinoma. *Tumour Biol. J. Int. Soc. Oncodev. Biol. Med.* **2014**, *35*, 9707–9716. [CrossRef] [PubMed]

15. Sun, G.G.; Lu, Y.F.; Cheng, Y.J.; Hu, W.N. The expression of BTG1 is downregulated in NSCLC and possibly associated with tumor metastasis. *Tumour Biol. J. Int. Soc. Oncodev. Biol. Med.* **2014**, *35*, 2949–2957. [CrossRef] [PubMed]

16. Sun, G.G.; Wang, Y.D.; Cheng, Y.J.; Hu, W.N. The expression of BTG1 is downregulated in nasopharyngeal carcinoma and possibly associated with tumour metastasis. *Mol. Biol. Rep.* **2014**, *41*, 5979–5988. [CrossRef] [PubMed]

17. Liu, C.; Tao, T.; Xu, B.; Lu, K.; Zhang, L.; Jiang, L.; Chen, S.; Liu, D.; Zhang, X.; Cao, N.; et al. BTG1 potentiates apoptosis and suppresses proliferation in renal cell carcinoma by interacting with PRMT1. *Oncol. Lett.* **2015**, *10*, 619–624. [CrossRef] [PubMed]

18. Zhu, R.; Zou, S.T.; Wan, J.M.; Li, W.; Li, X.L.; Zhu, W. BTG1 inhibits breast cancer cell growth through induction of cell cycle arrest and apoptosis. *Oncol. Rep.* **2013**, *30*, 2137–2144. [CrossRef] [PubMed]

19. Kim, J.Y.; Do, S.I.; Bae, G.E.; Kim, H.S. B-cell translocation gene 1 is downregulated by promoter methylation in ovarian carcinoma. *J. Cancer* **2017**, *8*, 2669–2675. [CrossRef] [PubMed]

20. Aznavoorian, S.; Murphy, A.N.; Stetler-Stevenson, W.G.; Liotta, L.A. Molecular aspects of tumor cell invasion and metastasis. *Cancer* **1993**, *71*, 1368–1383. [CrossRef]

21. Di Nezza, L.A.; Misajon, A.; Zhang, J.; Jobling, T.; Quinn, M.A.; Ostor, A.G.; Nie, G.; Lopata, A.; Salamonsen, L.A. Presence of active gelatinases in endometrial carcinoma and correlation of matrix metalloproteinase expression with increasing tumor grade and invasion. *Cancer* **2002**, *94*, 1466–1475. [CrossRef]

22. Shaco-Levy, R.; Sharabi, S.; Benharroch, D.; Piura, B.; Sion-Vardy, N. Matrix metalloproteinases 2 and 9, E-cadherin, and beta-catenin expression in endometriosis, low-grade endometrial carcinoma and non-neoplastic eutopic endometrium. *Eur. J. Obstet. Gynecol. Reprod. Biol.* **2008**, *139*, 226–232. [CrossRef] [PubMed]

23. Talbi, S.; Hamilton, A.E.; Vo, K.C.; Tulac, S.; Overgaard, M.T.; Dosiou, C.; Le Shay, N.; Nezhat, C.N.; Kempson, R.; Lessey, B.A.; et al. Molecular phenotyping of human endometrium distinguishes menstrual cycle phases and underlying biological processes in normo-ovulatory women. *Endocrinology* **2006**, *147*, 1097–1121. [CrossRef] [PubMed]

24. Weigel, M.T.; Kramer, J.; Schem, C.; Wenners, A.; Alkatout, I.; Jonat, W.; Maass, N.; Mundhenke, C. Differential expression of MMP-2, MMP-9 and PCNA in endometriosis and endometrial carcinoma. *Eur. J. Obstet. Gynecol. Reprod. Biol.* **2012**, *160*, 74–78. [CrossRef]

25. Liu, H.; Wang, J.; Wang, H.; Tang, N.; Li, Y.; Zhang, Y.; Hao, T. Correlation between matrix metalloproteinase-9 and endometriosis. *Int. J. Clin. Exp. Pathol.* **2015**, *8*, 13399–13404.

26. Collette, T.; Maheux, R.; Mailloux, J.; Akoum, A. Increased expression of matrix metalloproteinase-9 in the eutopic endometrial tissue of women with endometriosis. *Hum. Reprod.* **2006**, *21*, 3059–3067. [CrossRef]

27. Emonard, H.; Grimaud, J.A. Matrix metalloproteinases. A review. *Cell. Mol. Biol.* **1990**, *36*, 131–153. [PubMed]

28. Nahta, R.; Esteva, F.J. Bcl-2 antisense oligonucleotides: A potential novel strategy for the treatment of breast cancer. *Semin. Oncol.* **2003**, *30*, 143–149. [CrossRef]

29. Ghobrial, I.M.; Witzig, T.E.; Adjei, A.A. Targeting apoptosis pathways in cancer therapy. *CA A Cancer J. Clin.* **2005**, *55*, 178–194. [CrossRef]

30. Cohen, G.M. Caspases: The executioners of apoptosis. *Biochem. J.* **1997**, *326 Pt 1*, 1–16. [CrossRef]

31. Thornberry, N.A.; Lazebnik, Y. Caspases: Enemies within. *Science* **1998**, *281*, 1312–1316. [CrossRef] [PubMed]

32. Kymionis, G.D.; Dimitrakakis, C.E.; Konstadoulakis, M.M.; Arzimanoglou, I.; Leandros, E.; Chalkiadakis, G.; Keramopoulos, A.; Michalas, S. Can expression of apoptosis genes, bcl-2 and bax, predict survival and responsiveness to chemotherapy in node-negative breast cancer patients? *J. Surg. Res.* **2001**, *99*, 161–168. [CrossRef] [PubMed]

33. Canis, M.; Donnez, J.G.; Guzick, D.S.; Halme, J.K.; Rock, J.A.; Schenken, R.S.; Vernon, M.W. Revised American Society for Reproductive Medicine classification of endometriosis: 1996. *Fertil. Steril.* **1997**, *67*, 817–821.

34. Bourdel, N.; Alves, J.; Pickering, G.; Ramilo, I.; Roman, H.; Canis, M. Systematic review of endometriosis pain assessment: How to choose a scale? *Hum. Reprod. Update* **2015**, *21*, 136–152. [CrossRef] [PubMed]

35. Cho, S.; Mutlu, L.; Zhou, Y.; Taylor, H.S. Aromatase inhibitor regulates let-7 expression and let-7f-induced cell migration in endometrial cells from women with endometriosis. *Fertil. Steril.* **2016**, *106*, 673–680. [CrossRef] [PubMed]

36. Cho, S.; Ahn, Y.S.; Choi, Y.S.; Seo, S.K.; Nam, A.; Kim, H.Y.; Kim, J.H.; Park, K.H.; Cho, D.J.; Lee, B.S. Endometrial osteopontin mRNA expression and plasma osteopontin levels are increased in patients with endometriosis. *Am. J. Reprod. Immunol.* **2009**, *61*, 286–293. [CrossRef] [PubMed]

37. Grewal, S.; Carver, J.G.; Ridley, A.J.; Mardon, H.J. Implantation of the human embryo requires Rac1-dependent endometrial stromal cell migration. *Proc. Natl. Acad. Sci. USA* **2008**, *105*, 16189–16194. [CrossRef] [PubMed]

Endometriosis in Menopause—Renewed Attention on a Controversial Disease

Cristina Secosan [1], Ligia Balulescu [1,*], Simona Brasoveanu [1], Oana Balint [1], Paul Pirtea [2], Grigoraş Dorin [1] and Laurentiu Pirtea [1]

[1] Department of Obstetrics and Gynecology, University of Medicine and Pharmacy "Victor Babeş", 300041 Timişoara, Romania; cristina.secosan@gmail.com (C.S.); brasoveanu_simona@yahoo.com (S.B.); oana.balint@gmail.com (O.B.); grigorasdorin@ymail.com (G.D.); laurentiupirtea@gmail.com (L.P.)

[2] Department of Ob Gyn and Reproductive Medicine, Hopital Foch—Faculté de Medicine Paris Ouest (UVSQ), 92151 Suresnes, France; paulpirtea@gmail.com

* Correspondence: ligia_balulescu@yahoo.com

Abstract: Endometriosis, an estrogen-dependent inflammatory disease characterized by the ectopic presence of endometrial tissue, has been the topic of renewed research and debate in recent years. The paradigm shift from the belief that endometriosis only affects women of reproductive age has drawn attention to endometriosis in both premenarchal and postmenopausal patients. There is still scarce information in literature regarding postmenopausal endometriosis, the mostly studied and reported being the prevalence in postmenopausal women. Yet, other important issues also need to be addressed concerning diagnosis, pathophysiology, and management. We aimed at summarizing the currently available data in literature in order to provide a concise and precise update regarding information available on postmenopausal endometriosis.

Keywords: endometriosis; menopause; diagnosis; management; malignancy

1. Introduction

The concept that endometriosis is a disease that only affects women of reproductive age has prevailed since 1942, when the first case of endometriosis in a postmenopausal patient was reported by Edgar Haydon [1].

In spite of this early report, endometriosis has also been described in premenarchal patients and is a common occurrence in adolescents [2–4].

The recurrence of endometriosis lesions in patients with a prior diagnosis of endometriosis during the premenopausal period or the de novo appearance of endometriosis in postmenopausal patients with no prior history of endometriosis-related complaints has been however well documented in numerous case series, case reports, and retrospective studies [5–9].

The management of endometriosis in postmenopause and hormone replacement therapy (HRT) in patients with a history of endometriosis remains controversial.

2. Prevalence

The incidence of postmenopausal endometriosis reported in literature is of approximately 2–5%. It commonly represents a side effect of HRT, rarely occurring in patients without a history of HRT or Tamoxifen treatment [10]. In a few cases, postmenopausal endometriosis has been described in women who had no history of endometriosis on imaging or surgery prior to menopause [11].

In order to evaluate the prevalence of postmenopausal endometriosis, Haas et al. performed a retrospective epidemiological study on 42,079 women admitted for surgical treatment with histologically confirmed endometriosis. Patients were sorted in 5 years age groups and also in premenopausal, perimenopausal, and postmenopausal subgroups. The results showed that 33,814 patients (80.36%) were in the premenopausal group (age 0–45 years), with 23 patients (0.05%) being younger than 15 years; of the remaining patients, 7191 (17.09%) were in the perimenopausal (45–55 years), and 1074 patients (2.55%) in the postmenopausal group, respectively [6].

3. Pathophysiology

Endometriosis is an estrogen-dependent inflammatory disease characterized by the presence of ectopic endometrial tissue. The pathogenesis of endometriosis remains enigmatic [12].

Postmenopausal endometriosis is considered to have an even more complex pathophysiology than premenopausal endometriosis. It is still unclear whether this represents a recurrence or continuation of a previous disease or a de novo condition. Excess estrogen, in general, represents a promoting factor for endometriosis. The arrest of estrogen production at the level of the ovaries at the time of menopause is counterbalanced by peripheral estrogen production from conversion of androgens (especially in the adipose tissue and skin). The leading estrogen found in these patients is estrone.

An attractive theory regarding the pathogenic mechanism of postmenopausal endometriosis involves the "estrogen threshold", i.e., when a certain estrogen level is reached or surpassed in postmenopausal patients it activates undetected or "transient" foci of endometriosis.

In addition to the peripheral estrogen production, a high circulating level of estrogen may be of external source, especially in the form of phytoestrogens and HRT. Phytoestrogens appear to exert estrogenic effects on the uterus, breast, and pituitary and could also support the growth of endometriotic lesions [13–15].

Despite the fact that postmenopausal endometriosis has the same immunochemical profile as premenopausal endometriosis and has the potential to reactivate under estrogen stimulation, endometriosis lesions in the postmenopausal period seem to be less common, less extensive, and less active in most cases [16].

4. Symptomatology

The clinical presentation of endometriosis in menopausal patients is unspecific, such as pelvic pain, ovarian cysts, or intestinal symptoms. Given the age of the patients, they are often suspected of a neoplastic process. As a general consideration, all postmenopausal patients should be evaluated for malignancy if a new suspicious structure is found on ultrasound examination.

In menopausal women with a history of endometriosis, the drop in estrogen levels after menopause relieves the endometriosis-related symptoms but generates specific menopausal ones, such as mood swings, hot flushes, vaginal atrophy, and night sweats [5,17]. The clinical grim reality is that the severity of the disease is not necessarily reflected in the degree of discomfort. Commonly, the complaints of pelvic pain underestimate the disease's severity in both premenopausal and postmenopausal endometriosis.

5. Diagnosis

Despite intensive research conducted in the last decades, endometriosis remains a disease with a delayed diagnosis, especially in older patients. This results from the lack of noninvasive tools available for early stage diagnosis. For many years, there has been a long-standing myth that endometriosis is a disease that affects only adult women of reproductive age. However, in recent years, focus has turned to the diagnosis of endometriosis in postmenopausal patients, given that the onset of pain can start after the onset of menopause, with reports of endometriosis occurring even in 80-year-old patients [1,5].

The ovaries are the most common location of endometriotic lesions in postmenopausal patients (79.2% of cases) [18].

Distinction between endometriosis lesions and cancer is complicated by the fact that some of the risk factors are similar, such as low parity rate, infertility, late childbearing age, and a short duration of oral contraceptive use [19].

Currently, laparoscopy and biopsy for histological confirmation of suspicious lesions is the gold standard for diagnosis of endometriosis, irrespective of age. Laparoscopy, the standard technique for inspecting the pelvis, can provide simultaneous diagnosis and treatment of lesions. Additional tools are needed for a noninvasive diagnostic and classification. To this date, no serum marker or test is available for reliably diagnosing endometriosis [20,21]. Regarding imaging investigations, MRI and ultrasound are important, but findings are more difficult to interpret in menopausal patients than in younger patients due to the higher suspicion for neoplastic lesions and the polymorphic aspect of endometriosis.

5.1. Clinical Examination

The patient's medical history, clinical examination, or preoperative symptoms have a limited role in determining the extent of endometriosis lesions as there is no direct relationship between symptoms and the anatomic-surgical characteristics of endometriotic lesions [22]. Also, there is usually a discrepancy between the severity of symptoms and the extent of lesions with many patients whose severe lesions remain asymptomatic. This is an important factor contributing to a delay of approximately 6 to 8 years from onset of symptoms to diagnosis in premenopausal and postmenopausal patients alike [23].

Pelvic vaginal and rectal examination is useful in identifying endometriosis nodules in the lower posterior compartment, but clinical examination may be normal in many patients with deep infiltrating endometriosis [23].

5.2. Imaging

While diagnostic laparoscopy remains the gold standard, it is often not the first line of diagnosis any more, as noninvasive testing for early diagnosis and progression of endometriosis is being preferred [24]. Yet, no imaging method can definitively confirm the diagnosis of endometriosis, being notably inconclusive in case of peritoneal implants [25].

Deep infiltrating endometriosis (DIE) can be investigated through several imaging techniques, including transvaginal sonography (TVS), magnetic resonance imaging (MRI), computerized tomography, rectal endoscopic sonography, and three-dimensional (3D) ultrasound [23].

TVS has gained interest in recent years and is starting to be recommended as the first-line investigation technique in endometriosis because it allows extensive exploration of the pelvis, is widely available, cost efficient, and well tolerated [26–28].

TVS has the benefit of a lack of exposure to radiation and is the main method for the evaluation of adnexal masses, but remains limited for the diagnosis of other kinds of endometriosis. Endometriomas have distinct characteristics on ultrasound: unilocular cysts, most often of homogenous "ground glass" appearance. The identification of an endometrioma should alert the clinician to the possibility of moderate-to-advanced stage disease. An important exception is postmenopausal women, in whom ovarian cysts with a "ground glass" appearance are associated with a 44% risk of malignancy. In addition, TVS may have a role in assessing disease involving the bladder and rectum [29].

Computed tomography (CT) plays a major role in the diagnosis of bowel endometriosis in the presence of colon distension. Genitourinary tract involvement should be taken into consideration in case of hydronephrosis or hydroureter diagnosed on CT scan, especially in patients with a history of chronic pelvic pain or in patients with a history of endometriosis. Radiation exposure should be taken into consideration [29].

MRI is a noninvasive diagnostic method of DIE that offers the possibility to fully investigate the pelvic cavity with a high accuracy, but increased costs [30]. Nevertheless, MRI has limited indication in the diagnosis of endometriosis. It can confirm the diagnosis of endometrioma in the presence of an adnexal mass when TVS is uncertain. MRI can also be used as an investigation method when involvement of the ureter is suspected, and may be beneficial in the evaluation of anatomy when expanded pelvic adhesions are suspected [29].

Sonovaginography using saline solution (saline contrast sonovaginography (SCSV)) or gel infusion sonovaginography is a new diagnostic method in DIE. First described by Dessole et al., it consists of TVS combined with the introduction of saline solution or gel infusion into the vagina, which offers the benefit of a more complete view of the vaginal walls and fornix, pouch Douglas, uterosacral ligaments, and rectovaginal septum [22]. The data available in literature is limited, with only a few reports from Brazil, Italy, Romania, and Australia, but the methods seems beneficial in the diagnosis of posterior deep infiltrating endometriosis. Up to date, no studies have reported its use in postmenopausal patients [22,31–33].

The role of double-contrast barium enema (DCBE) in the evaluation of rectovaginal endometriosis is controversial. Some studies have reported high accuracy in predicting the need for intestinal surgery in endometriosis cases. The superiority of DCBE over rectal ultrasound or MRI is not well established, the results reported in literature being scarce and contradictory. However, certain studies have demonstrated a lower sensitivity of DCBE for rectovaginal disease. DCBE does not allow the examination of the entire intestinal wall thickness and does not provide information regarding the depth of infiltration, but may provide useful information for preoperative planning when severe disease is suspected [29].

5.3. Biomarkers

To this date, no specific markers for the diagnosis of endometriosis have been identified. A change in levels of proteins, microRNAs, and other markers corresponding to a disease state could be the basis for identifying novel biomarkers. Endometriosis patients often show modified ranges of CA-125 (Cancer Antigen 125), cytokines, angiogenic and growth factors compared with normal women, but all of these biomarkers are frequently encountered in various other pathologies and are not specific enough for diagnosing endometriosis. A combination of biomarkers may improve the sensitivity and specificity over single biomarker measurements. Moreover, stem cell, proteomic, and genomic studies could contribute to the development of new high-sensitivity biomarkers in the diagnosis of endometriosis in the future [24].

Many authors have studied the role of biomarkers for diagnosis of endometriosis and concluded that, to date, endometrial tissue, menstrual or uterine fluids, and immunologic markers in blood or urine are not recommended for clinical use for diagnosis of endometriosis [24].

Regarding the differential diagnosis between endometriomas and malignant ovarian tumors in postmenopausal patients, we have not found any information in the literature that supports the use of any novel tests, such as OVA1 (Ovarian Malignancy Algorithm), ROMA (risk of ovarian malignancy algorithm), circulating miRs, etc. Despite the potential clinical utility of these biomarkers in the diagnosis of malignant ovarian tumors in premenopausal patients, the costs implied, the lack of easy availability, and the decreased incidence of endometriomas in older patients make the usefulness of novel biomarkers difficult to assess [34–36].

5.4. Minimally Invasive Surgery: Laparoscopy and Robot Assistance

Because of the lack of specific and efficient noninvasive tests for endometriosis, there is often a significant delay in diagnosis of this disease, especially in older patients. The gold standard for the diagnosis of endometriosis remains visual inspection by laparoscopy, preferably with histological confirmation. A positive histological examination confirms the diagnosis, but negative histology does not exclude it, in the presence of pathognomonic lesions [23].

Whether histology should be obtained if peritoneal disease alone is present is controversial: a visual inspection of the pelvis should be enough, but histological confirmation of at least one lesion is ideal. In some cases, histology should be obtained to identify endometriosis and to exclude malignant disease. For example, in ovarian endometriomas (>3 cm in diameter) and in deeply infiltrating disease, a histological confirmation to exclude a rare instance of malignancy is necessary [37].

Laparoscopy is used for the diagnosis and treatment of DIE and serves to eradicate all visible endometriosis implants, especially in postmenopausal patients due to the risk of malignant transformation. Several studies have shown a significant improvement of symptoms and a decreased risk of malignancy in postmenopausal women after complete resection of all visible lesions. Precise preoperative imaging may help guide surgical therapeutic approaches and aid to obtain the best postoperative results [23]. In the last years, the da Vinci surgical system started to be used in the diagnosis and treatment of endometriosis. Three-dimensional (3D) vision offers the advantage of improved depth perception and accuracy in the performance of robotic surgery, particularly for complex surgical tasks such as identifying suspected implants. However, the robotic platform has the distinct disadvantage of offering only a unidirectional view within the abdominal cavity. Authors recommend for the first instance to undertake a diagnostic laparoscopy to exclude a suspected lesion of endometriosis in the upper abdomen, liver, diaphragm, and appendix before using the da Vinci robotic system in the pelvis. Another disadvantage is the loss of haptic feedback to identify fibrotic lesions which are characteristic of deeply infiltrating disease. However, the da Vinci robot may offer improved ease by avoiding hand and more instinctual movement of the wristed instruments in the treatment of endometriosis. The cost related to the procedure also make it unavailable at a large scale [29].

6. Management

6.1. The Impact of Hormone Replacement Therapy in Women with a History of Endometriosis

The recently published guidelines on menopause management have no statements of endometriosis symptoms [38]. The use of HRT raises concerns about disease reactivation and recurrence of pain and need for surgical treatment, and even malignant transformation of residual endometriosis. The risk of recurrence with HRT is considered to be linked to residual disease after surgery. The data regarding hormone therapy regimens is scarce. Continuous combined estrogen–progesterone treatment or tibolone, in patients with or without hysterectomy, is considered to carry a lower risk of disease recurrence, compared with estrogen-only regimens, but larger studies are required in order to prove the safety and efficacy. Management of potential recurrence is best monitored by awareness of the possibility of symptom recurrence. Patients with contraindication or who refuse hormonal treatment should be offered alternative pharmacological treatment for menopausal symptoms and for skeletal protection, if indicated. Herbal products should be avoided as some may contain estrogenic compounds and their efficacy is uncertain [39–41]. The risk of malignant transformation of endometriosis in women with a history of endometriosis who received HRT remains a matter of debate. Long-term follow-up studies are needed to evaluate the risk of an adverse outcome. Further studies are mandatory in order to determine the optimal management of menopause in women with endometriosis [15].

6.2. The Management of De Novo Endometriosis in Postmenopausal Patients and Pain Management

"De novo" endometriosis appears especially after unopposed estrogen therapy or obesity, which has an additional effect for increasing the risk of endometriosis development.

Postmenopausal women with symptomatic endometriosis should be managed surgically with removal of all visible endometriotic tissue because of the higher risk of recurrence and the risk of malignancy [41]. A similar approach is recommended by current ESHRE (European Society of Human Reproduction and Embryology) recommendations. Medical therapy can be used in case of pain recurrence after surgery or if surgery is contraindicated. Co-morbidities represent an additional risk to contraindicate surgery and include advanced age or pelvic adhesions from previous surgery [38,41]. Approximately 12% of all endometriosis cases will finally require a hysterectomy with or without oophorectomy [42,43]. To prevent recurrences, to restore bowel, urinary, or sexual function or to alleviate pain it is now recommended to remove all the implants [38].

Progesterone administration (oral or intrauterine system) has been proposed as a reliable alternative treatment in patients with contraindication for surgery, but, up to date, no extensive data is available and further studies are needed regarding progesterone use in postmenopausal endometriosis [44,45].

Aromatase inhibitors act by decreasing extra-ovarian estrogen production and by blocking the feed-forward stimulation loop between inflammation and aromatase within endometriosis lesions. Only six case reports of aromatase inhibitors administration in postmenopausal patients with a history of endometriosis have been published so far. In 1998, Kayama presented a 57-year-old patient who had presented with recurrent endometriosis with a painful vaginal polypoid mass. The use of Anastrozole reduced the volume of the vaginal mass. Other studies concluded that Letrozole has a similar efficacy to Anastrozole [46–48]. The most important risk of this treatment is osteoporosis and related fractures. Aromatase inhibitors impair bone mineral density and need to be associated with bisphosphonate therapy.

7. Tamoxifen and Postmenopausal Endometriosis

Tamoxifen represents a hormonal substitution therapy used in postmenopausal women with breast cancer. Tamoxifen has antiestrogenic effects on breast tissues but promotes endometriosis through unknown mechanisms. In 1993, the first case of tamoxifen-related endometriosis was reported in a woman who received tamoxifen for 2 years due to breast cancer [49]. In the next year, it was reported another case of operated breast cancer and adjuvant tamoxifen [50]. During the next years, many authors reported cases of ovarian and endometrioid carcinoma in the women who had used tamoxifen [51–54]. Considering that there is no significant statistical evidence, the relation between tamoxifen and malignant transformation may be coincidental [43].

8. Risk of Malignant Transformation

The possible transformation of endometriosis lesions into malignant lesions and their dissemination in the ovaries, bowel, and even lungs has been described. The risk of malignant transformation of endometrioma into an ovarian cancer is estimated at 2% or 3% [41,55], and may be higher in patients receiving estrogen therapy. Furthermore, patients with endometriosis have an increased risk of other malignancies, apart from ovarian cancer [41].

Differential diagnosis of benign from malignant tumors in postmenopausal women is difficult. We must take into account that some endometriosis lesions may have a similar appearance to malignant disease and can cause local and distant metastases and can infiltrate adjacent tissues and organs. Age is an important risk factor for many malignancies, thus it may be questioned whether the postmenopausal endometriosis increases the risk for malignancy [41].

In 1997, Brinton et al. showed that patients with endometriosis seem to have an increased overall cancer risk [56]. Some authors indicate an increased risk of ovarian cancer, calculated to be around 35% for clear cell carcinoma and 19% for endometrioid type carcinoma in women with endometriosis [57].

On the other hand, Somigliana et al. concluded that there is evidence to support that endometriosis should be considered a medical condition associated with a clinically relevant risk of any specific cancer [58].

Regarding the relationship between endometriosis and breast cancer, Bertelsen et al. published a study which followed around 115,000 Danish women over a period of 30 years. Authors concluded that the risk for breast cancer increased with age (<40 years) at diagnosis of endometriosis and it is around 0.97%. The increased risk associated with endometriosis among postmenopausal women may be due to common risk factors between postmenopausal endometriosis and breast cancer or an altered endogenous estrogen [59].

Because endometriosis and ovarian malignancy have some common risk factors, including low parity rate, infertility, late childbearing age, and short duration of oral contraceptive use, in clinical practice is very difficult to discriminate a benign from a malignant tumor in postmenopausal women [60].

In postmenopausal women who underwent surgery for endometriosis, hormonal therapy remains controversial. Unopposed estrogen stimulation is associated with an increased risk of endometrial cancer. Some studies show that exogenous estrogens are increasing the risk of malignancy transformation of endometriosis lesions. In a retrospective study which followed 31 women with cancer developing from endometriosis, Zanetta et al. concluded that prevalence of endometriosis associated with co-existing risk factors (obesity and unopposed estrogen therapy) represents a significant risk factor for the development of cancer in endometriotic lesions [61].

The indication for initiating hormone therapy in women with endometriosis must be carefully evaluated. In premenopausal women who underwent total hysterectomy and bilateral salpingo-oophorectomy due to endometriosis, the benefits of hormone therapy outweigh the risks. Postmenopausal hormone therapy may increase the risk of malignant transformation or recurrence of endometriosis [41,62]. More data are needed to confirm this.

9. Extrapelvic Endometriosis

Extrapelvic endometriosis is a rare clinical condition in postmenopausal women. It affects a slightly older population due to the fact that it takes several years for pelvic endometriosis to metastasize outside the pelvis. Statistical data regarding menopausal patients are limited. The most common location of extrapelvic endometriosis is the gastrointestinal tract, followed by the urinary system. Bladder and ureteral endometriosis are the most common sites for urinary tract involvement [63]. Regarding the gastrointestinal tract, the sigmoid colon is the most commonly involved, followed by the rectum, ileum, appendix, and caecum [64,65]. Extremely rare locations that have been reported include the gallbladder, the Meckel diverticulum, stomach, and endometriosis cysts of the pancreas and liver [63].

Flyckt et al. presented a 59-year-old woman with a periaortic mass with ureteral obstruction. A computed tomography was performed, and a surgical management was necessary to resect the mass. The pathology exam confirmed endometriosis invasion of the inferior vena cava [66].

9.1. Gastrointestinal Tract Endometriosis

In postmenopausal women with low estrogen levels, a vascular transport or metaplasia of intestinal tissue should be considered for the etiology of gastrointestinal tract endometriosis [65]. The intestinal involvement in endometriosis after menopause is a rare phenomenon and it has been described in literature only in case reports (Figure 1).

Figure 1. Sigmoid colon endometriosis—macroscopic aspect of the piece after laparoscopic resection using a circular stapler (personal collection, L. Pirtea).

Snyder et al. presented the case of a woman with iron-deficiency anemia, who underwent total hysterectomy with bilateral salpingo-oophorectomy. During the surgical procedure, an endometrial implant at the hepatic flexure was discovered, a rare location for endometriosis. The patient was treated with conjugated estrogen–bazedoxifen to antagonize the effects of estrogen. No evidence of lesion was found at colonoscopy after five months of therapy [11].

Popoutchi reported a rare case of postmenopausal intestinal endometriosis simulating a malignant lesion in a woman who previously underwent hysterectomy with bilateral salpingo-oophorectomy, with no hormone replacement treatment. She was treated by rectosigmoidectomy with colostomy [65].

It is difficult to diagnose bowel endometriosis by colonoscopy because most cases do not infiltrate beyond the serosa and very few infiltrate the mucosa [67]. Deep endometriosis is a very complicated disease to diagnose and treat, especially in older patients [43,68].

Jones et al. reported a case of a surgical menopause for deep rectovaginal endometriosis, with estrogen replacement therapy. A polyp was detected on colonoscopy and the biopsy confirmed a malignant transformation of endometriosis to adenocarcinoma [69].

9.2. Urinary Tract Endometriosis

Urinary tract endometriosis is an uncommon pathology and a silent cause of monolateral or bilateral kidney dysfunction. The diagnosis of urinary tract endometriosis is difficult since the disease is associated with nonspecific symptoms, regardless of the hormonal status [70] (Figure 2).

Figure 2. Urinary tract endometriosis—laparoscopic resection of a bladder endometriosis nodule infiltrating the bladder mucosa (personal collection, L. Pirtea).

A few case reports have been published regarding bladder endometriosis in postmenopausal women. Stewart reported a case of bladder endometriosis extending into the bowel in a postmenopausal woman. He concluded that it was due to reactivation of the endometrial implants under exogenous estrogen stimulation [71]. Also, a case of a 68-year-old postmenopausal woman, with no exogenous estrogen therapy, with an abnormal mass of the bladder that turned out to be an endometriosis lesion, was reported. This case suggests that endometriosis may persist even after years of a hormonally castrated state [72].

10. Conclusions

The paradigm shift from the belief that endometriosis only affects women of reproductive age has drawn attention to endometriosis in both premenarchal and postmenopausal patients. Despite its relatively low incidence, physicians should consider endometriosis in cases of unclear pelvic pain in postmenopausal patients, even if the patient has no prior history of endometriosis lesions.

Postmenopausal endometriosis seems to expose the patient to a higher risk of malignant transformation. Due to the lack of high-quality studies, it remains unclear how to advise women with a history of endometriosis regarding the management of menopausal symptoms. The absolute risk of disease recurrence and malignant transformation cannot be quantified, and the impact of HRT use on these outcomes is not known. Multicenter randomized trials or large observational studies are urgently needed to inform clinicians and patients alike.

Author Contributions: L.B., C.S. and S.B. were responsible for drafting the article, L.B. and O.B. performed the data collection, data analysis and contributed to the interpretation of the results. L.B., P.P. and G.D. participated in the conception and the design of the study. L.P. and C.S. were responsible for the critical revision of the article and approved the final version to be published. All authors have read and agreed to the published version of the manuscript.

References

1.   Guy, J.M.; Edgar, H. (1859–1942): General practitioner and radium pioneer. *J. Med. Biogr.* **2009**, *17*, 127–134. [CrossRef] [PubMed]

2.   Laufer, M.R.; Sanfilippo, J.; Rose, G. Adolescent endometriosis: Diagnosis and treatment approaches. *J. Pediatr. Adolesc. Gynecol.* **2003**, *16*, S3–S11. [CrossRef]

3.   Janssen, E.B.; Rijkers, A.C.M.; Hoppenbrouwers, K.; Meuleman, C.; D'Hooghe, T.M. Prevalence of endometriosis diagnosed by laparoscopy in adolescents with dysmenorrhea or chronic pelvic pain: A systematic review. *Hum. Reprod. Update* **2013**, *19*, 570–582. [CrossRef] [PubMed]

4.   Dowlut-McElroy, T.; Strickland, J.L. Endometriosis in adolescents. *Curr. Opin. Obstet. Gynecol.* **2017**, *29*, 306–309. [CrossRef] [PubMed]

5.   Suchońska, B.; Gajewska, M.; Zyguła, A.; Wielgoś, M. Endometriosis resembling endometrial cancer in a postmenopausal patient. *Climacteric* **2018**, *21*, 88–91. [CrossRef] [PubMed]

6.   Haas, D.; Chvatal, R.; Reichert, B.; Renner, S.; Shebl, O.; Binder, H.; Wurm, P.; Oppelt, P. Endometriosis: A premenopausal disease? Age pattern in 42,079 patients with endometriosis. *Arch. Gynecol. Obstet.* **2012**, *286*, 667–670. [CrossRef]

7.   Henriksen, E. Endometriosis. *Am. J. Surg.* **1955**, *90*, 331–337. [CrossRef]

8.   Ranney, B.E., III. Complete operations. *Am. J. Obstet. Gynecol.* **1971**, *109*, 1137–1144. [CrossRef]

9.   Nikkanen, V.; Punnonen, R. External endometriosis in 801 operated patients. *Acta Obstet. Gynecol. Scand.* **1984**, *63*, 699–701. [CrossRef]

10. Dong-Su, J.; Tae-Hee, K. Endometriosis in a Postmenopausal Woman on Hormonal Replacement Therapy. *J. Menopausal Med.* **2013**, *19*, 151–153.

11. Benjamin, M. Snyder Postmenopausal Deep Infiltrating Endometriosis of the Colon: Rare Location and Novel Medical Therapy. *Hindawi Case Rep. Gastrointest. Med.* **2018**, *2018*, 5.

12. Palep-Singh, M.; Gupta, S. Endometriosis: Associations with menopause, hormone replacement therapy and cancer. *Menopause Int.* **2009**, *15*, 169–174. [CrossRef] [PubMed]

13. Abdallah, A.A. Gastric wall endometriosis in a postmenopausal woman. *Egypt. J. Radiol. Nucl. Med.* **2016**, *47*, 1783–1786.

14. Asencio, F.; Ribeiro, H.A.; Ribeiro, P.A.; Malzoni, M.; Adamyan, L.; Ussia, A.; Gomel, V.; Martin, D.C.; Koninckx, P.R. Symptomatic endometriosis developing several years after menopause in the absence of increased circulating estrogen concentrations: A systematic review and seven case reports. *Gynecol. Surg.* **2019**, *3*, 16.

15. Streuli, I.; Gaitzsch, H.; Wenger, J.M.; Petignat, P. Endometriosis after menopause: Physiopathology and management of an uncommon condition. *Climacteric* **2017**, *20*, 138–143. [CrossRef]

16. Cumiskey, J.; Whyte, P.; Kelehan, P.; Kelehan, P.; Gibbons, D. A detailed morphologic and immunohistochemical comparison of pre- and postmenopausal endometriosis. *J. Clin. Pathol.* **2008**, *61*, 455–459. [CrossRef]

17. Kempers, R.D.; Dockerty, M.B.; Hunt, A.B.; Symmonds, R.E. Significant postmenopausal endometriosis. *Surg. Gynecol. Obstet.* **1960**, *111*, 348–356.

18. Morotti, M.; Remorgida, V.; Venturini, P.L.; Ferrero, S. Endometriosis in menopause: A single institution experience. *Arch. Gynecol. Obstet.* **2012**, *286*, 1571–1575. [CrossRef]

19. Manero, M.G.; Royo, P. Endometriosis in a postmenopausal woman without previous hormonal therapy: A case report. *J. Med. Case Rep.* **2009**, *3*, 135. [CrossRef]

20. Mehedintu, C.; Plotogea, M.N. Endometriosis still a challenge. *J. Med. Life* **2014**, *7*, 349–357.

21. Rolla, E. Writing–Review & Editing Endometriosis: Advances and controversies in classification, pathogenesis, diagnosis, and treatment. *F1000Research* **2019**, 8. [CrossRef]

22. Saccardi, C.; Cosmi, E.; Borghero, A.; Tregnaghi, A.; Dessole, S.; Litta, P. Comparison between transvaginal sonography, saline contrast sonovaginography and magnetic resonance imaging in the diagnosis of posterior deep infiltrating endometriosis. *Ultrasound Obstet. Gynecol.* **2012**, *40*, 464–469. [CrossRef]

23. Vimercatti, A.; Achilarre, M.T.; Scardapane, A.; Lorusso, F.; Ceci, O.; Mangiatordi, G.; Angelelli, G.; Herendael, B.V.; Selvaggi, L.; Bettocchi, S. Accuracy of transvaginal sonography and contrast-enhanced magnetic resonance-colonography for the presurgical staging of deep infiltrating endometriosis. *Ultrasound Obstet. Gynecol.* **2012**, *40*, 592–603. [CrossRef] [PubMed]

24. Parveen, P.; Pinar, O.; Terry, K.L. Endometriosis: Epidemiology, Diagnosis and Clinical Management. *Curr. Obstet. Gynecol. Rep.* **2017**, *6*, 34–41.

25. Ulrich, U.; Buchweitz, O.; Greb, R.; Keckstein, J.; von Leffern, I.; Oppelt, P.; Renner, S.P.; Sillem, M.; Stummvoll, W.; De Wilde, R.L.; et al. National German Guideline (S2k): Guideline for the Diagnosis and Treatment of Endometriosis: Long Version -AWMF Registry No. 015-045. *Geburtshilfe Frauenheilkd* **2014**, *74*, 1104–1118. [PubMed]

26. Armstrong, C. ACOG updates guideline on diagnosis and treatment of endometriosis. *Am. Fam. Physician* **2011**, *1*, 83–84.

27. Kuznetsov, L.; Dworzynski, K.; Davies, M.; Overton, C. Guideline Committee. Diagnosis and management of endometriosis: Summary of NICE guidance. *BMJ* **2017**, *358*, j3935. [CrossRef]

28. Dunselman, G.A.; Vermeulen, N.; Becker, C.; Calhaz-Jorge, C.; D'Hooghe, T.; De Bie, B. ESHRE guideline: Management of women with endometriosis. *Hum. Reprod.* **2014**, *29*, 400–412. [CrossRef]

29. Schipper, E.; Nezhat, C. Video-assisted laparoscopy for the detection and diagnosis of endometriosis: Safety, reliability, and invasiveness. *Int. J. Womens Health* **2012**, *4*, 383–393.

30. Alborzi, S.; Rasekhi, A.; Shomali, Z.; Madadi, G.; Alborzi, M.; Kazemi, M.; Nohandani, A.H. Diagnostic accuracy of magnetic resonance imaging, transvaginal, and transrectal ultrasonography in deep infiltrating endometriosis. *Medicine (Baltim.)* **2018**, *97*, e9536. [CrossRef]

31. Bratila, E.; Comandaşu, D.E.; Coroleucă, C.; Cîrstoiu, M.M.; Berceanu, C.; Mehedintu, C.; Bratila, P.; Vladareanu, S. Diagnosis of endometriotic lesions by sonovaginography with ultrasound gel. *Med. Ultrason* **2016**, *18*, 469–474. [CrossRef]

32. Cossi, P.; Schor, E.; Gonçalves, L.F.; Werner, H. Assessment of rectovaginal endometriosis using three-dimensional gel-infusion sonovaginography. *Ultrasound Obstet. Gynecol* **2019**, *53*, 558–560. [CrossRef]

33. Reid, S.; Lu, C.; Hardy, N.; Casikar, I.; Reid, G.; Cario, G.; Chou, D.; Almashat, D.; Condous, G. Office gel sonovaginography for the prediction of posterior deep infiltrating endometriosis: A multicenter prospective observational study. *Ultrasound Obstet. Gynecol.* **2014**, *44*, 710–718. [CrossRef] [PubMed]

34. Han, C.; Bellone, S.; Siegel, E.R.; Altwerger, G.; Menderes, G.; Bonazzoli, E.; Egkata-Takata, T.; Pettinella, F.; Bianchi, A.; Riccio, F.; et al. A novel multiple biomarker panel for the early detection of high-grade serous ovarian carcinoma. *Gynecol. Oncol.* **2018**, *149*, 585–591. [CrossRef] [PubMed]

35. Rai, N.; Champaneria, R.; Snell, K.; Mallett, S.; Bayliss, S.E.; Neal, R.D.; Balogun, M.; Kehoe, S.; Deeks, J.J.; Sundar, S.; et al. Symptoms, ultrasound imaging and biochemical markers alone or in combination for the diagnosis of ovarian cancer in women with symptoms suspicious of ovarian cancer. *Cochrane Database Syst. Rev.* **2015**, *2015*, CD011964. [CrossRef]

36. Dorien, F.O.; Fassbender, A.; Van Bree, R.; Laenen, A.; Peterse, D.P.; Vanhie, A.; Waelkens, E.; D'Hooghe, T.M. Technical Verification and Assessment of Independent Validation of Biomarker Models for Endometriosis. *Biomed. Res. Int.* **2019**, *2019*, 3673060.

37. Kennedy, S.; Bergvist, A.; Chapron, C.; D'Hooghe, T.; Dunselman, G.; Greb, R.; Hummelshoj, L.; Prentice, A. ESHRE guideline for the diagnosis and treatment of endometriosis. *Hum. Reprod.* **2005**, *20*, 2698–2704. [CrossRef]

38. Ozyurek, E.S.; Yoldemir, T.; Kalkan, U. Surgical challenges in the treatment of perimenopausal and postmenopausal endometriosis. *Climacteric* **2018**, *4*, 385–390. [CrossRef]

39. Moen, M.H.; Rees, M.; Brincat, M.; Erel, T.; Gambacciani, M.; Lambrinoudaki, I.; Schenck-Gustafsson, K.; Tremollieres, F.; Vujovic, S.; Rozenberg, S. European Menopause and Andropause Society. EMAS position statement: Managing the menopause in women with a past history of endometriosis. *Maturitas* **2010**, *67*, 94–97. [CrossRef]

40. Gemmell, L.C.; Webster, K.E.; Kirtley, S.; Vincent, K.; Zondervan, K.T.; Becker, C.M. The management of menopause in women with a history of endometriosis: A systematic review. *Hum. Reprod. Update* **2017**, *23*, 481–500. [CrossRef]

41. Oxholm, D.; Knudsen, U.B.; Kryger-Baggesen, N.; Ravn, P. Postmenopausal endometriosis. *Acta Obstet. Gynecol. Scand.* **2007**, *86*, 1158–1164. [CrossRef] [PubMed]

42. Tan, D.A.; Almaria, M.J.G. Postmenopausal endometriosis: Drawing a clearer clinical picture. *Climacteric* **2018**, *21*, 249–255. [CrossRef] [PubMed]

43. Inceboz, U. Endometriosis after menopause. *Womens Health (Lond.)* **2015**, *11*, 711–715. [CrossRef] [PubMed]

44. Somboonporn, W.; Panna, S.; Temtanakitpaisan, T.; Kaewrudee, S.; Soontrapa, S. Effects of the levonorgestrel-releasing intrauterine system plus estrogen therapy in perimenopausal and postmenopausal women: Systematic review and meta-analysis. *Menopause* **2011**, *18*, 1060–1066. [CrossRef] [PubMed]

45. Zanello, M.; Borghese, G.; Manzara, F.; Esposti, E.D.; Moro, E.; Raimondo, D.; Abdullahi, L.O.; Arena, A.; Terzano, P.; Meriggiola, M.C.; et al. Hormonal Replacement Therapy in Menopausal Women with History of Endometriosis: A Review of Literature. *Medcine* **2019**, *55*, 477. [CrossRef] [PubMed]

46. Takayama, K.; Zeitoun, K.; Gunby, R.T.; Sasano, H.; Carr, B.R.; Bulun, S.E. Treatment of severe postmenopausal endometriosis with an aromatase inhibitor. *Fertil. Steril.* **1998**, *69*, 709–713. [CrossRef]

47. Bulun, S.E.; Yang, S.; Fang, Z.; Gurates, B.; Tamura, M.; Sebastian, S. Estrogen production and metabolism in endometriosis. *Ann. N. Y. Acad. Sci.* **2002**, *955*, 75–85. [CrossRef]

48. Słopien, R.; Męczekalski, B. Aromatase inhibitors in the treatment of endometriosis. *Prz. Menopauzalny Menopause Rev.* **2016**, *15*, 43–47. [CrossRef]

49. Hajjar, L.R.; Kim, W.; Nolan, G.H.; Turner, S.; Raju, U.R. Intestinal and pelvic endometriosis presenting as a tumor and associated with tamoxifen therapy: Report of a case. *Obstet. Gynecol.* **1993**, *82* (Suppl. S2), 642–644.

50. Bardi, M.; Arnoldi, E.; Pizzocchero, G.; Pezzica, E.; Mattioni, D.; Perotti, M. Endometrioid carcinoma in pelvic endometriosis in a postmenopausal woman with tamoxifen adjuvant therapy for breast cancer: A case report. *Eur. J. Gynaecol. Oncol.* **1994**, *15*, 393–395.

51. Cohen, I.; Altaras, M.M.; Lew, S.; Tepper, R.; Beyth, Y.; Ben-Baruch, G. Ovarian endometrioid carcinoma and endometriosis developing in a postmenopausal breast cancer patient during tamoxifen therapy: A case report and review of the literature. *Gynecol. Oncol.* **1994**, *55*, 443–447. [CrossRef] [PubMed]

52. Schlesinger, C.; Silverberg, S.G. Tamoxifen-associated polyps (basalomas) arising in multiple endometriotic foci: A case report and review of the literature. *Gynecol. Oncol.* **1999**, *73*, 305–311. [CrossRef] [PubMed]

53. Okugawa, K.; Hirakawa, T.; Ogawa, S.; Kaku, T.; Nakano, H. Ovarian endometrioid adenocarcinoma arising from an endometriotic cyst in a postmenopausal woman under tamoxifen therapy for breast cancer: A case report. *Gynecol. Oncol.* **2002**, *87*, 231–234. [CrossRef] [PubMed]

54. Bese, T.; Simsek, Y.; Bese, N.; Ilvan, S.; Arvas, M. Extensive pelvic endometriosis with malignant change in tamoxifen-treated postmenopausal women. *Int. J. Gynecol. Cancer* **2003**, *13*, 376–380. [CrossRef]

55. Marie-Scemama, L.; Even, M.; De La Joliniere, J.B.; Ayoubi, J.M. Endometriosis and the menopause: Why the question merits our full attention. *Horm. Mol. Biol. Clin. Investig.* **2019**, *37*, 1. [CrossRef]

56. Brinton, L.A.; Gridley, G.; Persson, I.; Baron, J.; Bergqvist, A. Cancer risk after a hospital discharge diagnosis of endometriosis. *Am. J. Obstet. Gynecol.* **1997**, *176*, 572–579. [CrossRef]

57. Van Gorp, T.; Amant, F.; Neven, P.; Vergote, I.; Moerman, P. Endometriosis and the development of malignant tumours of the pelvis. A review of literature. *Best Pract. Res. Clin. Obstet. Gynaecol.* **2004**, *18*, 349–371. [CrossRef]

58. Somigliana, E.; Vigano, P.; Parazzini, F.; Stoppelli, S.; Giambattista, E.; Vercellini, P. Association between endometriosis and cancer: A comprehensive review and critical analysis of clinical epidemiological evidence. *Gynecol. Oncol.* **2006**, *101*, 331–341. [CrossRef]

59. Bertelsen, L.; Mellemkjær, L.; Frederiksen, K.; Kjær, S.K.; Brinton, L.A.; Sakoda, L.C.; van Valkengoed, I.; Olsen, J.H. Risk for breast cancer among women with endometriosis. *Int. J. Cancer* **2006**, *120*, 1372–1375. [CrossRef]

60. Ness, R.B. Endometriosis and ovarian cancer: Thoughts on shared pathophysiology. *Am. J. Obstet. Gynecol.* **2003**, *189*, 280–294. [CrossRef]

61. Zanetta, G.M.; Webb, M.J.; Li, H.; Keeney, G.L. Hyperestrogenism: A relevant risk factor for the development of cancer from endometriosis. *Gynecol. Oncol.* **2000**, *79*, 18–22. [CrossRef] [PubMed]

62. Mathey, M.P.; de Jolinière, J.B.; Major, A.; Pugin, F.; Monnard, E.; Fiche, M.; Sandmeier, D.; Khomsi, F.; Feki, A. Endometriotic Mass after Hysterectomy in a 61 Year Old Post-menopausal Woman: A Case Report and Update. *Front. Surg.* **2019**, *6*, 14. [CrossRef] [PubMed]

63. Charatsi, D.; Koukoura, O.; Ntavela, I.G. Gastrointestinal and Urinary Tract Endometriosis: A Review on the Commonest Locations of Extrapelvic Endometriosis. *Adv. Med.* **2018**, *2018*, 3461209. [CrossRef] [PubMed]

64. Bergqvist, A. Extragenital endometriosis: A review. *Eur. J. Surg.* **1992**, *158*, 7–12. [PubMed]

65. Popoutchi, P.; Reis Lemos, C.R.; Silva, J.C.; Nogueira, A.A.; Feres, O.; Ribeiro da Rocha, J.J. Postmenopausal intestinal obstructive endometriosis: Case report and review of the literature. *Sao Paulo Med. J.* **2008**, *126*, 190–193. [CrossRef] [PubMed]

66. Flyckt, R.; Lyden, S.; Roma, A.; Falcone, T. Post-menopausal endometriosis with inferior vena cava invasion requiring surgical management. *Hum. Reprod.* **2011**, *26*, 2709–2712. [CrossRef] [PubMed]

67. Milone, M.; Mollo, A.; Musella, M.; Maietta, P.; Fernandez, L.M.S.; Shatalova, O.; Conforti, A.; Barone, G.; De Placide, G.; Milone, F. Role of colonoscopy in the diagnostic work-up of bowel endometriosis. *World J. Gastroenterol.* **2015**, *21*, 4997–5001. [CrossRef]

68. Thomsen, L.H.; Schnack, T.H.; Buchardi, K.; Hummelshoj, L.; Missmer, S.A.; Forman, A.; Blaakaer, J. Risk factors of epithelial ovarian carcinomas among women with endometriosis: A systematic review. *Acta Obstet. Gynecol. Scand.* **2017**, *96*, 761–778. [CrossRef]

69. Jones, K.D.; Owen, E.; Berresford, A.; Sutton, C. Endometrial adenocarcinoma arising from endometriosis of the rectosigmoid colon. *Gynecol. Oncol.* **2002**, *86*, 220–222. [CrossRef]

70. Ponticelli, C.; Graziani, G.; Montanari, E. Ureteral Endometriosis: A Rare and Underdiagnosed Cause of Kidney Dysfunction. *Nephron Clin. Pract.* **2010**, *114*, c89–c94. [CrossRef]

71. Stewart, W.W.; Ireland, G.W. Vesical endometriosis in a postmenopausal woman: A case report. *J. Urol.* **1977**, *118*, 480–481. [CrossRef]

72. Habuchi, T.; Okagaki, T.; Miyakawa, M. Endometriosis of Bladder after Menopause. *J. Urol.* **1991**, *145*, 361–363. [CrossRef]

The Pathogenesis of Endometriosis: Molecular and Cell Biology Insights

Antonio Simone Laganà [1,*,†], **Simone Garzon** [1,†], **Martin Götte** [2], **Paola Viganò** [3], **Massimo Franchi** [4], **Fabio Ghezzi** [1] **and Dan C. Martin** [5,6]

1   Department of Obstetrics and Gynecology, "Filippo Del Ponte" Hospital, University of Insubria, Piazza Biroldi 1, 21100 Varese, Italy; simone.garzon@univr.it (S.G.); fabio.ghezzi@uninsubria.it (F.G.)
2   Department of Gynecology and Obstetrics, Münster University Hospital, D-48149 Münster, Germany; mgotte@uni-muenster.de
3   Reproductive Sciences Laboratory, Division of Genetics and Cell Biology, San Raffaele Scientific Institute, Via Olgettina 60, 20136 Milan, Italy; vigano.paola@hsr.it
4   Department of Obstetrics and Gynecology, AOUI Verona, University of Verona, Piazzale Aristide Stefani 1, 37126 Verona, Italy; massimo.franchi@univr.it
5   School of Medicine, University of Tennessee Health Science Center, 910 Madison Ave, Memphis, TN 38163, USA; danmartin46@gmail.com
6   Virginia Commonwealth University, 907 Floyd Ave, Richmond, VA 23284, USA
*   Correspondence: antoniosimone.lagana@uninsubria.it
†   Equal contributions (joint first authors).

Abstract: The etiopathogenesis of endometriosis is a multifactorial process resulting in a heterogeneous disease. Considering that endometriosis etiology and pathogenesis are still far from being fully elucidated, the current review aims to offer a comprehensive summary of the available evidence. We performed a narrative review synthesizing the findings of the English literature retrieved from computerized databases from inception to June 2019, using the Medical Subject Headings (MeSH) unique ID term "Endometriosis" (ID:D004715) with "Etiology" (ID:Q000209), "Immunology" (ID:Q000276), "Genetics" (ID:D005823) and "Epigenesis, Genetic" (ID:D044127). Endometriosis may origin from Müllerian or non-Müllerian stem cells including those from the endometrial basal layer, Müllerian remnants, bone marrow, or the peritoneum. The innate ability of endometrial stem cells to regenerate cyclically seems to play a key role, as well as the dysregulated hormonal pathways. The presence of such cells in the peritoneal cavity and what leads to the development of endometriosis is a complex process with a large number of interconnected factors, potentially both inherited and acquired. Genetic predisposition is complex and related to the combined action of several genes with limited influence. The epigenetic mechanisms control many of the processes involved in the immunologic, immunohistochemical, histological, and biological aberrations that characterize the eutopic and ectopic endometrium in affected patients. However, what triggers such alterations is not clear and may be both genetically and epigenetically inherited, or it may be acquired by the particular combination of several elements such as the persistent peritoneal menstrual reflux as well as exogenous factors. The heterogeneity of endometriosis and the different contexts in which it develops suggest that a single etiopathogenetic model is not sufficient to explain its complex pathobiology.

Keywords: endometriosis; pathogenesis; genetics; epigenetics; immunology

1. Introduction

The etiopathogenesis of endometriosis is a multifactorial process resulting in a heterogeneous disease [1]. Its origin may be from Müllerian or non-Müllerian stem cells. These could include stem cells of the endometrial basal layer, Müllerian remnants, bone marrow, or the peritoneum. Furthermore, the innate ability of endometrial stem cells to regenerate cyclically under the influence of estrogen followed by estrogen/progesterone stimulation and then hormonal withdrawal seems to play a key role. The presence of such cells in the peritoneal cavity and what leads to the development of endometriosis is a complex process with a large number of interconnected factors potentially both inherited and acquired [2]. Genetic studies have confirmed a complex genetic nature [3]. At the same time, the epigenetic mechanisms underlying endometriosis support the processes that promote the acquisition and maintenance of immunologic, immunohistochemical, histological, and biological aberrations that characterize both the eutopic and ectopic endometrium in patients affected by endometriosis. This may be related to the particular combination of factors linked menstrual reflux into the peritoneal cavity as well as exogenous factors [4]. Once started, the process is variable and can lead to the development of endometriosis or can reach a limit to its growth and then stabilize or regress. As a result, the heterogeneity of endometriosis and the different phenotypes suggest that a single etiopathogenetic explaining model is not sufficient.

What is Endometriosis?

Endometriosis is a common, benign, inflammatory, generally gynecologic disease that includes the presence and growth of dysfunctional endometrial-like glands and stroma often with reactive fibrosis and muscular metaplasia outside the uterus [5]. It is associated with pelvic pain and subfertility in reproductive age women and can severely compromise the quality of life of affected women [6–11] and require extensive surgery when more conservative treatment options fail [12,13]. The prevalence rate of symptomatic endometriosis is estimated to be 10% with an incidence of about 2-7/1000 women per year and a further 11% of undiagnosed cases, although there are only a few studies with well-estimated prevalence and incidence of endometriosis in the general population [14–16] and some suggesting that many, if not all, women have endometriosis as a transient phenomenon [17,18].

Since the introduction of the term "endometriosis" and its pathogenesis theories by Sampson [19–21], extensive basic and clinical research concerning the etiopathogenesis of endometriosis has been carried out. However, the exact origin and mechanism of endometriosis development remain theoretical. The growing body of evidence confirms the multifactorial nature of endometriosis that is the result of the combined contribution of anatomical, hormonal, immunological, reactive, estrogenic, genetic, epigenetic, and environmental factors in affected women [7]. These multiple interconnected factors may explain the complex and heterogeneous presentations of the disease with different locations, appearances, developments, and hormone responsiveness. The heterogeneity and differences among the three main classes of endometriosis presentation (peritoneal, ovarian, and deep infiltrating endometriosis) are such as to suggest different pathogenetic pathways [22,23]. Moreover, a generally accepted hypothesis is that endometriosis is a phenomenon that may occur intermittently in all women during menstrual cycles, but that develops in a disabling disease only in a subset of women [17,18,24,25]. Understanding the multiple pathogenetic pathways underlining the development of endometriosis is of paramount importance, as they may have implications in the prevention, diagnosis, treatment, and prognosis of the disease [6].

2. Theories on the Origin of Endometriosis

The first question about the pathogenesis of endometriosis was about the origin of the endometrial-like glands and stroma that constitute the disease. Several hypotheses have been proposed since 1870 [26], some of only historical interest and some that are now considered the most plausible; nevertheless, none is able to completely explain the pathogenesis of endometriosis and all the different presentations of the disease [27]. Overall, all the proposed hypotheses for the cell origin can be categorized into two main theories: the in-situ theory and the transplantation theory.

2.1. The in Situ Theory

All the hypotheses belonging to this category are based on the concept that stroma and glands of endometrial-like tissue of endometriosis originate in-situ from the local tissues by metaplasia or by embryological origin. This hypothesis was proposed by Waldeyer in 1870 [26], who suggested that endometriosis develops from the germinal epithelium of the ovary by "metaplasia". Later, Von Recklinghausen in 1895 and Russell in 1899 introduced the concept of embryological origin from mesonephric/Wolffian remnants and Müllerian remnants, respectively [27].

The terms metaplasia and differentiation, whether these refer to the endometrium, to endometriotic cells, or pluripotent stem cells to endometriotic cells [28], are both used in this manuscript based on the original source document. We do not attempt to distinguish the differences between those two terms with overlapping meanings.

The Müllerian remnants hypothesis explains endometrial-like tissue as having developed from differentiation and proliferation of embryonic cell rests that are constituted by misplaced cells of primitive endometrial tissue along the migratory pathway of Müllerian ducts [29,30]. The cells spread across the posterior pelvic floor due to aberrant migration and differentiation during organogenesis of the female genital tract. Based on this hypothesis, "Müllerianosis" and "Secondary Müllerian system" theories were proposed as theoretical explanations of cell origin and dissemination of Müllerian-type epithelium outside the expected area of Müllerian duct development, including endometriosis, adenomyosis, endosalpingiosis, and endocervicosis [29,30]. However, embryological studies support the presence of Müllerian rests near the normal deep cul-de-sac area and not in other sites such as the ovary, sigmoid colon, appendix, or more distal sites such as the diaphragm and pleura [31].

The "Müllerianosis" hypothesis might explain that endometriosis is often found in the cul-de-sac, uterosacral ligaments, and medial broad ligaments; that peritoneal pockets with and without endometriosis have been associated with congenital tract malformations; and that endometriosis seems to have higher prevalence even in women with non-obstructive Müllerian abnormalities [32]. Moreover, this hypothesis is supported by the fact that is able to explain the presence of endometriosis in women with Mayer–Rokitansky–Küster–Hauser syndrome, in adolescents before or shortly after menarche , and in human female fetuses; where organoid structures outside uterine cavity resembling primitive endometrium were reported [31,33–35]. As previously noted, Signorile et al. [31] found CD10 positive remnants in the deep cul-de-sac only. Finally, Müllerian remnants or coelomic metaplasia in prostate and utricle may explain rare cases of endometriosis reported in males, after long-term high doses of estrogens for prostate carcinoma [36,37]. Immunohistochemical studies in men support both Müllerianosis and metaplasia theories [37].

Coelomic metaplasia or the stem cell differentiation hypothesis is based on the fact that, in the embryonic phase, the coelomic epithelium gives rise to both mesothelium of serosae and the epithelium lining of the cavity of Müllerian ducts, which forms the endometrium in the uterine body. This hypothesis explains endometriosis as developing from the metaplastic transformation of germinal ovarian epithelium and/or peritoneum serosa [38,39]. These metaplastic changes are supposed to occur secondary to hormonal influences [40,41], inflammatory processes [42,43], or the action of one or several endogenous biochemical or immunological factors derived from eutopic endometrium, based on the "induction" theory [44,45]. The induction theory is based on animal model studies suggesting that specific cell-free endometrial products were capable of inducing the metaplasia of undifferentiated mesenchyme into endometrial epithelium and glands, although no endometrial stroma was found. On that basis, it was supposed that these substances, released by uterine endometrium, may diffuse into the lymphatic and bloodstream and induce the formation of endometriosis in distant parts of the body [44,45]. The coelomic metaplasia hypothesis and the Müllerian remnants hypothesis may explain endometriosis in the absence of menstruation; and, additionally, it may explain the presence of endometriosis outside the pelvis such as in the chest, diaphragm, pleura, and lungs [36,46], although direct infiltration through the diaphragm or dissemination through diaphragmatic fenestrations or perforations are retrograde possibilities.

The main strength of in-situ theories is that they are able to explain endometriosis in women without menses or endometrium. Nevertheless, several factors are against in-situ theories. If peritoneal cells can easily undergo metaplastic transformation, endometriosis should be observed more frequently in men, in the thoracic cavity, and with a uniform distribution in the peritoneum. Moreover, if coelomic metaplasia resembles common metaplasia, the incidence of endometriosis should increase with advancing age. Finally, although some evidence suggests that endometriosis has a higher prevalence even in women with non-obstructive Müllerian abnormalities [32], other studies reported endometriosis to be more frequent in patients with Müllerian anomalies and outflow obstruction, and not in Müllerian anomalies as a whole [47,48].

2.2. The Transplantation Theory

In this category, the hypotheses are based on the concept that the stroma and glands of endometriosis originate from the eutopic endometrium. Endometriosis is proposed as benign metastasis of eutopic endometrium, which is displaced from the uterine cavity to another location inside the body through different routes. Hematogenous, lymphatic, and iatrogenic (mechanical) spread of endometrial or endometriotic cells can explain all uncommon extraperitoneal locations [49]. However, the most popular theory was introduced by Sampson in 1927 based on clinical and anatomical observations. Sampson proposed the retrograde menstruation theory that concludes that most endometriosis derives from the reflux of eutopic endometrial fragments through the fallopian tubes during menstruation, with subsequent implantation, transition from endometrium to endometriosis, and growth on and into the peritoneum and the ovary [19–21]. In addition, Sampson recognized that retrograde menstruation could not explain all forms of endometriosis and suggested venous dissemination or metaplasia as alternate theories [19,20].

Over the years, a growing body of evidence has supported the "retrograde menstruation" theory, and it is now the most accepted hypothesis for most forms of endometriosis. The most important step was the demonstration that the tubal reflux of menstrual tissue is a common event in women with patent fallopian tubes documented in 76-90% of women [6]. Blood was found in peritoneal fluid by laparoscopy in 90% of women with patent tubes and only in 15% with occluded tubes during the peri-menstrual period [50], and endometrial epithelial cells have been isolated in the peritoneal fluid of women during the early proliferative phase [51]. The second step was the identification of viable endometrium, single cells, and glandular structures in the shed menstrual tissue [52]. The demonstration that reflux of viable endometrium in the peritoneal cavity is a common event in fertile age women was essential to consider the "retrograde menstruation" theory plausible.

Moreover, the anatomical distribution of endometriosis in the pelvis with higher prevalence in the left side than in the right side, that is compatible with anatomical differences between the right and left hemipelvis [53], and the distribution in the abdomen with higher prevalence in the right diaphragm than in the left following the counter-clockwise distribution of peritoneal fluid [54], further supports the "retrograde menstruation" theory [53–55].

However, the transplantation theories are unable to explain endometriosis in women with Mayer–Rokitansky–Küster–Hauser syndrome, in adolescents before or shortly after menarche, and in males [19,31,33–35,37]. Moreover, available evidence suggests that endometriosis is not simply a transplanted normal endometrium. Numerous differences in hormone receptor levels, as well as histological, morphological, and biological characteristics, were reported when comparing endometriosis with eutopic endometrium, with only limited similarities. Although Sampson recognized that endometriosis was different from endometrium "both in structure and in function" and noted a transition from one to the other [19,20], his 1920s observations of a transition do not include all of the inflammatory, chemical, immunologic, epigenetic and genetic changes that have been discovered the last 40 years. Those changes require additional understanding of the transformation of any Müllerian (endometrial or rest) or non-Müllerian cell to endometriosis. Furthermore, eutopic endometrium of affected women is reported to have similar alterations of endometriotic lesions, that are not found in the eutopic endometrium of healthy women. This supports the hypothesis that the primary defect might be rooted in eutopic endometrium of women with endometriosis, although the gap between the incidence of refluxed menstruation and the incidence of endometriosis highlights the presence of further mechanisms [2].

3. Behind the Origins of Endometriosis

Although the origin of endometrial-like tissue that constitutes endometriosis is theoretical and debated, it is generally agreed that endometriosis is a phenomenon that may occur in all women during reproductive age, close laparoscopic examination of otherwise healthy peritoneum and microscopic examination of resected bowel can reveal almost microscopic or minimal peritoneal lesions [56–58], and many, if not most, of the small lesions tend to resolve or become inactive spontaneously. Therefore, only a subset of women with endometriosis develops a disabling disease regardless of the tissue origin [17,18,24,25]. To understand the origin of endometriosis and the mechanisms that explain the development of endometriosis as a disabling disease instead of spontaneous resolution, in vitro and in vivo studies and immunohistochemical, genetic, and epigenetic analysis were conducted [59–61]. Some studies, typically based on in vitro and in vivo models, were developed to investigate the stepwise formation of endometriotic lesions in order to test different specific hypotheses of the origin of endometriosis and to identify mechanisms that allow endometriotic lesion development [59,60]. Conversely, other studies, typically immunohistochemical, genetic, and epigenetic analysis, focused the investigation on the identification of prerequisites for the development of the disease instead of spontaneous resolution, comparing ectopic with eutopic endometrium in affected women or comparing parameters between affected and unaffected women [54,62–64]. Overall, this growing body of evidence suggests that endometriosis is not simply ectopic endometrium, with many reported differences between the endometrial-like tissue of endometriosis and eutopic endometrium in affected women [65]. However, this data has not clarified when replanted endometrium or Müllerian remnants begin the transition from ectopic Müllerian tissue to endometriosis, or when non-Müllerian stem cells are committed to differentiate into endometriosis. At the same time, when women with symptomatic endometriosis are compared with women without or minimal disease, the differences were reported not only at the level of endometriosis implants but even at the level of eutopic endometrium [66], uterus [67], and peritoneal environment [68].

3.1. Comprehensive Models on the Origin of Endometriosis

The induction theory was tested by in vivo studies on rabbit models. Endometrium was implanted in the abdominal cavity, and tissue was histologically evaluated for seven days [44]. Endometrial implants degenerated during the first four days, and cysts and endometrium-like differentiation were observed in the next three days in the surrounding connective tissue. If the tissue was dissociated before implantation, better results were obtained. These findings were further confirmed in a study in which viable and ischemic endometrial tissue was implanted intraperitoneally in rabbits within Millipore filters, that allowed only chemical substances to pass due to the small pore size [45]. Endometrium-like epithelium and glands were observed in the connective tissue adjacent to the implants. Although these changes did not include stroma, these observations support the hypothesis that endometrial tissue liberates specific substances inducing undifferentiated mesenchyme to develop into endometrial tissue.

Conversely, investigating the possibility that retrograde menstruation of shed endometrium is the origin of endometriosis, a chicken chorioallantoic membrane (CAM) model, an in vitro model that uses the membrane covering the chicken embryo, was used to study the stepwise endometriotic lesion formation involved in this process [69]. Tissue can be transplanted onto CAM and interventions can be carried out, allowing the behavior of the tissue and the consequences of interventions to be observed. In order to visualize the different steps of "retrograde menstruation" theory, human menstrual endometrial fragments were collected and were transplanted onto the CAM. After 24, 48, and 72 hours, cross-sections of the CAMs were cut and immunohistochemically stained. After 24 hours, direct contact was present between menstrual tissue fragments and the CAM mesenchyme. After 48 h, the menstrual endometrium was reorganized inside the CAM mesenchyme, and after 72 hours, a complete endometrium with glands and stroma was present in the CAM mesenchyme. Moreover, blood vessels attracted from the CAM were present inside the endometrium fragment. This model showed that viable endometrium is necessary to form an endometriotic lesion, and that stroma and glands of shed menstrual endometrium are able to adhere to and degrade the matrix and to induce neo-angiogenesis in order to survive [70].

3.2. Role of Hormones

Why a transplanted or congenital ectopic endometrium develops into endometriosis is the source of much research. The causes of this development include research on the role of estrogen and estrogen receptors (ERs), the estrogen-dependent physiologic and molecular changes [71], the local levels of estrogen [71,72], the role of estrogen in macrophage-nerve interaction [72], the effects of environmental toxicants on estrogen signaling [73], and the intracellular estrogen production related to aromatase activity. In addition, the normal control of cyclic estrogen and progesterone requires activation and crosstalk of cAMP and progesterone mediated signaling pathways [74].

Intracellular production of estrogens has a key role in the pathogenesis of endometriosis, particularly in post-menopausal women [75], as well as of other benign and malignant diseases of the female reproductive tract. Aromatase P450 catalyzes the conversion of androgens to estrogens and is physiologically expressed in different human tissues, including ovaries and adipose tissue, but usually not in the endometrium [76,77].

In women with endometriosis, this enzyme has been found in both endometriotic tissue and eutopic endometrium [77,78]. Moreover, in endometriosis the protective action of 17β-hydroxysteroid dehydrogenase (17β-HSD) type 2 is lost due to enzymatic deficiency. 17β-HSD lowers the level of the strong 17β-estradiol, converting it into the weak estrone, modulating the exposure to estrogens action [79]. The local production of estrogens and the loss of protective mechanisms determine a higher estradiol level that characterizes both endometriosis and eutopic endometrium of affected women, as demonstrated by the higher estradiol level of menstrual effluent in women with endometriosis as compared to controls [80]. Moreover, the increased estrogen production in endometriotic lesions and eutopic endometrium determines a positive feedback loop resulting in further estrogen production through the induction of cyclo-oxygenase type 2 (COX-2) enzyme. The subsequently elevated levels of prostaglandin E2 further stimulates the aromatase activity [78,81].

Of interest, the local production of estrogen was reported as a result of the activation of tissue injury and repair (TIAR) mechanisms induced by microtrauma at the level of basal endometrial layer. The basal endometrial layer has stem cell characteristics and exhibits the potential for dislocation and proliferation, that was reported enhanced in women with endometriosis [82,83]. The fragments of basal endometrium dislocated into the peritoneal cavity may induce chronic inflammation and TIAR mechanisms, that activate local production of estrogen, proliferation, and infiltrative growth resulting in endometriosis [67,84].

The estrogenic microenvironment was reported able to activate macrophages into peritoneum with the consequent secretion of pro-inflammatory cytokines such as tumor necrosis factor-α (TNF-α) and interleukin-1β (IL-1β) that stimulate the activation of NFkB. Moreover, these mechanisms induce vascular endothelial growth factor (VEGF) expression, cell cycle activation, and activation of the anti-apoptotic gene Bcl-2 [7,85] (Figure 1).

The key role of estrogens in endometriotic tissue survival and development is mediated by ERs. Endometriotic tissue development was reported suppressed by ER-selective modulators inhibiting estrogen receptor alfa (ERα) or beta (ERβ) [86], as well as ectopic implants did not develop normally in ERα- or ERβ-knockout mice [87,88]. ERs have similar affinity for estrogens and are transcriptional factors for similar subset of genes. Nevertheless, the differences between target genes, estrogen affinity, and tissue distribution of ERα and ERβ homodimers as well as ERα/ERβ heterodimer explain the reciprocal inhibitory and regulatory functions, as well as the different roles [89]. Although ERα was historical investigated due to his higher prevalence in the uterus and the supposed inhibitory effect of ERβ in the eutopic endometrium [90], in the endometriotic tissue ERα was reported having a normal expression level as compared to normal endometrium. Conversely, ERβ was reported overexpressed, determining an inversion of ERβ to ERα ratio as compared to eutopic endometrium [91]. On that basis, it was supposed that both the high estrogens concentration and the overexpression of ERβ are involved in the estrogen-based ectopic tissue survival and development. At the cytoplasmatic level, ERβ was reported involved in the inhibition and disruption of TNF-α-induced apoptosis signaling [88]. At nuclear level, ERβ was identified involved in the direct activation of the NFkB pathway and the radical oxygen species detoxification system, that are able to improve cell survival and cell escaping from immune clearance [92]. At the same time, ERβ was related to the upregulation of hypoxia-induced signaling, epithelial mesenchymal transition signaling, and cytoskeleton components, that are all involved in the invasion and progression of endometriotic implants [92].

The synergistic counterpart of estrogen overproduction and ERs overexpression is the progesterone resistance in endometriotic tissue, that impedes to modulate genes involved in the decidualization, cell cycle regulation, and estrogen response inhibition [93]. The progesterone resistance is a characteristic of the endometriotic tissue as compared to the eutopic endometrium, although it was identified in the eutopic endometrium of affected women as compared to controls [94].

The main mechanism involved in the progesterone resistance is the downregulation of progesterone receptor (PR) in the ectopic tissue, that determines a variation in the expression of progesterone target genes, such as the gene coding the 17β-HSD [93,95].

The pathways potentially underlining the PR suppression are multiple. The concentration of pro-inflammatory cytokines, such as TNF-α and IL-1β involved in the chronic inflammation and TIAR mechanisms, is reported directly correlated with PR expression [96]. The activation of NFkB pathway by inflammation signaling determines a direct interaction with PR thorough an antagonist effect [97]. Similarly, the persistent phosphorylation of AKT determined by inflammation is involved in the inhibition of PR expression [98].

These mechanisms explain the progesterone resistance as an acquired characteristic of the endometriotic tissue versus an individual predisposition. This is further supported by the inconsistent results provided by genetic studies [99] and the involvement of epigenetic mechanisms, such as the methylation of the gene and related promoter coding for the PR [100], and the higher expression of miRNAs blocking the estrogen-dependent PR expression [101].

Figure 1. Summary of the mechanisms underlining the key role of estrogens in the pathogenesis of endometriosis. Tissue injury and repair (TIAR); Tumor necrosis factor (TNF); Interleukins (IL); Vascular endothelial growth factor (VEGF); Antiapoptotic protein B cell lymphoma 2 (Bcl-2); 17β-hydroxysteroid dehydrogenase (17β-HSD).

3.3. The Peritoneal Microenvironment and the Role of Immune Surveillance

The peritoneal fluid is produced by peritoneal and, mainly, ovarian exudation. It is a microenvironment that contains different cells, such as immune cells, endometrial cells, and red blood cells, which produce and secrete growth factors, angiogenic factors, and cytokines, that are able to affect processes in the abdominal cavity [102]. Of note, studies reported shed endometrial cells differing from eutopic cells; this may be explained by the different environments of bloodstream as compared to the peritoneal fluid [2]. In the abdominal cavity, the menstrual effluent determines an inflammatory response, of which physiological role is to clear the ectopic cells and tissue. Neutrophils, phagocytic leukocytes, and chemotactic leukocytes are attracted from the circulation, where an increased influx of bone marrow-derived cells is physiologically observed before the menstruation onset. Approximately 70-80% are macrophages CD14+, 20% are natural killer cells (NK cells) CD56+, and 10% are T-cells CD3+. This system is suggested to be overwhelmed or insufficient in women with endometriosis [103–105]. Shorter intervals and longer menstrual periods with heavy blood flow, that are often reported in women with endometriosis, may result in larger amounts of endometrial tissue collected in the abdominal cavity that overwhelms this system of cleansing [106,107]. Larger endometrial tissue fragments may provide protection from enzymatic and phagocytic activity to cells residing inside, that continue to produce angiogenic factors due to continued hypoxia. Moreover, the overwhelmed capacity to clean the peritoneum due to excessive refluxed endometrium may explain the higher prevalence of some anatomical defects reported in women with endometriosis, such as uterine malformations that prevent or disturb normal antegrade menstruation or that determine dysfunctional retrograde contractions [47,48,108,109].

Moreover, in women with endometriosis, endometrial cells were more resistant to the cytolytic action of autologous peritoneal macrophages than in healthy controls [110]. The cytotoxicity of NK cells against endometrial cells was reported as decreased with an inverse correlation with the stage of the disease [111]. Protection against the cytotoxicity of peritoneal NK cells seems to be provided by an altered antigenicity due to the overexpression of human leukocyte antigen class I [62,112]. Additionally, the eutopic endometrium of women with endometriosis releases higher levels of the soluble form of intercellular adhesion molecule-1 (sICAM-1) than those of women without endometriosis; and the ectopic endometrial cells express higher levels of sICAM-1 when compared to their eutopic endometrium. sICAM-1 modulates the cytotoxic activity of NK and CD8+ cells competing with ICAM-1 to bind leukocyte function antigen-1 (LFA-1). Binding of sICAM-1 to LFA-1 impedes leukocytes to bind ICAM-1 on the surface of target cells, preventing leukocyte activation [113–115]. The inflammatory response in endometriosis is further accentuated by the increased expression and activity of COX- 2, interleukins, and oxidative stress that act through the mitogen-activated protein kinase (MAPK) pathways. The subsequent dysregulation of MAPK signaling pathways increases inflammation, thereby recruiting immune cells and amplifying the inflammatory response. Moreover, MAPK signaling increases expression of growth factors, determines the development of pain and hypersensitivity to pain, and induces antiapoptotic signals. Of note, the dysregulation of apoptotic pathways and subsequent resistance to apoptosis contribute to the failure of immune clearance [116,117].

The failure to remove fragments of menstrual effluent from the abdominal cavity induces excessive local inflammation with further and persistent activation of macrophages, which may secrete an altered pattern of cytokines and chemokines. Evidence suggests that the number and activity level of peritoneal macrophages are higher in women with endometriosis, but their cytotoxic power is reduced [118–120]. Compared to physiology, macrophages in the peritoneum of affected women are not destroyed after completing their functions due to overexpression of the antiapoptotic protein Bcl-2, which protects them from apoptosis [121]. Peritoneal macrophages imbalance in M1 and M2 macrophages was reported in both eutopic and ectopic endometrium with upregulation of M2 type as compared to M1 type. Compared to M1 macrophages, which produce inflammatory cytokines and eliminate microorganisms and defective cells, the M2 macrophages modulate adaptive immune response, scavenge cellular debris, induce tissue repair, and induce angiogenesis. On that basis and experiments with macrophage depletion, M2 macrophages are supposed to have a key role in endometriosis development [116,122]. Moreover, smaller amounts of pro-inflammatory cytokines modulating the activation of macrophages (IL-6, IL-13, and IL-10 family) were produced and liberated in the eutopic endometrium of women with endometriosis as compared to the endometrium of healthy controls, reducing their cytotoxic capacity in the endometrium [120,123]. Production of IL-6 and MAPK activation in endometriotic cells are furthermore regulated by the proteoglycan Syndecan-1 (CD138), which also acts as a modulator of leukocyte and dendritic cell recruitment in mouse models of inflammation [124–126]. Studies reported that pro-inflammatory cytokines of Th1 profile are prevalent in the early stages, while these change to a Th2 profile in late stages, exerting an immunosuppressive effect and activating tissue injury-repair mechanisms [127]. This is consistent with data reporting reduced activity of cytotoxic T cells, a relative reduction of Th1 cell numbers, and a higher CD4/CD8 ratio in women affected by endometriosis as compared to healthy controls. Moreover, women with endometriosis were reported with both increased number and activation of B cells with an associated higher production of antibodies and higher numbers of regulatory T cells [116,128,129]. It is supposed that this altered inflammatory response may favor survival and implantation of ectopic endometrium with extracellular matrix (ECM) remodeling and angiogenesis as well as may cause metaplasia of the peritoneum or the development of Müllerian remnants, particularly overexpression of IL-1, IL-8, TNF-α [6,7]. Of interest, it is still unclear whether this altered peritoneal microenvironment is a cause or a consequence of endometriosis. Moreover, the presence of this altered inflammatory microenvironment could favor the implantation and development of endometriosis from refluxed endometrium or induce coelomic metaplasia of in situ mesothelium [20].

3.4. Apoptosis Defects

Cell turnover in human endometrium is regulated by apoptosis, which eliminates senescent cells from the functional layer during menses. Although apoptosis is regulated by several genes with variable expression during the menstrual cycle (bax, c-myc, and P53 induce it, while sentrin, B-cell lymphoma/leukemia-xL, and Bcl-2 inhibit it), the variation of endometrial apoptosis in the menstrual cycle seems to be primarily modulated by ovarian steroids through the up- and downregulation of Bcl-2 and bax expression, from the expression level of bax depends on the Bcl-2 action. Bcl-2 maximum expression was reported during the proliferative phase when the estrogens production and the expression of receptors in glandular cells is greatest [85,130–132].

In women with endometriosis, the eutopic endometrium is reported to exhibit significantly reduced apoptosis compared to women without endometriosis, particularly in the late secretory, menstrual, and early proliferative cycle phases. This may explain a reduced percentage of apoptotic cells and a greater number of surviving cells entering the peritoneal cavity, which is a prerequisite for the development of endometriosis [85,133–135]. The resistance to apoptosis could be related to different mechanisms. Inappropriate signal transduction was related to the dysregulated expression of proteins involved in the modulation of apoptosis, such as the increased expression of Bcl-2, that along with bax represent the key proteins of apoptosis regulation in endometriosis [85]. Compared to the cyclical activity of mTOR in eutopic endometrium, mTOR in endometriosis is constantly activated with persistent inhibition of cell autophagy and apoptosis [136]. Further studies identified the altered and excessive expression of the soluble-FasL in women with endometriosis, with subsequent dysregulated interaction between Fas and FasL that represent a possible cause of apoptosis resistance in endometriotic cells, in addition to immunoescaping. Of note, concomitant induced expression of FasL in stromal cells seems to mediate apoptosis of activated immune cells [116,137]. A constant source of TNF-α that initiates and modulates apoptosis during menses, and the absence of apoptosis induced by signals from adhesion receptors in cells that do not adhere to the peritoneal mesothelium, such as the E-cadherin suppression, are further mechanisms reported related to escape from apoptosis in endometriosis [131,135]. Of note, accumulating evidence suggests that apoptotic resistance has a key role in the "immunoescaping" of endometriotic cells from immune homeostasis of the peritoneal microenvironment [136] (Figure 2).

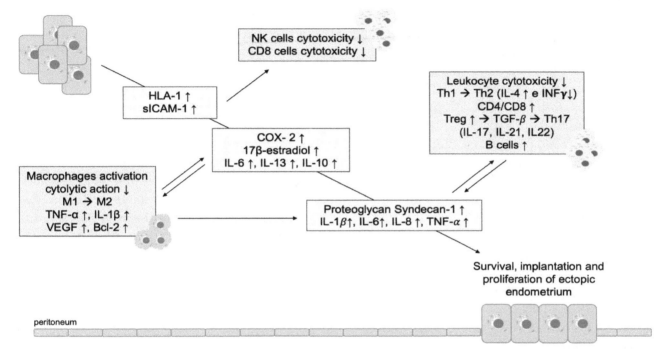

Figure 2. Immunoescaping mechanisms involved in the etiopathogenesis of endometriosis. Human leukocyte antigen class I (HLA-1); Intercellular adhesion molecule-1 (sICAM-1); Natural killer (NK); Cyclo-oxygenase type 2 (COX-2); Interleukins (IL); Tumor necrosis factor (TNF); Vascular endothelial growth factor (VEGF); Antiapoptotic protein B cell lymphoma 2 (Bcl-2); Interferon (INF); transforming growth factor-β (TGF-β).

3.5. Cell-Matrix and Cell-Cell Adhesion

Dysregulated cell-cell and cell-matrix adhesion has a role in the development of endometriosis [138]. Endometrial cells derived from proliferative and secretory endometrial fragments, as well as menstrual endometrial fragments, are able to adhere to where the peritoneal mesothelium is damaged and the basement membrane or the interstitial ECM are exposed. Although an intact mesothelial lining may prevent adhesion and implantation of menstrual endometrial fragments, mesothelium can easily be damaged by surgery, inflammatory cells, and menstrual endometrium [139–142]. Some studies reported that isolated cells from menstrual endometrial fragments as well as non-cellular medium prepared from menstrual effluent are able to induce morphological alterations in the mesothelium, from an epithelial to a mesenchymal phenotype, and to damage it, creating its own adhesion sites at the mesothelial lining [143–147].

Adhesion of retrograde menstrual endometrium to the peritoneum is mediated by adhesion molecules that modulate cell-matrix and cell-cell attachments and are expressed by endometrial cells, including cadherins, integrins, proteoglycans such as syndecans, laminin-binding proteins, the immunoglobulin superfamily, and CD44. Integrins, syndecans, cadherins, CD44, and CD44's binding partner hyaluronan have been studied extensively in endometrium and in endometriosis [138].

The integrins are transmembrane glycoproteins that modulate cell-matrix attachment and are involved in cell motility and invasion. The endometrial expression of integrins changes during the menstrual cycle under hormonal regulation. Altered patterns of expression that have been associated with endometriosis are able to express or to not express certain integrins independently of the hormones without cyclical modifications. Endometriosis is reported to have an overall highly variable and aberrant integrin expression as compared with eutopic endometrium. Fibronectin receptors were identified in glands of endometriosis implants but not in eutopic endometrial glands, suggesting that fibronectin receptors may contribute to the adhesion of endometriotic cells during menstruation [148–152].

Moreover, differences were observed between the eutopic endometrium of affected women and healthy women. The αvβ3 integrin is expressed in the endometrium at the time of implantation from 19-20 days of the menstrual cycle, and its absence suggests out of phase endometrium. In women with endometriosis, αvβ3 integrin is constantly absent in the eutopic endometrium although in the presence of in-phase histological features. This defect was associated with nulliparity and inversely related to the stage of disease [152,153].

Another family of ECM receptors is formed by the syndecans, four transmembrane-anchored proteoglycans that are expressed in the endometrium in a menstrual cycle-dependent manner [154]. Notably, the most ubiquitous member of the family, syndecan-4, was shown to be upregulated in the eutopic endometrium of endometriosis patients compared to an IVF control collective, and functional studies in an endometriotic cell line revealed that experimental syndecan-4 downregulation resulted in reduced invasiveness in vitro, and reduced expression of the cytoskeletal modulator Rac1, the transcription factor ATF-2, and MMP3 [155]. In addition, functional studies revealed a similar invasion-modulating role for the epithelial member of the syndecans family, syndecan-1: siRNA knockdown of this proteoglycan in endometriotic cells resulted in a substantial inhibition of Matrigel invasiveness, which was accompanied by a reduction of IL-6 secretion, MMP9 expression and MMP2 activity, and upregulation of plasminogen activator inhibitor-1 protein [124]. Overall, these data suggest that syndecans dysregulation in endometriosis contributes mechanistically to proteolytic remodeling, alterations in cell motility, and the inflammatory microenvironment, thus promoting invasive growth of endometriotic lesions.

Cadherins belong to a large family of transmembrane glycoproteins that mediate cell-cell adhesion and may suppress invasion inhibiting the escape of cells from their primary site. In vitro, tumor cells that express E-cadherin are retained by cell-cell adhesions, but when tumor cells do not express E-cadherin are no longer constrained and can invade. Therefore, E-cadherin is considered a central player in the development of cancer metastasis [156–159]. Immunohistochemical studies have reported that epithelial-glandular cells of menstrual effluent, eutopic endometrium, peritoneal fluid, peritoneum, and endometriosis express epithelial cadherin (E-cadherin), suggesting a role of E-cadherin in the maintenance of the endometrial epithelial architecture [151,160]. Endometriosis cells may share molecular mechanisms of invasion and metastasis with carcinoma cells that are related to the level of E-cadherin expression [156,157].

Finally, expression of the transmembrane adhesion molecule and stem cell marker CD44 is dysregulated in endometriosis [161], as exemplified by the correlation of high levels of soluble CD44 in the serum and peritoneal fluid of endometriosis patients with the severity of the disease. Indeed, preclinical data from animal models suggest that interference with CD44 function or with its binding partner, the ECM carbohydrate hyaluronan, may be a worthwhile therapeutic approach [162]. For example, inhibition of CD44 glycosylation was shown to decrease the attachment of endometrial cell lines to peritoneal mesothelial cells [163], and transplantation of endometrium from CD44-deficient mice into wild-type mice and vice versa resulting in a decreased formation of endometriotic lesions in vitro [164], suggesting an important role of CD44 in the adhesion of endometriotic cells to ectopic sites. Finally, pharmacological inhibition of biosynthesis of the CD44 substrate hyaluronan by 4-methylumbelliferone reduced angiogenesis in an in vivo mouse model of endometriosis [165], suggesting that interference with the CD44-hyaluronan axis may represent an approach that synchronously targets multiple molecular mechanisms of endometriosis.

3.6. Extracellular Matrix Remodeling and Matrix Metalloproteinases

The CAM models demonstrate that endometrium is able to adhere and subsequently degrade the ECM, suggesting that endometriotic lesion development requires ECM breakdown. The breakdown and remodeling of the ECM are mainly modulated by matrix metalloproteinases (MMPs) that degrade

ECM components and are reported to be expressed by fragments of endometrium. MMPs are secreted in a latent preform requiring activation to acquire proteolytic activity and are inhibited by specific tissue inhibitors of MMPs (TIMPs). MMPs are structurally related but have different substrate specificity, cellular sources, and inducibility. Based on their substrate specificity, MMPs can be classified into collagenases, gelatinases, stromelysins, membrane-type MMPs, and other MMPs [166].

The activity of MMPs is modulated at the level of gene expression, at the level of latent proenzymes activation, and at the level of the inhibitory activity of TIMPs. Gene expression is modulated by hormones, growth factors, and inflammatory cytokines including IL-6, IL-1, epidermal growth factor, TNF-α, basic fibroblast growth factor (bFGF), and platelet-derived growth factor. Secreted latent proenzymes are activated by the stepwise activation of plasmin, which is considered the most potent activator in vivo, and by the activity of membrane-type MMPs, that are present at the cell surface and intracellularly. TIMPs are expressed by different types of cells and are present in the majority of tissues and body fluids [167–169].

MMPs are involved with highly regulated activity in many reproductive processes, including menstruation, ovulation, and embryo implantation [170,171]. The endometrial expression of MMPs is low during the proliferative phase, declines further during the early secretory phase and increases in the late secretory phase. Although MMPs activity in the endometrium is regulated by different hormones, cytokines, and growth factors, progesterone is a potent repressor both in vitro and in vivo. Progesterone might regulate MMP expression indirectly through the plasminogen activator pathway, increasing the levels of plasminogen activator inhibitor (PAI)-1 and thus reducing the plasmin-mediated activation of latent MMPs [172–174]. Moreover, locally produced retinoic acid and transforming growth factor-β (TGF-β) seem to be mediators of the progesterone suppression enhancing expression of TIMPs. Nevertheless, prematurely decreased progesterone levels not consistent with the peri-menstrual increased expression of MMPs and tissue degradation at focal points rather than throughout the different expression and regulation of MMPs entire endometrium are more likely than progesterone to be the primary modulator of endometrial collagenase activity [175–177].

After the initial attachment, the development of endometriotic lesion requires the invasion of adjacent tissues through the ECM degradation regulated by MMPs activity. This role of MMPs in the pathogenesis of endometriosis was proposed after finding ECM breakdown products in the peritoneal fluid of affected women [174]. Later, studies with artificial induced endometriosis, in mice and in the CAM, reported that endometriotic lesion development could be prevented by inhibiting the activity of MMPs [178,179]. Moreover, different expression and regulation of MMPs were demonstrated in women without and with endometriosis. This included an altered expression of specific MMPs and related TIMPs with an increased MMP/TIMP ratio in women affected by endometriosis as compared to healthy controls [63,166,180–186]. Specifically, in women with endometriosis, as compared to healthy controls, the expression of MMPs was reported enhanced in the secretory phase dominated by progesterone. In vitro studies reported an increased MMP-3 and MMP-7mRNA expression in the eutopic endometrium of women affected by endometriosis in the secretory phase. These results suggest that a contribution to the development of endometriosis comes from a defect in the response to the suppressing action of progesterone, a form of progesterone insensitivity [187].

Furthermore, evidence suggests that MMPs cleave not only ECM components but may also be implicated in the degradation of cytokines and growth factors, regulating tissue organization, angiogenesis, and cell survival. Therefore, MMP activity seems to be able to influence the initial lesion development as well as lesion survival and maintenance [188].

3.7. Angiogenesis

In CAM models, after 72 hours, a complete endometrium with glands and stroma was present in the CAM mesenchyme, and blood vessels were attracted from the CAM inside the endometrium fragment. These studies demonstrated that human endometrium is highly angiogenic and able to attract blood vessels from the surrounding tissue [189]. Angiogenesis is induced when vascular growth factors exceed inhibiting factors, and, although it is reported altered in pathological conditions such as cancer, chronic inflammation, and endometriosis, it is essential in a physiological process such as wound healing, growth, pregnancy and menstrual cycle [190,191]. Therefore, endometrial cells have physiologically angiogenic potential. In the eutopic endometrium during the menstrual cycle, angiogenesis is modulated by many factors, of which VEGF appears to be the most important for its ability to induce proliferation and migration of endothelial cell, vasodilation, and increased vascular permeability [190]. In the proliferative phase, estradiol induces VEGF-A production in endometrium resulting increased in the secretory phase and further increased prior to menstruation when endometrium becomes hypoxic as a result of vasoconstriction [192,193].

Increased endothelial cell proliferation, increased micro-vessel density, and higher levels of VEGF-A and angiopoietin-1 and -2mRNA expression were detected in the eutopic endometrium of patients with endometriosis than in the eutopic endometrium of disease-free women. These factors suggest a dysregulated angiogenic activity in the eutopic endometrium of women affected by endometriosis [64,191,194–196].

Focused studies on the vascularization of endometriotic lesions compared the vascular density and vessel diameter between white, black, and red lesions as well as between deep infiltrating lesions and endometriomas. No differences in the numbers of vessels were reported between different types of lesions, but red lesions have more vessels with a small diameter (<10 μm), whereas black lesions have more vessels with a larger diameter (>20 μm) [197]. The observations of endothelial cell proliferation with the development of blood vessels without smooth muscle in endometriotic lesions suggest that VEGF-A and angiogenesis are of significant value, particularly in early lesions. This was further suggested by studies investigating the soluble VEGF receptor sflt-1 that antagonizes VEGF-A action and was reported able to reduce the number of lesions formed in mice after intraperitoneal injection of endometrium [198]. More support to antiangiogenic therapy as effective in preventing the development of endometriosis has been provided by CAM model studies, in which anti-human VEGF factors administered to the CAM significantly decreased the vascular density of the CAM and prevented endometriosis-like lesion formation after the transplantation of human endometrium [199]. Moreover, after endometriotic lesions had been induced by transplanting human endometrium intraperitoneally, antiangiogenic agents resulted in a significant reduction of the number of endometriotic lesions in treated mice compared to control. The reduction in lesion number was related to a reduction of newly developed vessels, with mature vessels remaining unchanged [200,201]. Although VEGF is the key angiogenetic factor in endometriosis, further factors were reported involved in the angiogenesis of endometriotic lesions, including TGF-α, TGF-β, bFGF, angiopoietin, and hepatocyte growth factor [202–204]. Furthermore, recent results have indicated a role of the stem cell-related notch signaling pathway in sprouting angiogenesis of endometriotic lesions in an in vivo model [205].

3.8. Endometrial Stem Cells

More recently, endometrial stem progenitor cells were proposed as cells that give rise to the origin of endometriotic lesions, both ectopic or transplanted cells [206]. The human endometrium is subject to profound changes in tissue structure and function during the menstrual cycle, and the recovery of epithelial glands and stroma is produced by the endometrial progenitor stem cells within the basal layer, although some studies have suggested the origin may also be from bone marrow [206–208]. Endometrial stem cells demonstrated a high plastic capacity of differentiation by the characterization of several lines of cells with a different expression pattern of cell surface markers, endometrial localization, and clonal efficiency [209]. Recent evidence suggests the monoclonal origin of endometriotic cells within ovarian endometriomas, while peritoneal implants were reported to be polyclonal [210–212]. Moreover, as previously reported, the cells that give rise to endometriotic implants must undergo migration, adhesion, proliferation, and induction of angiogenesis. The endometrial stem cells have demonstrated the ability to activate all these characteristics [213]. As previously reported, it is proposed that physical and biochemical injuries caused by inflammatory cytokines and reactive oxygen species trigger the activation of endometrial stem cells inducing local production of estrogen and tissue injury-repair mechanisms such as cell cycle activation. On that basis, endometrial stem progenitor cells may be involved in the etiopathogenesis of benign and malignant endometrial aberrations such as endometriosis, endometrial hyperplasia, and endometrial cancer [214]. In general, endometrial stem progenitor cells have a long lifespan and trigger epigenetic mechanisms of protection from stress and senescence. They express genes such as Wnt/β-catenin, anti-apoptotic Bcl-2, cell cycle regulatory genes, and enzymes to repair DNA damage [206,209]. For all these characteristics, endometrial stem cells are supposed to be the cells that give rise to endometriotic implants instead of differentiated endometrial tissue fragments [7]. Of interest, endometrial stem progenitor cells can find their potential source from refluxed menstrual endometrium, Müllerian remnants from embryogenesis, as well as an hematogenic origin from the recruitment of circulating stem cell of bone marrow [215]. Notably, several stemness-associated molecular markers have been shown to be upregulated in the eutopic endometrium and ectopic lesions of endometriosis patients, including Msi1, SOX2, notch and numb [82,216,217], supporting the hypothesis of an involvement of stem cells in the pathogenetic process. Preclinical studies demonstrated that the microRNAs miR-145 and miR-200b were suitable tools to alter stemness-related properties of endometriotic cells, opening new therapeutic perspectives [218,219].

4. The Genetics of Endometriosis

The etiopathogenesis of endometriosis is still undefined and debated. To better understand the mechanism leading to the development of endometriosis as a disabling disease instead of spontaneous resolution of peritoneal implants, genetic studies offer an approach of paramount importance [3,220–222]. The evidence for a genetic contribution to the development of endometriosis comes from epidemiological studies that reported familial aggregation of the disease in humans [223–227] and primates [228]. Both hospital- and population-based studies reported higher rates of endometriosis among the relatives of affected women compared to healthy controls [224,225,229]. A study based on siblings, twins and familiars of affected woman reported a higher relative recurrence risk of 2.3 times as compared to the risk in the general population, although it is difficult to perform an accurate estimation because the prevalence in the general population is unknown and there is bias in the surgical diagnosis of endometriosis in siblings [226] and in the daughters of endometriosis patients (personal observation of D.C.M.). A genetic background for endometriosis was further supported by evidence that comes from larger studies in twins and in the population of Iceland [225,226,230–232]. Monozygotic twins show higher concordance for endometriosis than dizygotic twins [230,231], with intra-pair correlation rates of 0.52 versus 0.19 [232]. This data suggest that genetic factors influence about half of the risk for endometriosis development and estimate a heritability of 51% [232]. Further evidence comes from studies in the rhesus macaque animal model, that reported a familial aggregation of spontaneous endometriosis with a significantly higher coefficient of recurrence risk for full siblings (0.75) as compared to maternal (0.26) and paternal (0.18) half-siblings [228].

Although the familial aggregation of confounding risk factors, such as age at menarche, questioned the real role of genetic background in endometriosis risk [233], current evidence supports the genetic contribution to endometriosis development, and genetic approaches can be used to identify genes having a role in endometriosis risk, allowing a better definition of the etiopathogenetic pathways. Moreover, the identification of genetic markers may allow the development of more informative risk predictors as compared to family history, a better understanding of the pathogenesis providing new opportunities for drug discovery, and genetic profiles allow identification of co-morbidity, that may improve diagnosis and treatments.

4.1. Candidate Gene Studies

A general approach to investigate the role of genes in the etiopathogenesis of diseases is the study of specific candidate genes chosen based on the biological mechanisms known as contributors to the disease [234–238]. Nevertheless, for endometriosis, the definition of candidate genes is problematic because of the limited knowledge of etiopathogenetic mechanisms that may involve many genetic pathways and many genes.

Studies have investigated genes involved in sex steroid pathways, detoxification pathways, cytokine signaling pathways, adhesion, and cell cycle regulation molecules and enzymes of the ECM [234,238]. Based on the estrogen-dependent nature of endometriosis, genes from pathways of sex hormones signaling and biosynthesis have been studied. These investigations provided limited evidence supporting the association between either PR or ERα and endometriosis [237], although a further large family-based study failed to demonstrate any association between endometriosis and PR [99]. Similarly, conflicting results were reported for the association between the gene expression of cytochrome P450 and endometriosis [239,240].

Detoxification pathways were investigated based on the supposed role of environmental estrogens in the etiopathogenesis of endometriosis, reporting questionable evidence [73,241]. Glutathione S-transferase enzymes are involved in the detoxification of different toxic compounds and carcinogens. Different studies investigated gene polymorphisms and reported evidence for an increased risk of endometriosis in the presence of specific enzyme variants. Nevertheless, significant heterogeneity between studies and publication bias suggests caution [235]. Similarly, a meta-analysis of studies that investigated the association between polymorphisms in the detoxification enzyme N-acetyltransferase 2 and endometriosis reported no association [236].

In general, many factors have contributed to the failure of candidate gene studies to provide new insights into the pathogenesis of endometriosis. A few of the reported associations have been investigated in an independent sample, as it is suggested before accepting the association with a disease, and the majority of replications failed to confirm previous results [238]. Study power is another cause of concerns both for initial and replication studies [242,243]. In complex diseases such as endometriosis, many genes, as well as environmental factors, may contribute to the etiopathogenesis; therefore, the effect size for the majority of common risk alleles is expected to be low, with odds ratios having a range of 1.1–1.5 [244–246]. On that basis, large sample sizes are required, and most candidate gene studies investigated small samples with inadequate power to detect the small contribution of all genes contributing to the risk of endometriosis [238,247,248]. Moreover, publication bias of significant compared to negative results [242,249], statistical and technical issues, and problems in experimental design provides further concerns [237]. In general, many gene variants with small effects can be considered associated with an increased risk of endometriosis [238].

4.2. Linkage and Association Studies

Linkage studies are performed in families with multiple cases and search for genomic regions shared more frequently than expected between relatives affected by the disease. These regions likely carry gene variants increasing the risk of developing the disease. These studies provided important results in disease related to single-gene mutations with Mendelian segregation [250–252]. Due to the high prevalence of endometriosis, the low recurrence in familiars, and the difficulties in ascertaining the healthy subjects, the best design was to analyze pairs of sisters both affected [252].

A genome analysis of DNA samples from 1176 sister-pair with both laparoscopically confirmed endometriosis and family members from Australian and UK was performed [253]. The study was designed with a power of 80% to detect a region with a recurrence risk to sisters of 1.35 [226]. The analysis identified significant linkage on chromosome 10 and on chromosome 20, although evidence for linkage was confirmed only in chromosome 10 for both Australian and UK families. A separate linkage study was conducted in families with three or more affected women and identified a significant linkage peak on chromosome 7p [254–256]. This suggests that in high-risk families, a locus with high penetrance for endometriosis risk may be located in this region.

Nevertheless, linkage studies are limited by the ability to identify a genomic region of interest but not a specific gene locus. Therefore, association studies are required to identify specific gene variants.

Association studies, with or without family-based designs, compare gene variants frequency in women with endometriosis versus healthy controls. Because most human genome variants are single-base differences, methods to genotype large numbers of single nucleotide polymorphisms (SNPs) are now used for both linkage and association studies. Of interest, common SNPs (with a population frequency > 0.01) that are located close together are not independently inherited (linkage disequilibrium or LD) [257]. Therefore, a SNP can act as a marker for others, allowing the identification of the common variation in a particular region by typing a limited number of SNPs. With this technique, association studies investigated chromosome seven and 10 linkage regions identifying several genes implicated in endometriosis and endometrial cancer such as PTEN, homeobox protein EMX2, and the FGF receptor 2 gene (FGFR2). EMX2 is a transcription factor involved in the development of the reproductive tract and in the cyclicity of eutopic endometrium [258–260]. PTEN regulates proliferation and survival of cells and it is inactivated in the early events of endometrial hyperplasia development and ovarian and endometrial cancer pathogenesis [261]. FGFR2 has been associated with endometrial and breast cancer development [262,263]. Nevertheless, SNP studies, investigating common variants and variants related to endometrial or breast cancer of these three genes, suggested that the linkage signal is not related to these common variants, demonstrating no evidence for any association with the endometriosis [258,264]. However, a role for other unknown variants of these genes in the development of endometriosis cannot be completely excluded. Moreover, the hypothesis that different families may have different mutations of the same gene reduces the probability of identifying these specific variants. It is suggested that the results of linkage studies may be caused by multiple different variants of the same gene; the variant is the same across a single-family but is rare in the general population. Conversely, association studies require that investigated variants are common in the general population [258,264].

4.3. Genome-Wide Association Studies

The complex and multifactorial etiopathogenesis of endometriosis contributes to the failure of candidate gene, association, and linkage studies [245]. Genome-wide association (GWA) provided a new tool to identify genetic variants related to complex human diseases, with the use of genetic markers that include most of the common gene variants (up to 1 million SNPs) and can be screened in a single analysis [257].

Nevertheless, study design, particularly the definition of characteristics, traits of the disease being studied, and the choice of population controls, remains of paramount importance [265]. Moreover, cases and controls need to be well matched for ethnicity to reduce the false-positive rate, and standard, rigorous, and quality control procedures are required to reduce bias. Association results are reported as significant for every SNP that show a significant association as points above a stringent threshold determining the probability of finding a false positive. Once a genetic association is identified, replication provides an important safeguard against false-positive results and gives an independent and better estimate of the effect size [266]. The identified region can be subsequently examined to locate the genes relative to association signals and analyze the variation pattern because SNPs statistically associated with disease are probably not the causal variants, that usually are absent on the gene chip used for SNP detection, but correlate with the common variants genotyped on the chip. The causal variants probably lie near the regions of SNPs statistically associated with disease for the LD [267]. Of note, signals could identify both areas of the genome with genes and intragenic regions identifying regulatory regions of gene expression [244].

Well-powered endometriosis case-control GWA studies identified several genes as possible candidates in the pathogenesis of endometriosis. A Japanese GWA study identified a significant association with LD blocks of chromosome 1 near the cyclin-dependent kinase inhibitor 2B antisense RNA (CDKN2BAS) and the wingless-type MMTV integration site family 4 (WNT4) gene [268]. A smaller Japanese GWA study reported a significant association with LD blocks near IL-1 alpha proprotein. Notably, IL-1α has been shown to be elevated in both the peritoneal fluid and the serum of infertile women with endometriosis compared to healthy controls [269,270]. In a United States

GWA study, SNP-association with endometriosis was reported with LD blocks near nuclear factor erythroid-derived 2-like 3 gene, typically expressed in placenta, and HOXA10 and HOXA11 genes, two candidate genes of the homeobox A transcription factors family. HOXA10 and HOXA11 have key roles in uterine embryogenesis and are expressed at high levels during the luteal phase. Of interest, studies reported that HOXA10 levels were not increased in women affected by endometriosis leading to infertility [271]. A meta-analysis incorporating available data about SNP-association reported different SNPs in the gene of interest between European descents and Japanese, likely reflecting the different genetic backgrounds of investigated populations. Nevertheless, WNT4 was confirmed as a candidate gene for endometriosis, with a signal that overlaps completely with an association signal for ovarian cancer, suggesting some common molecular pathways [220,222,271]. WNT4 is an interesting candidate involved in female reproductive tract embryogenesis, ovarian follicle development, and steroidogenesis. WNT4 was reported to be involved in numerous anomalies of the female genital tract. Moreover, the signaling pathway of WNT genes and WNT/β-catenin were reported to be associated in the control of different types of stem cells and in the resistance to apoptosis by the cell-cell interaction mediated by cadherins [268,272–274].

The International ENDOGENE Consortium, in addition to using SNP–disease associations, applied GWA data to investigate with statistical methods the percentage of disease risk variation attributable to genetic variants, and whether the disease status in an independent sample can be predicted by the disease status in another sample [226,275]. Analyses suggested that in moderate-to-severe endometriosis (Revised American Fertility Society (rAFS) classification stages III-IV) genetic load is higher than in minimal-to-mild disease (rAFS classification stages I-II) with strongest signals of SNP-association. This was subsequently confirmed by prediction analyses with SNP data from moderate-to-severe endometriosis of UK samples that predict moderate-to-severe disease in Australian samples better than data from all endometriosis cases. These results were confirmed by inverted analysis [226,275].

A recent meta-analysis incorporating available data from 11 GWA case-control studies, involving 17,045 endometriosis cases and 191,596 controls, identified five new loci significantly associated with endometriosis risk, that were reported involved in sex steroid hormones pathways. Overall, GWA case-control studies have identified 19 independent SNPs associated with endometriosis risk. Those include SNPs associated with endometriosis identified regions near the gene for ERα, regions upstream of the beta subunit of follicle-stimulating hormone (FSH), and the Growth Regulating Estrogen Receptor Binding 1 (GREB1), previously associated with breast cancer. Other regions identified genes involved in cell migration, adhesion, and proliferation, such as WNT4. Nevertheless, together, these identified SNPs are able to explain only 5.19% of the variance in endometriosis [220,222]. Therefore, the combined effects of all identified genes explain only a small fraction of the estimated 51% heritability of endometriosis [276]. This "missing" heritability may be explained, as reported for other complex diseases, by the small effect size of multiple single variants that contribute to disease risk and do not reach statistical significance. Additionally, SNPs on the current commercial chips may not tag well causal variants. Functional genetic variants that contribute to susceptibility for some common diseases, if rare, limit the performance of GWA studies that are designed to detect common variants and fail to identify low-frequency alleles [277–280].

5. The Epigenetics of Endometriosis

It has been demonstrated that a single lesion of endometriosis is monoclonal [210–212] and, based on gene expression profiling studies, a large number of genes are dysregulated in endometriosis [281–287]. Nevertheless, although the heritability of endometriosis is estimated to be 51% [232], it is difficult to identify specific genes consistently associated with endometriosis and with predictive power in identifying high-risk women [233,234]. During the development of endometriotic lesions from progenitor cells, it was proposed that the aberrations are acquired sequentially and usually without any change in the sequence of DNA (i.e., DNA mutations). Conversely, gene expression dysregulation in the cellular lineage is acquired and maintained by epigenetic processes in a heritable manner. Therefore, sequentially acquired and inherited changes at the level of gene transcription, post-transcriptional modulations, translation, and post-translational modifications are proposed as the common denominator explaining the hormonal, immunological, molecular, histological and cellular aberrations that characterize endometriosis. Furthermore, they may explain the SNPs-association with regulatory regions of gene expression instead of gene loci and the small effect of multiple single-gene variants in GWA studies [244]. At the same time, Bruner-Tran et al. [288] have investigated heritable epigenetic changes in mice in germ cells after exposure to 2,3,7,8-tetrachlorodibenzo-p-dioxin (TCDD) and demonstrated a transgenerational occurrence of several reproductive diseases that have been linked to endometriosis in women, although they could not determine if those changes lead to the development of endometriosis or were a consequence of the inflammatory nature of the disease. However, epigenetic markers occurring within the germline of mice are inheritable and can positively or negatively affect offspring [289,290]. These epigenetic changes potentially include a stable, heritable phenotype caused by chromosomal changes without DNA sequence alterations if they escape epigenetic reprogramming. If so, they are essential in tissue development and cell differentiation [291]. Moreover, epigenetic processes modulate phenomena such as genomic imprinting and X chromosome inactivation, and they are involved in aging and disease development [292–294]. Epigenetic processes involve dynamic changes in the chromatin structure influencing gene expression. Chromatin architecture is modulated by methylation of DNA (hypo- and hypermethylation correspond to gene expression and silencing, respectively), acetylation, ubiquitination, ADP-ribosylation and SUMOylation of histone proteins; and by non-histone proteins DNA-binding [295]. Moreover, epigenetic processes involve the expression of microRNAs (miRNAs). MiRNAs interact with mRNA, inhibiting translation, or inducing mRNA degradation [296–299]. In ectopic endometrial-like cells of endometriosis, the cellular identity and gene expression programs are defined and maintained by epigenetics that may have a key role in the pathogenesis. Of interest, these epigenetic aberrations are dynamic and reversible and may have potential implications for diagnosis, prognosis, and therapy of the disease. In summary, available evidence may suggest a role of epigenetics both in the development of endometriosis lesions and in the heritability of the disease.

5.1. Epigenetics in the Eutopic Endometrium

Epigenetic processes are involved in numerous mechanisms that modulate the gene expression in endometrial development during the menstrual cycle, resulting in coordinated functional and morphological changes [300]. The global methylation level of eutopic endometrium was reported higher in the proliferative phase as compared to the secretory phase of the menstrual cycle. This hypermethylation is consistent with the expression level of DNA methyltransferases 1 (DNMT1) that was reportedly higher in the proliferative and late secretory phase and lower in the mid-secretory phase. A similar expression level was reported for DNMT3A and DNMT3B, for which the gene expression levels were decreased by treatment with estrogen and progestin. Conversely, the expression level of DNMT1 was reported to be unchanged by hormones either due to technical limitations of the used method or because the estrogen and progestin act at the post-transcriptional level, reducing the stability of DNMT1 protein [301].

Similarly, histone modifications by acetylation seem to be involved in endometrial function, with histone acetylation levels reported as globally increased in the early proliferative phase and gradually reduced in the late proliferative phase until ovulation [300]. The histone deacetylase 1 (HDAC1), HDAC3, and two histone acetylases were reported to be constitutively expressed in the endometrium during the menstrual cycle, with HDAC1 having a reduced expression level in the secretory phase [302]. Of note, HDAC inhibitors (HDACIs) were able to determine a differentiation and morphological transformation in endometrium similar to the combined treatment with estrogen and progestin. These results suggest that histone modifications may play a role in the control of decidualization through the regulation of the function of ERs and PGE2-induced 17β-estradiol synthesis [4,303–305].

MiRNAs post-transcriptionally downregulate the expression of genes and seem to be involved in endometrium development during the menstrual cycle, similar to acetylation and methylation [306–308].

MiRNAs were identified in normal endometrium and in eutopic and ectopic endometrium of women affected by endometriosis [101]. An inverse correlation was reported between the expression level of specific miRNAs and the suppression of protein production derived from their target genes, such as aromatase and COX-2 [309]. Moreover, estrogen and progestins were reported able to modify the expression level of miRNAs in endometrial stromal and glandular epithelial cells. Progesterone may oppose estrogen action by fine-tuning gene expression modulating miRNAs, which seems to suppress genes involved in cycle progression and cell proliferation in the secretory-phase [309,310]. This involvement of miRNAs in endometrial cyclicity is consistent with data suggesting that miRNAs seem to have a role in embryo implantation and postnatal uterus development in the mouse [311,312].

5.2. Epigenetics in Endometriosis

Some forms of endometriosis could be considered an epigenetic disorder. A growing body of evidence suggests that epigenetics processes have a key role in the pathogenesis and pathophysiology of endometriosis [313]. Aberrant methylation, acetylation, post-translational modifications, and dysregulation of miRNAs expression were identified in eutopic as well as ectopic endometrium of affected woman and may have great potential as therapeutic targets or as biomarkers for diagnosis and recurrence risk prediction [314].

The first piece of evidence suggesting the role of epigenetic in the etiopathogenesis of endometriosis comes from studies reporting the hypermethylation of the HOXA10 gene promoter in eutopic endometrium of women with endometriosis as compared with healthy controls [315,316]. HOXA10 is a transcription factor belonging to the homeobox gene family and has a role in the development and function of the uterus. Eutopic endometrium expresses HOXA10 during the menstrual cycle with a high expression level in the mid-secretory phase. This high expression, corresponding to increased progesterone levels and to the time of implantation, suggests that HOXA10 may have a key role in establishing the conditions necessary for implantation [316]. Of interest, the hypermethylation of the HOXA10 gene promoter, which means gene silencing, is consistent with studies reporting that HOXA10 levels are reduced in the eutopic endometrium of women affected by endometriosis [271], which may be a cause of the impaired fertility of these women [316]. Animal models further confirmed the key role of HOXA10 gene silencing by promoter hypermethylation both in eutopic and ectopic endometrium [317]. Moreover, animal models suggest that aberrant methylation of the HOXA10 promoter can be induced by in utero exposure to endocrine-disrupting chemicals (EDC) such as diethylstilbestrol, with or without overexpression of DNMTs [318–320].

A growing body of evidence suggests that aberrant expression of interacting homeobox genes and WNT family genes, particularly the WNT/β-catenin pathway, may disrupt organogenesis of the urogenital tract, altering the cell differentiation/migration with ectopic implantation. The WNT/β-catenin signaling pathway is involved in stem cell function and maintenance. These pathways may support the Müllerian remnants hypothesis as well as may be implicated in the survival and implantation of transplanted endometrial stem progenitor cells [7]. Indeed, data suggest that estradiol supports disease progression by upregulating β-catenin, which is degraded when it does not bind E-cadherin. The inhibition of phosphorylation stabilizes β-catenin that reach the nucleus and interacts with transcription factors regulating proliferation and angiogenesis [61].

The epigenetic mechanism of methylation was identified as having a role in progesterone resistance of endometriosis. Studies demonstrated that the promoter of PR-B gene is hypermethylated in endometriosis and adenomyosis with subsequent reduced PR-B expression [321–323]. The relatively permanent nature of hypermethylation of PR-B promoter provides further explanation to the persistent PR-B downregulation and progesterone resistance in endometriosis.

Further evidence confirmed the role of dysregulated methylation in the etiopathogenesis of endometriosis. Genes coding for three DNA methyltransferases, DNMT1, DNMT3A, and DNMT3B, were reported to be overexpressed in endometriosis. The aberrant expression of these enzymes involved in maintenance, as well as de novo methylation, suggests that hypermethylation in endometriosis may be widespread [324–326]. For example, in endometriotic cell lines lacking E-cadherin, whose deregulation was associated with endometriotic cells invasiveness, the gene was hypermethylated, suggesting that methylation of E-cadherin provides invasive properties [327,328]. Notably, E-cadherin expression is also regulated by miR-200b expression, suggesting that this important anti-invasive adhesion molecule is subject to epigenetic regulation [219]. Of interest, both hypoxia and inflammation were reported distinctly able to modulate DNMTs expression and can cause aberrant DNA methylation patterns [4,329].

Endometriosis has both epigenetic mechanisms of hypermethylation as well as hypomethylation. The hypomethylation of specific genes and genes promoters that are hypermethylated in eutopic endometrium explains the altered expression in endometriosis of genes usually silenced in eutopic endometrium. Steroidogenic factor-1 (SF-1) is a transcriptional factor activating multiple genes for the biosynthesis of estrogen. SF-1 is not detected in stromal cells of eutopic endometrium because SF-1 promoter is usually hypermethylated. In endometriotic cells, the SF-1 promoter was reported to be hypomethylated, explaining the aberrant overexpression of SF-1 [330]. Similarly, the ER-β promoter and the aromatase gene were hypomethylated in endometriotic cells, while in eutopic endometrium, they are hypermethylated, providing an explanation as to why these genes are expressed in ectopic but not in normal endometrium. Consistently, the gene coding for 17β-HSD type 2 was reported hypermethylated. Moreover, the promoter of COX-2 was reported to be hypomethylated, explaining the higher expression of COX-2 and subsequent prostaglandin E2 synthesis, which in turn enhances 17β-estradiol production and elevate DNMT3A [4,314,331–333] (Figure 3).

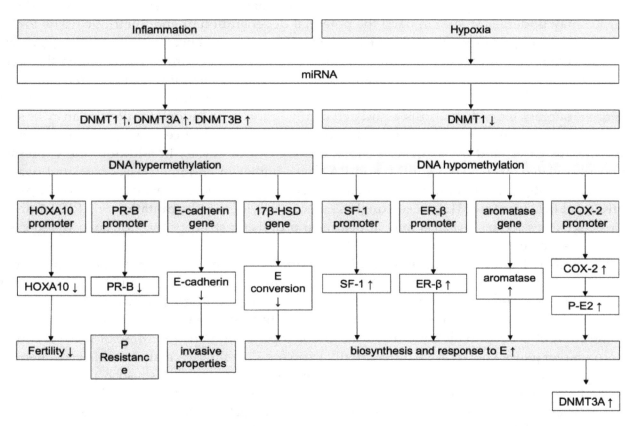

Figure 3. Epigenetic mechanisms of hypermethylation and hypomethylation involved in the etiopathogenesis of endometriosis. Hypoxia and inflammation regulate DNA methylation through microRNAs (miRNA), and genes coding for three DNA methyltransferases (DNMT) were reported overexpressed in endometriosis. microRNAs (miRNA); DNA methyltransferases (DNMT); Homeobox A transcription factor (HOXA10); Progesterone receptor B (PR-B); 17β-hydroxysteroid dehydrogenase (17β-HSD); Steroidogenic factor-1 (SF-1); Estrogen receptor β (ER-β); Cyclo-oxygenase type 2 (COX-2); Prostaglandin E2 (P-E2); Estrogen (E); Progesterone (P).

Regarding the epigenetic regulation by histone acetylation, the balance between the HDACs and histone acetyltransferase activity regulates the gene transcription. Gene expression is promoted by the acetylation of lysine residue by the histone acetyltransferase, whereas is inhibited trough the removal of acetyl group by the HDACs [334]. Endometriotic lesions as well as eutopic endometrium of affected women were reported globally hypoacetylated as compared to the eutopic endometrium of controls, with consequent gene silencing [335]. This observation was consistent with the reported higher expression of HDAC1 and HDAC2 genes and lower levels of SIRT1 in the endometriotic lesions. Moreover, the lost modulation of HDAC expression by estrogen and progesterone was reported in ectopic implants [335–337].

Different genes are known to be involved in the etiopathogenesis of endometriosis by the methylation of their promoters and subsequent downregulation. The same genes and others were reported having the promoter hypoacetylated as well, such as the genes coding ER-α, HOXA10, E-cadherin, and different proapoptotic proteins involved in the cell cycle regulation [335,338].

The global aberrant acetylation is able to explain the altered expression of different genes both for downregulation by hypoacetylation and upregulation by hyperacetylation of the promoter, such as the higher level of SF-1 and hypoxia-inducible factor-1α [335,339].

Interestingly, recent evidence founds not only somatic inactivating mutations of the tumor suppressor ARID1A but also the loss of its expression in endometriotic foci [340]. ARID1A is known to encode the protein BAF250a, which participates in forming SWI/SNF chromatin remodeling complexes. Considering that this gene is frequently mutated in ovarian clear cell and endometrioid carcinomas as well as in uterine endometrioid carcinomas, the epigenetic loss of expression of BAF250a may underlie (at least in part) the potential degeneration of endometriotic tissue toward carcinogenesis. In particular, the loss of expression of the protein encoded by ARID1A (BAF250a) can dysregulate the suppression of cellular proliferation, which is normally modulated through a p53-dependent transcription fashion of several tumor suppressors, including CDKN1A (encoding p21) and SMAD3 [341]. Indeed, published data highlighted that tissue samples from patients who had undergone surgery for endometriosis-associated ovarian cancers or endometriotic ovarian cysts show loss of BAF250a expression in 22% endometrioid cancers, 47% of clear cell cases, 44% of contiguous endometriosis cases, and 8% of benign endometriotic ovarian cysts; in addition, the expression of phosphorylated AKT, γH2AX, BIM, and BAX was higher in endometriosis-associated ovarian cancers and contiguous endometriosis than in benign endometriosis, whereas expression of pATM, pCHK2, and Bcl2 was low [342]. Based on these pieces of evidence, the mutation of ARID1A and/or the loss of expression of BAF250a may appear as a promising strategy for molecular diagnosis of endometriosis-associated ovarian cancer [343].

The epigenetic post-transcriptional mRNA modulation by miRNAs expression has a potential role in the etiopathogenesis of endometriosis [4]. MiRNAs interacting with the correspondent mRNAs downregulate gene expression. Different studies report progressively different expression of many specific miRNAs from eutopic endometrium of healthy women, paired eutopic and ectopic endometrium of women with endometriosis, and ectopic endometrium. Most of these identified miRNAs target genes known to be differentially expressed in eutopic versus ectopic endometrium. Identified miRNA target genes includes those involved in hormone metabolism such as aromatase, PR, ER-α, and ER-β [310]; modulators of the inflammatory response such as COX-2, IL-6, IL-6 receptor, IL-8, and TGF-β; and the induction of apoptosis and angiogenesis such as Bcl-2, cyclin-D, and VEGF [4,136]. The inverse correlation between the expression level of miRNAs and that of target genes supports the hypothesis that altered expression of these specific miRNAs is involved in the pathogenesis of endometriosis [344]. Both upregulated and downregulated expression of specific miRNAs were reported in ectopic endometrium as compared with eutopic endometrium of women with endometriosis [345], as well as in eutopic or ectopic endometrium of women affected by endometriosis as compared with eutopic endometrium of healthy controls [346]. Functional studies in preclinical cell models of endometriosis have confirmed a mechanistic involvement of selected microRNAs in pathogenetically relevant processes, including modulation of cell proliferation by miR-10b and miR-145, of invasive growth by miR-10b, miR-200b, and miR-145, and of stem cell properties, as exemplified by miR-145 and miR-200b [124,218,219]. Of interest, although there is a discrepancy between studies in the identification of miRNAs having altered expression, no miRNAs were "misclassified." These discrepancies can be explained by differences in study design and compared tissues. The comparison between eutopic and ectopic endometrium of affected women may not identify miRNAs associated with endometriosis that are aberrantly expressed in the same direction in both tissues. Finally, it should be noted that the role of miRNAs is more complex than a unidirectional negative regulation of gene expression. Evidence supports that many miRNAs are able to interact with transcription factors forming a network for gene regulation that yield negative as well as positive feedback loops [347]. Moreover, miRNAs have been reported to be both targets and regulators of other epigenetic mechanisms such as methylation and acetylation, and they resulted involved in hypoxia and inflammation signaling pathways [4,344].

5.3. Implications of Epigenetics in Diagnosis, Prognosis, and Therapy

The identification of epigenetic aberrations may provide promising tools for the diagnosis of endometriosis. DNA methylation markers, as well as other epigenetic aberrations that are present in the eutopic endometrium of women with endometriosis and absent in healthy controls, are present in the menstrual blood-derived from eutopic endometrium. The identification of these markers in the menstrual blood could provide high sensitivity and specificity in the identification of endometriosis with a minimally invasive approach [4,294]. These epigenetic markers may also provide prognostic information identifying patients at high risk of recurrence, allowing the tailoring of postoperative therapies and follow-up. For example, hypermethylation of the PR-B promoter identified in surgical tissue samples of endometriotic implants was related to a higher risk of recurrence [321,348].

The therapeutic implications are based on the reversible nature of epigenetic modifications. Therefore, enzymes involved in epigenetic mechanisms could be pharmacological targets. On that basis, HDACIs were investigated in vitro and in animal models as a potential therapy for endometriosis. In vitro, treatment with trichostatin A (TSA), an HDACI, elevated PR-B gene and protein expression, inhibited IL-1β-induced COX-2 expression, and inhibited cellular proliferation with cell cycle arrest in ectopic endometrial stromal cells, but not in eutopic cells [349–351]. In endometrial stromal cells, TSA upregulated Peroxisome proliferator-activated receptor (PPAR)γ expression which inhibits VEGF expression, angiogenesis, and TNF-induced IL-8 production [352–354]. Moreover, TSA attenuated invasion inducing E-cadherin expression [327]. In animal models with induced endometriosis, TSA represses endometriosis, reducing the size of ectopic implants as compared with no-treatment [59,355]. Treatments with other HDACIs and demethylation agents in both in vitro and in vivo studies provided similar promising results [59,323,356].

Data about the use of HDACI in humans derives from the use of Valproic Acid (VPA), an HDACI with known pharmacology. In women with adenomyosis, VPA reduces the amount of menses and dysmenorrhea. This could be explained by the fact that HDACIs suppress the expression of TNF-α-induced tissue factor and VEGF receptor as reported in both in vitro and in vivo studies. Both these pathways are involved in abnormal uterine bleeding and resulted in overexpressed in endometriosis [357–360]. VPA tested on patients was well tolerated, and after two months had reduced pain symptoms, reduced amount of menses, and reduced uterine size [361–363]. This evidence suggests that HDACIs have a potential role as therapy in endometriosis and/or adenomyosis [364].

6. Conclusions

The etiopathogenesis of endometriosis is a multifactorial process that leads to the development of an extremely heterogeneous disease characterized by the variable acquisition and loss of cellular functions. Its origin would appear to be from Müllerian or non-Müllerian stem cells with endometrial differentiation that can potentially originate from stem cells of the endometrial basal layer, present in Müllerian remnants, in the blood originating from bone marrow, or from the peritoneum. These stem cells have the ability of the endometrium to regenerate cyclically by mechanisms of tissue regeneration and angiogenesis in response to hypoxia, which seem to play a key role when they are dysregulated in the development of endometriosis. What determines the presence of such cells in the peritoneal cavity can occur during the development of the embryos as well as during each menstrual cycle, and what leads to the development of endometriosis is a complex process in which play a large number of interconnected factors potentially both inherited and acquired. Genetic studies have confirmed that endometriosis has a genetic nature, but at the same time, this predisposition is complex. It is constituted by the combined action of several genes with limited influence. At the same time, the epigenetic mechanisms underlying endometriosis control many of the processes of acquisition and maintenance of immunologic, immunohistochemical, histological and biological aberrations that characterize both the eutopic and ectopic endometrium in patients affected by endometriosis. However, what triggers such epigenetic alterations is not clear and may be both genetically and epigenetically inherited, or it may be acquired by the particular combination of several factors linked to the persistent presence of menstrual reflux in the peritoneal cavity as well as exogenous factors playing a critical role. Once started, the process is variable and can lead to the development of endometriosis through the progressive acquisition of alterations to the physiological processes of the endometrium, including the altered hormonal physiology, and modulating the interaction between endometriosis and the inflammatory response by subjugating it. However, the heterogeneity of endometriosis and the different contexts in which it develops suggests that a single etiopathogenetic explaining model is not sufficient.

Author Contributions: Conceptualization, A.S.L. and S.G.; methodology, M.F.; data curation, F.G.; writing—original draft preparation, A.S.L. and S.G.; writing—review and editing, M.G., D.C.M., and P.V.; project administration, A.S.L.

Acknowledgments: None.

Abbreviations

MeSH	Medical Subject Headings
CAM	Chorioallantoic membrane
17β-HSD	17β-hydroxysteroid dehydrogenase
COX-2	Cyclo-oxygenase type 2
TIAR	Tissue injury and repair
TNF	Tumor necrosis factor
IL	Interleukin
VEGF	Vascular endothelial growth factor
Bcl-2	Antiapoptotic protein B cell lymphoma 2
NK cells	Natural Killer cells
sICAM-1	Soluble form of intercellular adhesion molecule-1
LFA-1	Leukocyte function antigen-1
MAPK	Mitogen-activated protein kinase
ECM	Extracellular matrix
HLA-1	Human leukocyte antigen class I
INF	Interferon
TGF-β	Transforming growth factor-β
E-cadherin	Epithelial cadherin
MMPs	Matrix metalloproteinases
TIMPs	Tissue inhibitors of MMPs
bFGF	Basic fibroblast growth factor
PAI	Plasminogen activator inhibitor
PR	Progesterone receptor

ER	Estrogen receptor
SNPs	Single nucleotide polymorphisms
LD	Linkage disequilibrium
FGF	Fibroblast growth factor
FGFR2	FGF receptor 2 gene
GWA	Genome-wide association
CDKN2BAS	Cyclin-dependent kinase inhibitor 2B antisense RNA
MMTV	Mouse mammary tumor virus
WNT4	Wingless-type mouse mammary tumor virus integration site family 4
rAFS	Revised American Fertility Society
FSH	Follicle-stimulating hormone
GREB1	Growth Regulating Estrogen Receptor Binding 1
TCDD	2,3,7,8-tetrachlorodibenzo-p-dioxin
miRNAs	microRNAs
DNMT	DNA methyltransferase
HDAC	Histone deacetylase
HDACIs	Histone deacetylase inhibitors
EDC	Endocrine-disrupting chemicals
SF-1	Steroidogenic factor-1
HOXA10	Homeobox A transcription factor
P-E2	Prostaglandin E2
E	Estrogen
P	Progesterone
TSA	Trichostatin A
PPAR	Peroxisome proliferator-activated receptor
VPA	Valproic acid

References

1. Vercellini, P.; Viganò, P.; Somigliana, E.; Fedele, L. Endometriosis: Pathogenesis and treatment. *Nat. Rev. Endocrinol.* **2014**, *10*, 261–275. [CrossRef] [PubMed]

2. Garai, J.; Molnar, V.; Varga, T.; Koppan, M.; Torok, A.; Bodis, J. Endometriosis: Harmful survival of an ectopic tissue. *Front. Biosci. J. Virtual Libr.* **2006**, *11*, 595–619. [CrossRef] [PubMed]

3. Matalliotakis, M.; Zervou, M.I.; Matalliotaki, C.; Rahmioglu, N.; Koumantakis, G.; Kalogiannidis, I.; Prapas, I.; Zondervan, K.; Spandidos, D.A.; Matalliotakis, I.; et al. The role of gene polymorphisms in endometriosis. *Mol. Med. Rep.* **2017**, *16*, 5881–5886. [CrossRef] [PubMed]

4. Hsiao, K.; Wu, M.; Tsai, S. Epigenetic regulation of the pathological process in endometriosis. *Reprod. Med. Biol.* **2017**, *16*, 314–319. [CrossRef]

5. Clement, P.B. The pathology of endometriosis: A survey of the many faces of a common disease emphasizing diagnostic pitfalls and unusual and newly appreciated aspects. *Adv. Anat. Pathol.* **2007**, *14*, 241–260. [CrossRef]

6. Burney, R.O.; Giudice, L.C. Pathogenesis and pathophysiology of endometriosis. *Fertil. Steril.* **2012**, *98*, 511–519. [CrossRef]

7. Laganà, A.S.; Vitale, S.G.; Salmeri, F.M.; Triolo, O.; Ban Frangež, H.; Vrtačnik-Bokal, E.; Stojanovska, L.; Apostolopoulos, V.; Granese, R.; Sofo, V. Unus pro omnibus, omnes pro uno: A novel, evidence-based, unifying theory for the pathogenesis of endometriosis. *Med. Hypotheses* **2017**, *103*, 10–20. [CrossRef]

8. Laganà, A.S.; La Rosa, V.L.; Rapisarda, A.M.; Valenti, G.; Sapia, F.; Chiofalo, B.; Rossetti, D.; Ban Frangež, H.; Vrtačnik Bokal, E.; Vitale, S.G. Anxiety and depression in patients with endometriosis: Impact and management challenges. *Int. J. Womens Health* **2017**, *9*, 323–330. [CrossRef]

9. Laganà, A.S.; Condemi, I.; Retto, G.; Muscatello, M.R.A.; Bruno, A.; Zoccali, R.A.; Triolo, O.; Cedro, C. Analysis of psychopathological comorbidity behind the common symptoms and signs of endometriosis. *Eur. J. Obstet. Gynecol. Reprod. Biol.* **2015**, *194*, 30–33. [CrossRef]

10. Vitale, S.G.; Petrosino, B.; La Rosa, V.L.; Rapisarda, A.M.C.; Laganà, A.S. A Systematic Review of the Association Between Psychiatric Disturbances and Endometriosis. *J. Obstet. Gynaecol. Can.* **2016**, *38*, 1079–1080. [CrossRef]

11. Laganà, A.S.; La Rosa, V.; Petrosino, B.; Vitale, S.G. Comment on "Risk of developing major depression and anxiety disorders among women with endometriosis: A longitudinal follow-up study". *J. Affect. Disord.* **2017**, *208*, 672–673. [CrossRef] [PubMed]

12. Raffaelli, R.; Garzon, S.; Baggio, S.; Genna, M.; Pomini, P.; Laganà, A.S.; Ghezzi, F.; Franchi, M. Mesenteric vascular and nerve sparing surgery in laparoscopic segmental intestinal resection for deep infiltrating endometriosis. *Eur. J. Obstet. Gynecol. Reprod. Biol.* **2018**, *231*, 214–219. [CrossRef] [PubMed]

13. Baggio, S.; Pomini, P.; Zecchin, A.; Garzon, S.; Bonin, C.; Santi, L.; Festi, A.; Franchi, M.P. Delivery and pregnancy outcome in women with bowel resection for deep endometriosis: A retrospective cohort study. *Gynecol. Surg.* **2015**, *12*, 279–285. [CrossRef]

14. Viganò, P.; Parazzini, F.; Somigliana, E.; Vercellini, P. Endometriosis: Epidemiology and aetiological factors. *Best Pract. Res. Clin. Obstet. Gynaecol.* **2004**, *18*, 177–200. [CrossRef] [PubMed]

15. Buck Louis, G.M.; Hediger, M.L.; Peterson, C.M.; Croughan, M.; Sundaram, R.; Stanford, J.; Chen, Z.; Fujimoto, V.Y.; Varner, M.W.; Trumble, A.; et al. Incidence of endometriosis by study population and diagnostic method: The ENDO study. *Fertil. Steril.* **2011**, *96*, 360–365. [CrossRef] [PubMed]

16. Missmer, S.A.; Cramer, D.W. The epidemiology of endometriosis. *Obstet. Gynecol. Clin. North Am.* **2003**, *30*, 1–19. [CrossRef]

17. Evers, J.L. Endometriosis does not exist; all women have endometriosis. *Hum. Reprod. Oxf. Engl.* **1994**, *9*, 2206–2209. [CrossRef]

18. Evers, J.L. Is adolescent endometriosis a progressive disease that needs to be diagnosed and treated? *Hum. Reprod. Oxf. Engl.* **2013**, *28*, 2023. [CrossRef]

19. Sampson, J.A. Perforating hemorrhage (chocolate) cysts of the ovary: Their importance and especially their relation to pelvic adenomas of endometrial type ("adenomyoma" of the uterus, rectovaginal septum, sigmoid, etc.). *Arch. Surg.* **1921**, *3*, 245–323. [CrossRef]

20. Sampson, J.A. Peritoneal endometriosis due to the menstrual dissemination of endometrial tissue into the peritoneal cavity. *Am. J. Obstet. Gynecol.* **1927**, *14*, 422–469. [CrossRef]

21. Sampson, J.A. The development of the implantation theory for the origin of peritoneal endometriosis. *Am. J. Obstet. Gynecol.* **1940**, *40*, 549–557. [CrossRef]

22. Nisolle, M.; Donnez, J. Peritoneal endometriosis, ovarian endometriosis, and adenomyotic nodules of the rectovaginal septum are three different entities. *Fertil. Steril.* **1997**, *68*, 585–596. [CrossRef]

23. Koninckx, P.R.; Ussia, A.; Adamyan, L.; Wattiez, A.; Donnez, J. Deep endometriosis: Definition, diagnosis, and treatment. *Fertil. Steril.* **2012**, *98*, 564–571. [CrossRef] [PubMed]

24. Koninckx, P.R. Is mild endometriosis a disease?: Is mild endometriosis a condition occurring intermittently in all women? *Hum. Reprod.* **1994**, *9*, 2202–2205. [CrossRef]

25. Donnez, J.; Squifflet, J.; Casanas-Roux, F.; Pirard, C.; Jadoul, P.; Van, A.L. Typical and subtle atypical presentations of endometriosis. *Obstet. Gynecol. Clin. North Am.* **2003**, *30*, 83–93. [CrossRef]

26. Waldeyer, H. "Die epithelialen Eierstockgeschwülste." Ins besonders die Kystome (The epithelial ovarian tumors, especially the cystic tumors). *Arch Gynäkol* **1870**, *1*, 252–316. [CrossRef]

27. van der Linden, P.J. Theories on the pathogenesis of endometriosis. *Hum. Reprod. Oxf. Engl.* **1996**, *11* (Suppl. 3), 53–65. [CrossRef]

28. Miyazaki, K.; Dyson, M.T.; Coon V, J.S.; Furukawa, Y.; Yilmaz, B.D.; Maruyama, T.; Bulun, S.E. Generation of Progesterone-Responsive Endometrial Stromal Fibroblasts from Human Induced Pluripotent Stem Cells: Role of the WNT/CTNNB1 Pathway. *Stem Cell Rep.* **2018**, *11*, 1136–1155. [CrossRef]

29. Lauchlan, S.C. THE SECONDARY MÜLLERIAN SYSTEM. *Obstet. Gynecol. Surv.* **1972**, *27*, 133. [CrossRef]

30. Batt, R.E.; Smith, R.A.; Buck, G.L.; Martin, D.C.; Chapron, C.; Koninckx, P.R.; Yeh, J. Müllerianosis. *Histol. Histopathol.* **2007**, *22*, 1161–1166. [CrossRef]

31. Signorile, P.G.; Baldi, F.; Bussani, R.; D'Armiento, M.; De Falco, M.; Baldi, A. Ectopic endometrium in human foetuses is a common event and sustains the theory of müllerianosis in the pathogenesis of endometriosis, a disease that predisposes to cancer. *J. Exp. Clin. Cancer Res.* **2009**, *28*, 49. [CrossRef] [PubMed]

32. Nawroth, F.; Rahimi, G.; Nawroth, C.; Foth, D.; Ludwig, M.; Schmidt, T. Is there an association between septate uterus and endometriosis? *Hum. Reprod.* **2006**, *21*, 542–544. [CrossRef] [PubMed]

33. Mok-Lin, E.Y.; Wolfberg, A.; Hollinquist, H.; Laufer, M.R. Endometriosis in a Patient with Mayer-Rokitansky-Küster-Hauser Syndrome and Complete Uterine Agenesis: Evidence to Support the Theory of Coelomic Metaplasia. *J. Pediatr. Adolesc. Gynecol.* **2010**, *23*, e35–e37. [CrossRef] [PubMed]

34. Troncon, J.K.; Zani, A.C.T.; Vieira, A.D.D.; Poli-Neto, O.B.; Nogueira, A.A.; Rosa-E-Silva, J.C. Endometriosis in a patient with mayer-rokitansky-küster-hauser syndrome. *Case Rep. Obstet. Gynecol.* **2014**, *2014*, 376231. [CrossRef] [PubMed]

35. Batt, R.E.; Mitwally, M.F.M. Endometriosis from thelarche to midteens: Pathogenesis and prognosis, prevention and pedagogy. *J. Pediatr. Adolesc. Gynecol.* **2003**, *16*, 337–347. [CrossRef] [PubMed]

36. Suginami, H. A reappraisal of the coelomic metaplasia theory by reviewing, endometriosis occurring in unusual sites and instances. *Am. J. Obstet. Gynecol.* **1991**, *165*, 214–218. [CrossRef]

37. Rei, C.; Williams, T.; Feloney, M. Endometriosis in a Man as a Rare Source of Abdominal Pain: A Case Report and Review of the Literature. *Case Rep. Obstet. Gynecol.* **2018**, *2018*, 2083121. [CrossRef]

38. Cullen, T.S. *Adeno-myoma uteri diffusum benignum*; Johns Hopkins Press: Baltimore, Maryland, 1896.

39. Meyer, R. Über eine adenomatöse Wucherung der Serosa in einer Bauchnarbe. *Zeitschr Geburtsh Gynakol* **1903**, *49*, 32–41.

40. Novak, E. Pelvic endometriosis: Spontaneous rupture of endometrial cysts, with a report of three cases. *Am. J. Obstet. Gynecol.* **1931**, *22*, 826–837. [CrossRef]

41. Hu, Z.; Mamillapalli, R.; Taylor, H.S. Increased circulating miR-370-3p regulates steroidogenic factor 1 in endometriosis. *Am. J. Physiol. Endocrinol. Metab.* **2019**, *316*, E373–E382. [CrossRef]

42. Meyer, R. Uber den Stand der Frage der Adenomyositis und Adenomyome im allgeneinen und insbesondere uber Adenomyositis seroepithelialis und Adenomyometritis sarcomatosa. *Zentralbl Gynäkol* **1919**, *36*, 745–750.

43. Munrós, J.; Martínez-Zamora, M.-A.; Tàssies, D.; Reverter, J.C.; Rius, M.; Gracia, M.; Ros, C.; Carmona, F. Total Circulating Microparticle Levels After Laparoscopic Surgical Treatment for Endometrioma: A Pilot, Prospective, Randomized Study Comparing Stripping with CO2 Laser Vaporization. *J. Minim. Invasive Gynecol.* **2019**, *26*, 450–455. [CrossRef] [PubMed]

44. Levander, G.; Normann, P. The Pathogenesis of Endometriosis. *Acta Obstet. Gynecol. Scand.* **1955**, *34*, 366–398. [CrossRef] [PubMed]

45. Merrill, J.A. Endometrial induction of endometriosis across Millipore filters. *Am J Obstet Gynecol* **1966**, *94*, 780–790. [PubMed]

46. Maniglio, P.; Ricciardi, E.; Meli, F.; Vitale, S.G.; Noventa, M.; Vitagliano, A.; Valenti, G.; La Rosa, V.L.; Laganà, A.S.; Caserta, D. Catamenial pneumothorax caused by thoracic endometriosis. *Radiol. Case Rep.* **2018**, *13*, 81–85. [CrossRef] [PubMed]

47. Uğur, M.; Turan, C.; Mungan, T.; Kuşçu, E.; Şenöz, S.; Ağış, H.T.; Gökmen, O. Endometriosis in Association with Müllerian Anomalies. *Gynecol. Obstet. Investig.* **1995**, *40*, 261–264. [CrossRef] [PubMed]

48. Olive, D.L.; Henderson, D.Y. Endometriosis and mullerian anomalies. *Obstet. Gynecol.* **1987**, *69*, 412–415.

49. Javert, C.T. Pathogenesis of endometriosis based on endometrial homeoplasia, direct extension, exfoliation and implantation, lymphatic and hematogenous metastasis. Including five case reports of endometrial tissue in pelvic lymph nodes. *Cancer* **1949**, *2*, 399–410. [CrossRef]

50. Halme, J.; Hammond, M.G.; Hulka, J.F.; Raj, S.G.; Talbert, L.M. Retrograde menstruation in healthy women and in patients with endometriosis. *Obstet. Gynecol.* **1984**, *64*, 151–154.

51. Kruitwagen, R.F.; Poels, L.G.; Willemsen, W.N.; de Ronde, I.J.; Jap, P.H.; Rolland, R. Endometrial epithelial cells in peritoneal fluid during the early follicular phase. *Fertil. Steril.* **1991**, *55*, 297–303. [CrossRef]

52. Koks, C.A.M.; Dunselman, G.A.J.; de Goeij, A.F.P.M.; Arends, J.W.; Evers, J.L.H. Evaluation of a menstrual cup to collect shed endometrium for in vitro studies. *Fertil. Steril.* **1997**, *68*, 560–564. [CrossRef]

53. Vercellini, P.; Aimi, G.; De Giorgi, O.; Maddalena, S.; Carinelli, S.; Crosignani, P.G. Is cystic ovarian endometriosis an asymmetric disease? *Br. J. Obstet. Gynaecol.* **1998**, *105*, 1018–1021. [CrossRef] [PubMed]

54. Vercellini, P.; Abbiati, A.; Vigano, P.; Somigliana, E.D.; Daguati, R.; Meroni, F.; Crosignani, P.G. Asymmetry in distribution of diaphragmatic endometriotic lesions: Evidence in favour of the menstrual reflux theory. *Hum. Reprod.* **2007**, *22*, 2359–2367. [CrossRef] [PubMed]

55. Jenkins, S.; Olive, D.L.; Haney, A.F. Endometriosis: Pathogenetic implications of the anatomic distribution. *Obstet. Gynecol.* **1986**, *67*, 335–338.

56. Martin, D.C. Laparoscopic Appearance of Endometriosis. Available online: https://www.danmartinmd.com/files/lae1988.pdf (accessed on 15 September 2019).

57. Roman, H.; Hennetier, C.; Darwish, B.; Badescu, A.; Csanyi, M.; Aziz, M.; Tuech, J.-J.; Abo, C. Bowel occult microscopic endometriosis in resection margins in deep colorectal endometriosis specimens has no impact on short-term postoperative outcomes. *Fertil. Steril.* **2016**, *105*, 423–429. [CrossRef]

58. Badescu, A.; Roman, H.; Aziz, M.; Puscasiu, L.; Molnar, C.; Huet, E.; Sabourin, J.-C.; Stolnicu, S. Mapping of bowel occult microscopic endometriosis implants surrounding deep endometriosis nodules infiltrating the bowel. *Fertil. Steril.* **2016**, *105*, 430–434. [CrossRef]

59. Bruner-Tran, K.L.; Mokshagundam, S.; Herington, J.L.; Ding, T.; Osteen, K.G. Rodent Models of Experimental Endometriosis: Identifying Mechanisms of Disease and Therapeutic Targets. *Curr. Womens Health Rev.* **2018**, *14*, 173–188. [CrossRef]

60. Laganà, A.S.; Garzon, S.; Franchi, M.; Casarin, J.; Gullo, G.; Ghezzi, F. Translational animal models for endometriosis research: A long and windy road. *Ann. Transl. Med.* **2018**, *6*, 431. [CrossRef]

61. Klemmt, P.A.B.; Starzinski-Powitz, A. Molecular and Cellular Pathogenesis of Endometriosis. *Curr. Womens Health Rev.* **2018**, *14*, 106–116. [CrossRef]

62. Ota, H.; Igarashi, S. Expression of major histocompatibility complex class II antigen in endometriotic tissue in patients with endometriosis and adenomyosis. *Fertil. Steril.* **1993**, *60*, 834–838. [CrossRef]

63. Chung, H.W.; Wen, Y.; Chun, S.H.; Nezhat, C.; Woo, B.H.; Lake Polan, M. Matrix metalloproteinase-9 and tissue inhibitor of metalloproteinase-3 mRNA expression in ectopic and eutopic endometrium in women with endometriosis: A rationale for endometriotic invasiveness. *Fertil. Steril.* **2001**, *75*, 152–159. [CrossRef]

64. Di Carlo, C.; Bonifacio, M.; Tommaselli, G.A.; Bifulco, G.; Guerra, G.; Nappi, C. Metalloproteinases, vascular endothelial growth factor, and angiopoietin 1 and 2 in eutopic and ectopic endometrium. *Fertil. Steril.* **2009**, *91*, 2315–2323. [CrossRef] [PubMed]

65. Redwine, D.B. Was Sampson wrong? *Fertil. Steril.* **2002**, *78*, 686–693. [CrossRef]

66. Suda, K.; Nakaoka, H.; Yoshihara, K.; Ishiguro, T.; Tamura, R.; Mori, Y.; Yamawaki, K.; Adachi, S.; Takahashi, T.; Kase, H.; et al. Clonal Expansion and Diversification of Cancer-Associated Mutations in Endometriosis and Normal Endometrium. *Cell Rep.* **2018**, *24*, 1777–1789. [CrossRef] [PubMed]

67. Leyendecker, G.; Wildt, L.; Mall, G. The pathophysiology of endometriosis and adenomyosis: Tissue injury and repair. *Arch. Gynecol. Obstet.* **2009**, *280*, 529–538. [CrossRef] [PubMed]

68. Young, V.J.; Ahmad, S.F.; Duncan, W.C.; Horne, A.W. The role of TGF-β in the pathophysiology of peritoneal endometriosis. *Hum. Reprod. Update* **2017**, *23*, 548–559. [CrossRef] [PubMed]

69. Maas, J.W.; Groothuis, P.G.; Dunselman, G.A.; de Goeij, A.F.; Struijker-Boudier, H.A.; Evers, J.L. Development of endometriosis-like lesions after transplantation of human endometrial fragments onto the chick embryo chorioallantoic membrane. *Hum. Reprod.* **2001**, *16*, 627–631. [CrossRef]

70. Nap, A.W.; Groothuis, P.G.; Demir, A.Y.; Maas, J.W.; Dunselman, G.A.; de Goeij, A.F.; Evers, J.L. Tissue integrity is essential for ectopic implantation of human endometrium in the chicken chorioallantoic membrane. *Hum. Reprod.* **2003**, *18*, 30–34. [CrossRef]

71. Winterhager, E. Role of Steroid Hormones: Estrogen and Endometriosis. In *Endometriosis: Science and Practice*; John Wiley & Sons, Ltd.: Hoboken, NJ, USA, 2012; pp. 140–144. ISBN 978-1-4443-9851-9.

72. Liang, Y.; Xie, H.; Wu, J.; Liu, D.; Yao, S. Villainous role of estrogen in macrophage-nerve interaction in endometriosis. *Reprod. Biol. Endocrinol.* **2018**, *16*, 122. [CrossRef]

73. Rier, S.E.; Martin, D.C.; Bowman, R.E.; Becker, J.L. Immunoresponsiveness in endometriosis: Implications of estrogenic toxicants. *Environ. Health Perspect.* **1995**, *103*, 151–156.

74. Maruyama, T.; Yoshimura, Y. Molecular and cellular mechanisms for differentiation and regeneration of the uterine endometrium. *Endocr. J.* **2008**, *55*, 795–810. [CrossRef] [PubMed]

75. de Almeida Asencio, F.; Ribeiro, H.A.; Ayrosa Ribeiro, P.; Malzoni, M.; Adamyan, L.; Ussia, A.; Gomel, V.; Martin, D.C.; Koninckx, P.R. Symptomatic endometriosis developing several years after menopause in the absence of increased circulating estrogen concentrations: A systematic review and seven case reports. *Gynecol. Surg.* **2019**, *16*, 3. [CrossRef]

76. Kitawaki, J.; Noguchi, T.; Amatsu, T.; Maeda, K.; Tsukamoto, K.; Yamamoto, T.; Fushiki, S.; Osawa, Y.; Honjo, H. Expression of aromatase cytochrome P450 protein and messenger ribonucleic acid in human endometriotic and adenomyotic tissues but not in normal endometrium. *Biol. Reprod.* **1997**, *57*, 514–519. [CrossRef] [PubMed]

77. Noble, L.S.; Simpson, E.R.; Johns, A.; Bulun, S.E. Aromatase expression in endometriosis. *J. Clin. Endocrinol. Metab.* **1996**, *81*, 174–179. [PubMed]

78. Noble, L.S.; Takayama, K.; Zeitoun, K.M.; Putman, J.M.; Johns, D.A.; Hinshelwood, M.M.; Agarwal, V.R.; Zhao, Y.; Carr, B.R.; Bulun, S.E. Prostaglandin E2 stimulates aromatase expression in endometriosis-derived stromal cells. *J. Clin. Endocrinol. Metab.* **1997**, *82*, 600–606. [CrossRef]

79. Zeitoun, K.; Takayama, K.; Sasano, H.; Suzuki, T.; Moghrabi, N.; Andersson, S.; Johns, A.; Meng, L.; Putman, M.; Carr, B. Deficient 17β-hydroxysteroid dehydrogenase type 2 expression in endometriosis: Failure to metabolize 17β-estradiol. *J. Clin. Endocrinol. Metab.* **1998**, *83*, 4474–4480. [CrossRef]

80. TAKAHAsHI, K.; Nagata, H.; Kitao, M. Clinical usefulness of determination of estradiol level in the menstrual blood for patients with endometriosis. *Nippon Sanka Fujinka Gakkai Zasshi* **1989**, *41*, 1849–1850.

81. Bulun, S.E.; Yang, S.; Fang, Z.; Gurates, B.; Tamura, M.; Zhou, J.; Sebastian, S. Role of aromatase in endometrial disease. *J. Steroid Biochem. Mol. Biol.* **2001**, *79*, 19–25. [CrossRef]

82. Götte, M.; Wolf, M.; Staebler, A.; Buchweitz, O.; Kelsch, R.; Schüring, A.N.; Kiesel, L. Increased expression of the adult stem cell marker Musashi-1 in endometriosis and endometrial carcinoma. *J. Pathol.* **2008**, *215*, 317–329. [CrossRef]

83. Valentijn, A.J.; Palial, K.; Al-Lamee, H.; Tempest, N.; Drury, J.; Von Zglinicki, T.; Saretzki, G.; Murray, P.; Gargett, C.E.; Hapangama, D.K. SSEA-1 isolates human endometrial basal glandular epithelial cells: Phenotypic and functional characterization and implications in the pathogenesis of endometriosis. *Hum. Reprod. Oxf. Engl.* **2013**, *28*, 2695–2708. [CrossRef]

84. Leyendecker, G.; Herbertz, M.; Kunz, G.; Mall, G. Endometriosis results from the dislocation of basal endometrium. *Hum. Reprod.* **2002**, *17*, 2725–2736. [CrossRef] [PubMed]

85. Agic, A.; Djalali, S.; Diedrich, K.; Hornung, D. Apoptosis in endometriosis. *Gynecol. Obstet. Investig.* **2009**, *68*, 217–223. [CrossRef] [PubMed]

86. Zhao, Y.; Gong, P.; Chen, Y.; Nwachukwu, J.C.; Srinivasan, S.; Ko, C.; Bagchi, M.K.; Taylor, R.N.; Korach, K.S.; Nettles, K.W.; et al. Dual suppression of estrogenic and inflammatory activities for targeting of endometriosis. *Sci. Transl. Med.* **2015**, *7*, 271ra9. [CrossRef] [PubMed]

87. Burns, K.A.; Rodriguez, K.F.; Hewitt, S.C.; Janardhan, K.S.; Young, S.L.; Korach, K.S. Role of estrogen receptor signaling required for endometriosis-like lesion establishment in a mouse model. *Endocrinology* **2012**, *153*, 3960–3971. [CrossRef] [PubMed]

88. Han, S.J.; Jung, S.Y.; Wu, S.-P.; Hawkins, S.M.; Park, M.J.; Kyo, S.; Qin, J.; Lydon, J.P.; Tsai, S.Y.; Tsai, M.-J.; et al. Estrogen Receptor β Modulates Apoptosis Complexes and the Inflammasome to Drive the Pathogenesis of Endometriosis. *Cell* **2015**, *163*, 960–974. [CrossRef] [PubMed]

89. Simmen, R.C.M.; Kelley, A.S. Reversal of Fortune: Estrogen Receptor-Beta in Endometriosis. *J. Mol. Endocrinol.* **2016**, *57*, F23–F27. [CrossRef] [PubMed]

90. Hamilton, K.J.; Arao, Y.; Korach, K.S. Estrogen hormone physiology: Reproductive findings from estrogen receptor mutant mice. *Reprod. Biol.* **2014**, *14*, 3–8. [CrossRef]

91. Bulun, S.E.; Monsavais, D.; Pavone, M.E.; Dyson, M.; Xue, Q.; Attar, E.; Tokunaga, H.; Su, E.J. Role of Estrogen Receptor-β in Endometriosis. *Semin. Reprod. Med.* **2012**, *30*, 39–45. [CrossRef]

92. Han, S.J.; Lee, J.E.; Cho, Y.J.; Park, M.J.; O'Malley, B.W. Genomic Function of Estrogen Receptor β in Endometriosis. *Endocrinology* **2019**, *160*, 2495–2516. [CrossRef]

93. McKinnon, B.; Mueller, M.; Montgomery, G. Progesterone Resistance in Endometriosis: An Acquired Property? *Trends Endocrinol. Metab.* **2018**, *29*, 535–548. [CrossRef]

94. Patel, B.G.; Rudnicki, M.; Yu, J.; Shu, Y.; Taylor, R.N. Progesterone resistance in endometriosis: Origins, consequences and interventions. *Acta Obstet. Gynecol. Scand.* **2017**, *96*, 623–632. [CrossRef] [PubMed]

95. Bulun, S.E.; Cheng, Y.-H.; Yin, P.; Imir, G.; Utsunomiya, H.; Attar, E.; Innes, J.; Julie Kim, J. Progesterone resistance in endometriosis: Link to failure to metabolize estradiol. *Mol. Cell. Endocrinol.* **2006**, *248*, 94–103. [CrossRef] [PubMed]

96. Grandi, G.; Mueller, M.D.; Bersinger, N.A.; Facchinetti, F.; McKinnon, B.D. The association between progestins, nuclear receptors expression and inflammation in endometrial stromal cells from women with endometriosis. *Gynecol. Endocrinol. Off. J. Int. Soc. Gynecol. Endocrinol.* **2017**, *33*, 712–715. [CrossRef] [PubMed]

97. Allport, V.C.; Pieber, D.; Slater, D.M.; Newton, R.; White, J.O.; Bennett, P.R. Human labour is associated with nuclear factor-kappaB activity which mediates cyclo-oxygenase-2 expression and is involved with the "functional progesterone withdrawal". *Mol. Hum. Reprod.* **2001**, *7*, 581–586. [CrossRef] [PubMed]

98. Cinar, O.; Seval, Y.; Uz, Y.H.; Cakmak, H.; Ulukus, M.; Kayisli, U.A.; Arici, A. Differential regulation of Akt phosphorylation in endometriosis. *Reprod. Biomed. Online* **2009**, *19*, 864–871. [CrossRef] [PubMed]

99. Treloar, S.A.; Zhao, Z.Z.; Armitage, T.; Duffy, D.L.; Wicks, J.; O'Connor, D.T.; Martin, N.G.; Montgomery, G.W. Association between polymorphisms in the progesterone receptor gene and endometriosis. *Mol. Hum. Reprod.* **2005**, *11*, 641–647. [CrossRef]

100. Ren, Y.; Liu, X.; Ma, D.; Feng, Y.; Zhong, N. Down-regulation of the progesterone receptor by the methylation of progesterone receptor gene in endometrial cancer cells. *Cancer Genet. Cytogenet.* **2007**, *175*, 107–116. [CrossRef]

101. Teague, E.M.C.O.; Print, C.G.; Hull, M.L. The role of microRNAs in endometriosis and associated reproductive conditions. *Hum. Reprod. Update* **2010**, *16*, 142–165. [CrossRef]

102. Rižner, T.L. Diagnostic potential of peritoneal fluid biomarkers of endometriosis. *Expert Rev. Mol. Diagn.* **2015**, *15*, 557–580. [CrossRef]

103. Haney, A.F.; Muscato, J.J.; Weinberg, J.B. Peritoneal fluid cell populations in infertility patients. *Fertil. Steril.* **1981**, *35*, 696–698. [CrossRef]

104. Hill, J.A.; Faris, H.M.; Schiff, I.; Anderson, D.J. Characterization of leukocyte subpopulations in the peritoneal fluid of women with endometriosis. *Fertil. Steril.* **1988**, *50*, 216–222. [CrossRef]

105. Jones, R.K.; Bulmer, J.N.; Searle, R.F. Phenotypic and functional studies of leukocytes in human endometrium and endometriosis. *Hum. Reprod. Update* **1998**, *4*, 702–709. [CrossRef] [PubMed]

106. Darrow, S.L.; Vena, J.E.; Batt, R.E.; Zielezny, M.A.; Michalek, A.M.; Selman, S. Menstrual cycle characteristics and the risk of endometriosis. *Epidemiology* **1993**, 135–142. [CrossRef] [PubMed]

107. Vercellini, P.; De Giorgi, O.; Aimi, G.; Panazza, S.; Uglietti, A.; Crosignani, P.G. Menstrual characteristics in women with and without endometriosis. *Obstet. Gynecol.* **1997**, *90*, 264–268. [CrossRef]

108. Salamanca, A.; Beltrán, E. Subendometrial contractility in menstrual phase visualized by transvaginal sonography in patients with endometriosis. *Fertil. Steril.* **1995**, *64*, 193–195. [CrossRef]

109. Sanfilippo, J.S.; Wakim, N.G.; Schikler, K.N.; Yussman, M.A. Endometriosis in association with uterine anomaly. *Am. J. Obstet. Gynecol.* **1986**, *154*, 39–43. [CrossRef]

110. Oosterlynck, D.J.; Cornillie, F.J.; Waer, M.; Vandeputte, M.; Koninckx, P.R. Women with endometriosis show a defect in natural killer activity resulting in a decreased cytotoxicity to autologous endometrium. *Fertil. Steril.* **1991**, *56*, 45–51. [CrossRef]

111. Laganà, A.S.; Triolo, O.; Salmeri, F.M.; Granese, R.; Palmara, V.I.; Ban Frangež, H.; Vrtčnik Bokal, E.; Sofo, V. Natural Killer T cell subsets in eutopic and ectopic endometrium: A fresh look to a busy corner. *Arch. Gynecol. Obstet.* **2016**, *293*, 941–949. [CrossRef]

112. Semino, C.; Semino, A.; Pietra, G.; Mingari, M.C.; Barocci, S.; Venturini, P.L.; Ragni, N.; Melioli, G. Role of major histocompatibility complex class I expression and natural killer-like T cells in the genetic control of endometriosis*. *Fertil. Steril.* **1995**, *64*, 909–916. [CrossRef]

113. Somigliana, E.; Viganò, P.; Gaffuri, B.; Guarneri, D.; Busacca, M.; Vignali, M. Human endometrial stromal cells as a source of soluble intercellular adhesion molecule (ICAM)-1 molecules. *Hum. Reprod. Oxf. Engl.* **1996**, *11*, 1190–1194. [CrossRef]

114. Viganò, P.; Gaffuri, B.; Somigliana, E.; Busacca, M.; Di Blasio, A.M.; Vignali, M. Expression of intercellular adhesion molecule (ICAM)-1 mRNA and protein is enhanced in endometriosis versus endometrial stromal cells in culture. *Mol. Hum. Reprod.* **1998**, *4*, 1150–1156. [CrossRef] [PubMed]

115. Králíčková, M.; Vetvicka, V. Immunological aspects of endometriosis: A review. *Ann. Transl. Med.* **2015**, *3*, 153. [PubMed]

116. Riccio, L.D.G.C.; Santulli, P.; Marcellin, L.; Abrão, M.S.; Batteux, F.; Chapron, C. Immunology of endometriosis. *Best Pract. Res. Clin. Obstet. Gynaecol.* **2018**, *50*, 39–49. [CrossRef] [PubMed]

117. Santulli, P.; Marcellin, L.; Tosti, C.; Chouzenoux, S.; Cerles, O.; Borghese, B.; Batteux, F.; Chapron, C. MAP kinases and the inflammatory signaling cascade as targets for the treatment of endometriosis? *Expert Opin. Ther. Targets* **2015**, *19*, 1465–1483. [CrossRef]

118. Martínez-Román, S.; Balasch, J.; Creus, M.; Fábregues, F.; Carmona, F.; Vilella, R.; Vanrell, J.A. Transferrin Receptor (CD71) Expression in Peritoneal Macrophages from Fertile and Infertile Women With and Without Endometriosis. *Am. J. Reprod. Immunol.* **1997**, *38*, 413–417. [CrossRef]

119. Raiter-Tenenbaum, A.; Barañao, R.I.; Etchepareborda, J.J.; Meresman, G.F.; Rumi, L.S. Functional and phenotypic alterations in peritoneal macrophages from patients with early and advanced endometriosis. *Arch. Gynecol. Obstet.* **1998**, *261*, 147–157. [CrossRef]

120. Halme, J.; Becker, S.; Wing, R. Accentuated cyclic activation of peritoneal macrophages in patients with endometriosis. *Am. J. Obstet. Gynecol.* **1984**, *148*, 85–90. [CrossRef]

121. McLaren, J.; Prentice, A.; Charnock-Jones, D.S.; Sharkey, A.M.; Smith, S.K. Immunolocalization of the apoptosis regulating proteins Bcl-2 and Bax in human endometrium and isolated peritoneal fluid macrophages in endometriosis. *Hum. Reprod.* **1997**, *12*, 146–152. [CrossRef]

122. Bacci, M.; Capobianco, A.; Monno, A.; Cottone, L.; Di Puppo, F.; Camisa, B.; Mariani, M.; Brignole, C.; Ponzoni, M.; Ferrari, S.; et al. Macrophages Are Alternatively Activated in Patients with Endometriosis and Required for Growth and Vascularization of Lesions in a Mouse Model of Disease. *Am. J. Pathol.* **2009**, *175*, 547–556. [CrossRef]

123. McLaren, J.; Dealtry, G.; Prentice, A.; Charnock-Jones, D.S.; Smith, S.K. Decreased levels of the potent regulator of monocyte/macrophage activation, interleukin-13, in the peritoneal fluid of patients with endometriosis. *Hum. Reprod. Oxf. Engl.* **1997**, *12*, 1307–1310. [CrossRef]

124. Schneider, C.; Kässens, N.; Greve, B.; Hassan, H.; Schüring, A.N.; Starzinski-Powitz, A.; Kiesel, L.; Seidler, D.G.; Götte, M. Targeting of syndecan-1 by micro-ribonucleic acid miR-10b modulates invasiveness of endometriotic cells via dysregulation of the proteolytic milieu and interleukin-6 secretion. *Fertil. Steril.* **2013**, *99*, 871–881. [CrossRef] [PubMed]

125. Götte, M.; Joussen, A.M.; Klein, C.; Andre, P.; Wagner, D.D.; Hinkes, M.T.; Kirchhof, B.; Adamis, A.P.; Bernfield, M. Role of syndecan-1 in leukocyte-endothelial interactions in the ocular vasculature. *Investig. Ophthalmol. Vis. Sci.* **2002**, *43*, 1135–1141. [PubMed]

126. Averbeck, M.; Kuhn, S.; Bühligen, J.; Götte, M.; Simon, J.C.; Polte, T. Syndecan-1 regulates dendritic cell migration in cutaneous hypersensitivity to haptens. *Exp. Dermatol.* **2017**, *26*, 1060–1067. [CrossRef] [PubMed]

127. Pizzo, A.; Salmeri, F.M.; Ardita, F.V.; Sofo, V.; Tripepi, M.; Marsico, S. Behaviour of cytokine levels in serum and peritoneal fluid of women with endometriosis. *Gynecol. Obstet. Investig.* **2002**, *54*, 82–87. [CrossRef]

128. de Barros, I.B.L.; Malvezzi, H.; Gueuvoghlanian-Silva, B.Y.; Piccinato, C.A.; Rizzo, L.V.; Podgaec, S. "What do we know about regulatory T cells and endometriosis? A systematic review". *J. Reprod. Immunol.* **2017**, *120*, 48–55. [CrossRef]

129. Riccio, L.G.C.; Baracat, E.C.; Chapron, C.; Batteux, F.; Abrão, M.S. The role of the B lymphocytes in endometriosis: A systematic review. *J. Reprod. Immunol.* **2017**, *123*, 29–34. [CrossRef]

130. Sattler, M.; Liang, H.; Nettesheim, D.; Meadows, R.P.; Harlan, J.E.; Eberstadt, M.; Yoon, H.S.; Shuker, S.B.; Chang, B.S.; Minn, A.J.; et al. Structure of Bcl-xL-Bak peptide complex: Recognition between regulators of apoptosis. *Science* **1997**, *275*, 983–986. [CrossRef]

131. Tabibzadeh, S.; Zupi, E.; Babaknia, A.; Liu, R.; Marconi, D.; Romanini, C. Site and menstrual cycle-dependent expression of proteins of the tumour necrosis factor (TNF) receptor family, and BCL-2 oncoprotein and phase-specific production of TNF alpha in human endometrium. *Hum. Reprod. Oxf. Engl.* **1995**, *10*, 277–286. [CrossRef]

132. Taniguchi, F.; Kaponis, A.; Izawa, M.; Kiyama, T.; Deura, I.; Ito, M.; Iwabe, T.; Adonakis, G.; Terakawa, N.; Harada, T. Apoptosis and endometriosis. *Front. Biosci. Elite Ed.* **2011**, *3*, 648–662. [CrossRef]

133. Gebel, H.M.; Braun, D.P.; Tambur, A.; Frame, D.; Rana, N.; Dmowski, W.P. Spontaneous apoptosis of endometrial tissue is impaired in women with endometriosis. *Fertil. Steril.* **1998**, *69*, 1042–1047. [CrossRef]

134. Béliard, A.; Noël, A.; Foidart, J.-M. Reduction of apoptosis and proliferation in endometriosis. *Fertil. Steril.* **2004**, *82*, 80–85. [CrossRef] [PubMed]

135. Lac, V.; Verhoef, L.; Aguirre-Hernandez, R.; Nazeran, T.M.; Tessier-Cloutier, B.; Praetorius, T.; Orr, N.L.; Noga, H.; Lum, A.; Khattra, J.; et al. Iatrogenic endometriosis harbors somatic cancer-driver mutations. *Hum. Reprod. Oxf. Engl.* **2019**, *34*, 69–78. [CrossRef] [PubMed]

136. Vetvicka, V.; Laganà, A.S.; Salmeri, F.M.; Triolo, O.; Palmara, V.I.; Vitale, S.G.; Sofo, V.; Králíčková, M. Regulation of apoptotic pathways during endometriosis: From the molecular basis to the future perspectives. *Arch. Gynecol. Obstet.* **2016**, *294*, 897–904. [CrossRef] [PubMed]

137. Sturlese, E.; Salmeri, F.M.; Retto, G.; Pizzo, A.; De Dominici, R.; Ardita, F.V.; Borrielli, I.; Licata, N.; Laganà, A.S.; Sofo, V. Dysregulation of the Fas/FasL system in mononuclear cells recovered from peritoneal fluid of women with endometriosis. *J. Reprod. Immunol.* **2011**, *92*, 74–81. [CrossRef] [PubMed]

138. Rutherford, E.J.; Hill, A.D.K.; Hopkins, A.M. Adhesion in Physiological, Benign and Malignant Proliferative States of the Endometrium: Microenvironment and the Clinical Big Picture. *Cells* **2018**, *7*, e43. [CrossRef] [PubMed]

139. Groothuis, P.G.; Koks, C.A.; de Goeij, A.F.; Dunselman, G.A.; Arends, J.W.; Evers, J.L. Adhesion of human endometrial fragments to peritoneum in vitro. *Fertil. Steril.* **1999**, *71*, 1119–1124. [CrossRef]

140. Koks, C.A.; Groothuis, P.G.; Dunselman, G.A.; de Goeij, A.F.; Evers, J.L. Adhesion of shed menstrual tissue in an in-vitro model using amnion and peritoneum: A light and electron microscopic study. *Hum. Reprod. Oxf. Engl.* **1999**, *14*, 816–822. [CrossRef]

141. Dunselman, G.A.; Groothuis, P.G.; de Goeij, A.F.; Evers, J.L. The Mesothelium, Teflon or Velcro? Mesothelium in endometriosis pathogenesis. *Hum. Reprod. Oxf. Engl.* **2001**, *16*, 605–607. [CrossRef]

142. Canis, M.; Bourdel, N.; Houlle, C.; Gremeau, A.-S.; Botchorishvili, R.; Matsuzaki, S. Trauma and endometriosis. A review. May we explain surgical phenotypes and natural history of the disease? *J. Gynecol. Obstet. Hum. Reprod.* **2017**, *46*, 219–227. [CrossRef]

143. Koks, C.A.; Demir Weusten, A.Y.; Groothuis, P.G.; Dunselman, G.A.; de Goeij, A.F.; Evers, J.L. Menstruum induces changes in mesothelial cell morphology. *Gynecol. Obstet. Investig.* **2000**, *50*, 13–18. [CrossRef]

144. Demir Weusten, A.Y.; Groothuis, P.G.; Dunselman, G.A.; de Goeij, A.F.; Arends, J.W.; Evers, J.L. Morphological changes in mesothelial cells induced by shed menstrual endometrium in vitro are not primarily due to apoptosis or necrosis. *Hum. Reprod. Oxf. Engl.* **2000**, *15*, 1462–1468. [CrossRef] [PubMed]

145. Demir, A.Y.; Groothuis, P.G.; Nap, A.W.; Punyadeera, C.; de Goeij, A.F.P.M.; Evers, J.L.H.; Dunselman, G.A.J. Menstrual effluent induces epithelial-mesenchymal transitions in mesothelial cells. *Hum. Reprod. Oxf. Engl.* **2004**, *19*, 21–29. [CrossRef] [PubMed]

146. Bilyk, O.; Coatham, M.; Jewer, M.; Postovit, L.-M. Epithelial-to-Mesenchymal Transition in the Female Reproductive Tract: From Normal Functioning to Disease Pathology. *Front. Oncol.* **2017**, *5*, 145. [CrossRef] [PubMed]

147. Yang, Y.-M.; Yang, W.-X. Epithelial-to-mesenchymal transition in the development of endometriosis. *Oncotarget* **2017**, *8*, 41679–41689. [CrossRef]

148. Lessey, B.A.; Damjanovich, L.; Coutifaris, C.; Castelbaum, A.; Albelda, S.M.; Buck, C.A. Integrin adhesion molecules in the human endometrium. Correlation with the normal and abnormal menstrual cycle. *J. Clin. Investig.* **1992**, *90*, 188–195. [CrossRef]

149. Lessey, B.A. Endometrial integrins and the establishment of uterine receptivity. *Hum. Reprod.* **1998**, *13*, 247–258. [CrossRef]

150. Tabibzadeh, S. Patterns of expression of integrin molecules in human endometrium throughout the menstrual cycle. *Hum. Reprod.* **1992**, *7*, 876–882. [CrossRef]

151. van der Linden, P.J.Q.; de Goeij, A.F.P.M.; Dunselman, G.A.J.; Erkens, H.W.H.; Evers, J.L.H. Expression of cadherins and integrins in human endometrium throughout the menstrual cycle**Supported in part by a research grant from Organon International B.V., Oss, The Netherlands. *Fertil. Steril.* **1995**, *63*, 1210–1216. [CrossRef]

152. Lessey, B.A.; Castelbaum, A.J.; Sawin, S.W.; Buck, C.A.; Schinnar, R.; Bilker, W.; Strom, B.L. Aberrant integrin expression in the endometrium of women with endometriosis. *J. Clin. Endocrinol. Metab.* **1994**, *79*, 643–649.

153. Lessey, B.A.; Kim, J.J. Endometrial receptivity in the eutopic endometrium of women with endometriosis: It is affected, and let me show you why. *Fertil. Steril.* **2017**, *108*, 19–27. [CrossRef]

154. Germeyer, A.; Klinkert, M.S.; Huppertz, A.-G.; Clausmeyer, S.; Popovici, R.M.; Strowitzki, T.; von Wolff, M. Expression of syndecans, cell-cell interaction regulating heparan sulfate proteoglycans, within the human endometrium and their regulation throughout the menstrual cycle. *Fertil. Steril.* **2007**, *87*, 657–663. [CrossRef] [PubMed]

155. Chelariu-Raicu, A.; Wilke, C.; Brand, M.; Starzinski-Powitz, A.; Kiesel, L.; Schüring, A.N.; Götte, M. Syndecan-4 expression is upregulated in endometriosis and contributes to an invasive phenotype. *Fertil. Steril.* **2016**, *106*, 378–385. [CrossRef] [PubMed]

156. Starzinski-Powitz, A.; Handrow-Metzmacher, H.; Kotzian, S. The putative role of cell adhesion molecules in endometriosis: Can we learn from tumour metastasis? *Mol. Med. Today* **1999**, *5*, 304–309. [CrossRef]

157. Gaetje, R.; Kotzian, S.; Herrmann, G.; Baumann, R.; Starzinski-Powitz, A. Nonmalignant epithelial cells, potentially invasive in human endometriosis, lack the tumor suppressor molecule E-cadherin. *Am. J. Pathol.* **1997**, *150*, 461–467.

158. Guilford, P. E-cadherin downregulation in cancer: Fuel on the fire? *Mol. Med. Today* **1999**, *5*, 172–177. [CrossRef]

159. Wijnhoven, B.P.; Dinjens, W.N.; Pignatelli, M. E-cadherin-catenin cell-cell adhesion complex and human cancer. *Br. J. Surg.* **2000**, *87*, 992–1005. [CrossRef]

160. van der Linden, P.J.; de Goeij, A.F.; Dunselman, G.A.; van der Linden, E.P.; Ramaekers, F.C.; Evers, J.L. Expression of integrins and E-cadherin in cells from menstrual effluent, endometrium, peritoneal fluid, peritoneum, and endometriosis. *Fertil. Steril.* **1994**, *61*, 85–90. [CrossRef]

161. Mashayekhi, F.; Aryaee, H.; Mirzajani, E.; Yasin, A.A.; Fathi, A. Soluble CD44 concentration in the serum and peritoneal fluid samples of patients with different stages of endometriosis. *Arch. Gynecol. Obstet.* **2015**, *292*, 641–645. [CrossRef]

162. Karousou, E.; Misra, S.; Ghatak, S.; Dobra, K.; Götte, M.; Vigetti, D.; Passi, A.; Karamanos, N.K.; Skandalis, S.S. Roles and targeting of the HAS/hyaluronan/CD44 molecular system in cancer. *Matrix Biol. J. Int. Soc. Matrix Biol.* **2017**, *59*, 3–22. [CrossRef]

163. Rodgers, A.K.; Nair, A.; Binkley, P.A.; Tekmal, R.; Schenken, R.S. Inhibition of CD44 N- and O-linked glycosylation decreases endometrial cell lines attachment to peritoneal mesothelial cells. *Fertil. Steril.* **2011**, *95*, 823–825. [CrossRef]

164. Knudtson, J.F.; Tekmal, R.R.; Santos, M.T.; Binkley, P.A.; Krishnegowda, N.; Valente, P.; Schenken, R.S. Impaired Development of Early Endometriotic Lesions in CD44 Knockout Mice. *Reprod. Sci. Thousand Oaks Calif* **2016**, *23*, 87–91. [CrossRef] [PubMed]

165. Olivares, C.N.; Alaniz, L.D.; Menger, M.D.; Barañao, R.I.; Laschke, M.W.; Meresman, G.F. Inhibition of Hyaluronic Acid Synthesis Suppresses Angiogenesis in Developing Endometriotic Lesions. *PloS ONE* **2016**, *11*, e0152302. [CrossRef] [PubMed]

166. Bałkowiec, M.; Maksym, R.B.; Włodarski, P.K. The bimodal role of matrix metalloproteinases and their inhibitors in etiology and pathogenesis of endometriosis. *Mol. Med. Rep.* **2018**, *18*, 3123–3136. [CrossRef] [PubMed]

167. Murphy, G.; Willenbrock, F.; Crabbe, T.; O'Shea, M.; Ward, R.; Atkinson, S.; O'Connell, J.; Docherty, A. Regulation of matrix metalloproteinase activity. *Ann. N. Y. Acad. Sci.* **1994**, *732*, 31–41. [CrossRef]

168. Nagase, H. Activation mechanisms of matrix metalloproteinases. *Biol. Chem.* **1997**, *378*, 151–160.

169. Smigiel, K.S.; Parks, W.C. Matrix Metalloproteinases and Leukocyte Activation. *Prog. Mol. Biol. Transl. Sci.* **2017**, *147*, 167–195.

170. Marbaix, E.; Kokorine, I.; Henriet, P.; Donnez, J.; Courtoy, P.J.; Eeckhout, Y. The expression of interstitial collagenase in human endometrium is controlled by progesterone and by oestradiol and is related to menstruation. *Biochem. J.* **1995**, *305*, 1027–1030. [CrossRef]

171. Hulboy, D.L.; Rudolph, L.A.; Matrisian, L.M. Matrix metalloproteinases as mediators of reproductive function. *Mol. Hum. Reprod.* **1997**, *3*, 27–45. [CrossRef]

172. Rodgers, W.H.; Matrisian, L.M.; Giudice, L.C.; Dsupin, B.; Cannon, P.; Svitek, C.; Gorstein, F.; Osteen, K.G. Patterns of matrix metalloproteinase expression in cycling endometrium imply differential functions and regulation by steroid hormones. *J. Clin. Investig.* **1994**, *94*, 946–953. [CrossRef]

173. Bruner, K.L.; Eisenberg, E.; Gorstein, F.; Osteen, K.G. Progesterone and transforming growth factor-β coordinately regulate suppression of endometrial matrix metalloproteinases in a model of experimental endometriosis. *Steroids* **1999**, *64*, 648–653. [CrossRef]

174. Spuijbroek, M.D.; Dunselman, G.A.; Menheere, P.P.; Evers, J.L. Early endometriosis invades the extracellular matrix. *Fertil. Steril.* **1992**, *58*, 929–933. [CrossRef]

175. Osteen, K.G.; Bruner-Tran, K.L.; Keller, N.R.; Eisenberg, E. Progesterone-Mediated Endometrial Maturation Limits Matrix Metalloproteinase (MMP) Expression in an Inflammatory-like Environment. *Ann. N. Y. Acad. Sci.* **2002**, *955*, 37–47. [CrossRef] [PubMed]

176. Salamonsen, L.A.; Woolley, D.E. Matrix metalloproteinases in normal menstruation. *Hum. Reprod. Oxf. Engl.* **1996**, *11* (Suppl. 2), 124–133. [CrossRef]

177. Salamonsen, L.A.; Zhang, J.; Hampton, A.; Lathbury, L. Regulation of matrix metalloproteinases in human endometrium. *Hum. Reprod. Oxf. Engl.* **2000**, *15* (Suppl. 3), 112–119. [CrossRef]

178. Bruner, K.L.; Matrisian, L.M.; Rodgers, W.H.; Gorstein, F.; Osteen, K.G. Suppression of matrix metalloproteinases inhibits establishment of ectopic lesions by human endometrium in nude mice. *J. Clin. Investig.* **1997**, *99*, 2851–2857. [CrossRef] [PubMed]

179. Nap, A.W.; Dunselman, G.A.J.; de Goeij, A.F.P.M.; Evers, J.L.H.; Groothuis, P.G. Inhibiting MMP activity prevents the development of endometriosis in the chicken chorioallantoic membrane model. *Hum. Reprod.* **2004**, *19*, 2180–2187. [CrossRef] [PubMed]

180. Osteen, K.G.; Bruner, K.L.; Sharpe-Timms, K.L. Steroid and growth factor regulation of matrix metalloproteinase expression and endometriosis. *Semin. Reprod. Endocrinol.* **1996**, *14*, 247–255. [CrossRef] [PubMed]

181. Sillem, M.; Prifti, S.; Neher, M.; Runnebaum, B. Extracellular matrix remodelling in the endometrium and its possible relevance to the pathogenesis of endometriosis. *Hum. Reprod. Update* **1998**, *4*, 730–735. [CrossRef] [PubMed]

182. Sharpe-Timms, K.L.; Keisler, L.W.; McIntush, E.W.; Keisler, D.H. Tissue inhibitor of metalloproteinase-1 concentrations are attenuated in peritoneal fluid and sera of women with endometriosis and restored in sera by gonadotropin-releasing hormone agonist therapy. *Fertil. Steril.* **1998**, *69*, 1128–1134. [CrossRef]

183. Cox, K.E.; Piva, M.; Sharpe-Timms, K.L. Differential regulation of matrix metalloproteinase-3 gene expression in endometriotic lesions compared with endometrium. *Biol. Reprod.* **2001**, *65*, 1297–1303. [CrossRef]

184. Sharpe-Timms, K.L.; Cox, K.E. Paracrine regulation of matrix metalloproteinase expression in endometriosis. *Ann. N. Y. Acad. Sci.* **2002**, *955*, 147–156; discussion 157–158, 396–406. [CrossRef] [PubMed]

185. Pitsos, M.; Kanakas, N. The role of matrix metalloproteinases in the pathogenesis of endometriosis. *Reprod. Sci. Thousand Oaks Calif* **2009**, *16*, 717–726. [CrossRef] [PubMed]

186. Zhou, H.-E.; Nothnick, W.B. The relevancy of the matrix metalloproteinase system to the pathophysiology of endometriosis. *Front. Biosci. J. Virtual Libr.* **2005**, *10*, 569–575. [CrossRef] [PubMed]

187. Osteen, K.G.; Bruner-Tran, K.L.; Eisenberg, E. Reduced progesterone action during endometrial maturation: A potential risk factor for the development of endometriosis. *Fertil. Steril.* **2005**, *83*, 529–537. [CrossRef] [PubMed]

188. Stamenkovic, I. Extracellular matrix remodelling: The role of matrix metalloproteinases. *J. Pathol.* **2003**, *200*, 448–464. [CrossRef] [PubMed]

189. Maas, J.W.; Le Noble, F.A.; Dunselman, G.A.; de Goeij, A.F.; Struyker Boudier, H.A.; Evers, J.L. The chick embryo chorioallantoic membrane as a model to investigate the angiogenic properties of human endometrium. *Gynecol. Obstet. Investig.* **1999**, *48*, 108–112. [CrossRef]

190. Griffioen, A.W.; Molema, G. Angiogenesis: Potentials for pharmacologic intervention in the treatment of cancer, cardiovascular diseases, and chronic inflammation. *Pharmacol. Rev.* **2000**, *52*, 237–268.

191. McLaren, J. Vascular endothelial growth factor and endometriotic angiogenesis. *Hum. Reprod. Update* **2000**, *6*, 45–55. [CrossRef]

192. Charnock-Jones, D.S.; Sharkey, A.M.; Rajput-Williams, J.; Burch, D.; Schofield, J.P.; Fountain, S.A.; Boocock, C.A.; Smith, S.K. Identification and localization of alternately spliced mRNAs for vascular endothelial growth factor in human uterus and estrogen regulation in endometrial carcinoma cell lines. *Biol. Reprod.* **1993**, *48*, 1120–1128. [CrossRef]

193. Smith, S.K. Regulation of angiogenesis in the endometrium. *Trends Endocrinol. Metab. TEM* **2001**, *12*, 147–151. [CrossRef]

194. Donnez, J.; Smoes, P.; Gillerot, S.; Casanas-Roux, F.; Nisolle, M. Vascular endothelial growth factor (VEGF) in endometriosis. *Hum. Reprod. Oxf. Engl.* **1998**, *13*, 1686–1690. [CrossRef] [PubMed]

195. Wingfield, M.; Macpherson, A.; Healy, D.L.; Rogers, P.A. Cell proliferation is increased in the endometrium of women with endometriosis. *Fertil. Steril.* **1995**, *64*, 340–346. [CrossRef]

196. Bourlev, V.; Volkov, N.; Pavlovitch, S.; Lets, N.; Larsson, A.; Olovsson, M. The relationship between microvessel density, proliferative activity and expression of vascular endothelial growth factor-A and its receptors in eutopic endometrium and endometriotic lesions. *Reproduction* **2006**, *132*, 501–509. [CrossRef] [PubMed]

197. Matsuzaki, S.; Canis, M.; Murakami, T.; Dechelotte, P.; Bruhat, M.A.; Okamura, K. Immunohistochemical analysis of the role of angiogenic status in the vasculature of peritoneal endometriosis. *Fertil. Steril.* **2001**, *76*, 712–716. [CrossRef]

198. Hull, M.L.; Charnock-Jones, D.S.; Chan, C.L.K.; Bruner-Tran, K.L.; Osteen, K.G.; Tom, B.D.M.; Fan, T.-P.D.; Smith, S.K. Antiangiogenic agents are effective inhibitors of endometriosis. *J. Clin. Endocrinol. Metab.* **2003**, *88*, 2889–2899. [CrossRef]

199. Nap, A.W.; Dunselman, G.A.J.; Griffioen, A.W.; Mayo, K.H.; Evers, J.L.H.; Groothuis, P.G. Angiostatic agents prevent the development of endometriosis-like lesions in the chicken chorioallantoic membrane. *Fertil. Steril.* **2005**, *83*, 793–795. [CrossRef]

200. Nap, A.W.; Griffioen, A.W.; Dunselman, G.A.J.; Bouma-Ter Steege, J.C.A.; Thijssen, V.L.J.L.; Evers, J.L.H.; Groothuis, P.G. Antiangiogenesis therapy for endometriosis. *J. Clin. Endocrinol. Metab.* **2004**, *89*, 1089–1095. [CrossRef]

201. Van Langendonckt, A.; Donnez, J.; Defrère, S.; Dunselman, G.A.J.; Groothuis, P.G. Antiangiogenic and vascular-disrupting agents in endometriosis: Pitfalls and promises. *Mol. Hum. Reprod.* **2008**, *14*, 259–268. [CrossRef]

202. Becker, C.M.; D'Amato, R.J. Angiogenesis and antiangiogenic therapy in endometriosis. *Microvasc. Res.* **2007**, *74*, 121–130. [CrossRef]

203. May, K.; Becker, C.M. Endometriosis and angiogenesis. *Minerva Ginecol.* **2008**, *60*, 245–254.

204. Taylor, R.N.; Yu, J.; Torres, P.B.; Schickedanz, A.C.; Park, J.K.; Mueller, M.D.; Sidell, N. Mechanistic and Therapeutic Implications of Angiogenesis in Endometriosis. *Reprod. Sci. Thousand Oaks Calif* **2009**, *16*, 140–146. [CrossRef] [PubMed]

205. Körbel, C.; Gerstner, M.D.; Menger, M.D.; Laschke, M.W. Notch signaling controls sprouting angiogenesis of endometriotic lesions. *Angiogenesis* **2018**, *21*, 37–46. [CrossRef] [PubMed]

206. Maruyama, T.; Yoshimura, Y. Stem cell theory for the pathogenesis of endometriosis. *Front. Biosci. Elite Ed.* **2012**, *4*, 2754–2763. [CrossRef] [PubMed]

207. Gargett, C.E.; Masuda, H. Adult stem cells in the endometrium. *Mol. Hum. Reprod.* **2010**, *16*, 818–834. [CrossRef] [PubMed]

208. Taylor, H.S. Endometrial cells derived from donor stem cells in bone marrow transplant recipients. *JAMA* **2004**, *292*, 81–85. [CrossRef] [PubMed]

209. Masuda, H.; Matsuzaki, Y.; Hiratsu, E.; Ono, M.; Nagashima, T.; Kajitani, T.; Arase, T.; Oda, H.; Uchida, H.; Asada, H.; et al. Stem Cell-Like Properties of the Endometrial Side Population: Implication in Endometrial Regeneration. *PLoS ONE* **2010**, *5*, e10387. [CrossRef] [PubMed]

210. Wu, Y.; Basir, Z.; Kajdacsy-Balla, A.; Strawn, E.; Macias, V.; Montgomery, K.; Guo, S.-W. Resolution of clonal origins for endometriotic lesions using laser capture microdissection and the human androgen receptor (HUMARA) assay. *Fertil. Steril.* **2003**, *79*, 710–717. [CrossRef]

211. Nabeshima, H.; Murakami, T.; Yoshinaga, K.; Sato, K.; Terada, Y.; Okamura, K. Analysis of the clonality of ectopic glands in peritoneal endometriosis using laser microdissection. *Fertil. Steril.* **2003**, *80*, 1144–1150. [CrossRef]

212. Mayr, D.; Amann, G.; Siefert, C.; Diebold, J.; Anderegg, B. Does endometriosis really have premalignant potential? A clonal analysis of laser-microdissected tissue. *FASEB J.* **2003**, *17*, 693–695. [CrossRef]

213. Maruyama, T.; Masuda, H.; Ono, M.; Kajitani, T.; Yoshimura, Y. Human uterine stem/progenitor cells: Their possible role in uterine physiology and pathology. *Reprod. Camb. Engl.* **2010**, *140*, 11–22. [CrossRef]

214. Wang, Y.; Sacchetti, A.; van Dijk, M.R.; van der Zee, M.; van der Horst, P.H.; Joosten, R.; Burger, C.W.; Grootegoed, J.A.; Blok, L.J.; Fodde, R. Identification of Quiescent, Stem-Like Cells in the Distal Female Reproductive Tract. *PLOS ONE* **2012**, *7*, e40691. [CrossRef] [PubMed]

215. Laganà, A.S.; Salmeri, F.M.; Vitale, S.G.; Triolo, O.; Götte, M. Stem Cell Trafficking During Endometriosis: May Epigenetics Play a Pivotal Role? *Reprod. Sci. Thousand Oaks Calif* **2018**, *25*, 978–979. [CrossRef] [PubMed]

216. Schüring, A.N.; Dahlhues, B.; Korte, A.; Kiesel, L.; Titze, U.; Heitkötter, B.; Ruckert, C.; Götte, M. The endometrial stem cell markers notch-1 and numb are associated with endometriosis. *Reprod. Biomed. Online* **2018**, *36*, 294–301. [CrossRef] [PubMed]

217. Götte, M.; Wolf, M.; Staebler, A.; Buchweitz, O.; Kiesel, L.; Schüring, A.N. Aberrant expression of the pluripotency marker SOX-2 in endometriosis. *Fertil. Steril.* **2011**, *95*, 338–341. [CrossRef] [PubMed]

218. Adammek, M.; Greve, B.; Kässens, N.; Schneider, C.; Brüggemann, K.; Schüring, A.N.; Starzinski-Powitz, A.; Kiesel, L.; Götte, M. MicroRNA miR-145 inhibits proliferation, invasiveness, and stem cell phenotype of an in vitro endometriosis model by targeting multiple cytoskeletal elements and pluripotency factors. *Fertil. Steril.* **2013**, *99*, 1346–1355. [CrossRef]

219. Eggers, J.C.; Martino, V.; Reinbold, R.; Schäfer, S.D.; Kiesel, L.; Starzinski-Powitz, A.; Schüring, A.N.; Kemper, B.; Greve, B.; Götte, M. microRNA miR-200b affects proliferation, invasiveness and stemness of endometriotic cells by targeting ZEB1, ZEB2 and KLF4. *Reprod. Biomed. Online* **2016**, *32*, 434–445. [CrossRef]

220. Sapkota, Y.; Steinthorsdottir, V.; Morris, A.P.; Fassbender, A.; Rahmioglu, N.; De Vivo, I.; Buring, J.E.; Zhang, F.; Edwards, T.L.; Jones, S.; et al. Meta-analysis identifies five novel loci associated with endometriosis highlighting key genes involved in hormone metabolism. *Nat. Commun.* **2017**, *8*, 15539. [CrossRef]

221. Bouaziz, J.; Mashiach, R.; Cohen, S.; Kedem, A.; Baron, A.; Zajicek, M.; Feldman, I.; Seidman, D.; Soriano, D. How Artificial Intelligence Can Improve Our Understanding of the Genes Associated with Endometriosis: Natural Language Processing of the PubMed Database. *BioMed Res. Int.* **2018**, *2018*, 6217812. [CrossRef]

222. Gajbhiye, R.; Fung, J.N.; Montgomery, G.W. Complex genetics of female fertility. *NPJ Genomic Med.* **2018**, *3*, 29. [CrossRef]

223. Kennedy, S. The genetics of endometriosis. *J. Reprod. Med.* **1998**, *43*, 263–268.

224. Simpson, J.L.; Bischoff, F.Z. Heritability and molecular genetic studies of endometriosis. *Ann. N. Y. Acad. Sci.* **2002**, *955*, 239–251; discussion 293–295, 396–406. [CrossRef] [PubMed]

225. Stefansson, H.; Geirsson, R.T.; Steinthorsdottir, V.; Jonsson, H.; Manolescu, A.; Kong, A.; Ingadottir, G.; Gulcher, J.; Stefansson, K. Genetic factors contribute to the risk of developing endometriosis. *Hum. Reprod. Oxf. Engl.* **2002**, *17*, 555–559. [CrossRef] [PubMed]

226. Treloar, S.; Hadfield, R.; Montgomery, G.; Lambert, A.; Wicks, J.; Barlow, D.H.; O'Connor, D.T.; Kennedy, S.; International Endogene Study Group. The International Endogene Study: A collection of families for genetic research in endometriosis. *Fertil. Steril.* **2002**, *78*, 679–685. [CrossRef]

227. Zondervan, K.T.; Cardon, L.R.; Kennedy, S.H. The genetic basis of endometriosis. *Curr. Opin. Obstet. Gynecol.* **2001**, *13*, 309–314. [CrossRef]

228. Zondervan, K.T.; Weeks, D.E.; Colman, R.; Cardon, L.R.; Hadfield, R.; Schleffler, J.; Trainor, A.G.; Coe, C.L.; Kemnitz, J.W.; Kennedy, S.H. Familial aggregation of endometriosis in a large pedigree of rhesus macaques. *Hum. Reprod. Oxf. Engl.* **2004**, *19*, 448–455. [CrossRef]

229. Kennedy, S.; Mardon, H.; Barlow, D. Familial endometriosis. *J. Assist. Reprod. Genet.* **1995**, *12*, 32–34. [CrossRef]

230. Hadfield, R.M.; Mardon, H.J.; Barlow, D.H.; Kennedy, S.H. Endometriosis in monozygotic twins. *Fertil. Steril.* **1997**, *68*, 941–942. [CrossRef]

231. Moen, M.H. Endometriosis in monozygotic twins. *Acta Obstet. Gynecol. Scand.* **1994**, *73*, 59–62. [CrossRef]

232. Treloar, S.A.; O'Connor, D.T.; O'Connor, V.M.; Martin, N.G. Genetic influences on endometriosis in an Australian twin sample. *Fertil. Steril.* **1999**, *71*, 701–710. [CrossRef]

233. Di, W.; Guo, S.-W. The search for genetic variants predisposing women to endometriosis. *Curr. Opin. Obstet. Gynecol.* **2007**, *19*, 395–401. [CrossRef]

234. Falconer, H.; D'Hooghe, T.; Fried, G. Endometriosis and genetic polymorphisms. *Obstet. Gynecol. Surv.* **2007**, *62*, 616–628. [CrossRef] [PubMed]

235. Guo, S.-W. Glutathione S-transferases M1/T1 gene polymorphisms and endometriosis: A meta-analysis of genetic association studies. *Mol. Hum. Reprod.* **2005**, *11*, 729–743. [CrossRef] [PubMed]

236. Guo, S.-W. The association of endometriosis risk and genetic polymorphisms involving dioxin detoxification enzymes: A systematic review. *Eur. J. Obstet. Gynecol. Reprod. Biol.* **2006**, *124*, 134–143. [CrossRef] [PubMed]

237. Guo, S.-W. Association of endometriosis risk and genetic polymorphisms involving sex steroid biosynthesis and their receptors: A meta-analysis. *Gynecol. Obstet. Investig.* **2006**, *61*, 90–105. [CrossRef] [PubMed]

238. Montgomery, G.W.; Nyholt, D.R.; Zhao, Z.Z.; Treloar, S.A.; Painter, J.N.; Missmer, S.A.; Kennedy, S.H.; Zondervan, K.T. The search for genes contributing to endometriosis risk. *Hum. Reprod. Update* **2008**, *14*, 447–457. [CrossRef] [PubMed]

239. Çayan, F.; Ayaz, L.; Aban, M.; Dilek, S.; Gümüş, L.T. Role of CYP2C19 polymorphisms in patients with endometriosis. *Gynecol. Endocrinol.* **2009**, *25*, 530–535. [CrossRef] [PubMed]

240. Bozdag, G.; Alp, A.; Saribas, Z.; Tuncer, S.; Aksu, T.; Gurgan, T. CYP17 and CYP2C19 gene polymorphisms in patients with endometriosis. *Reprod. Biomed. Online* **2010**, *20*, 286–290. [CrossRef]

241. Guo, S.-W.; Simsa, P.; Kyama, C.M.; Mihályi, A.; Fülöp, V.; Othman, E.-E.R.; D'Hooghe, T.M. Reassessing the evidence for the link between dioxin and endometriosis: From molecular biology to clinical epidemiology. *MHR Basic Sci. Reprod. Med.* **2009**, *15*, 609–624. [CrossRef]

242. Ioannidis, J.P.A.; Ntzani, E.E.; Trikalinos, T.A.; Contopoulos-Ioannidis, D.G. Replication validity of genetic association studies. *Nat. Genet.* **2001**, *29*, 306–309. [CrossRef]

243. Lohmueller, K.E.; Pearce, C.L.; Pike, M.; Lander, E.S.; Hirschhorn, J.N. Meta-analysis of genetic association studies supports a contribution of common variants to susceptibility to common disease. *Nat. Genet.* **2003**, *33*, 177–182. [CrossRef]

244. Hindorff, L.A.; Sethupathy, P.; Junkins, H.A.; Ramos, E.M.; Mehta, J.P.; Collins, F.S.; Manolio, T.A. Potential etiologic and functional implications of genome-wide association loci for human diseases and traits. *Proc. Natl. Acad. Sci.* **2009**, *106*, 9362–9367. [CrossRef] [PubMed]

245. McCarthy, M.I.; Abecasis, G.R.; Cardon, L.R.; Goldstein, D.B.; Little, J.; Ioannidis, J.P.A.; Hirschhorn, J.N. Genome-wide association studies for complex traits: Consensus, uncertainty and challenges. *Nat. Rev. Genet.* **2008**, *9*, 356–369. [CrossRef] [PubMed]

246. Visscher, P.M.; Montgomery, G.W. Genome-wide association studies and human disease: From trickle to flood. *JAMA* **2009**, *302*, 2028–2029. [CrossRef] [PubMed]

247. Zondervan, K.; Cardon, L.; Desrosiers, R.; Hyde, D.; Kemnitz, J.; Mansfield, K.; Roberts, J.; Scheffler, J.; Weeks, D.E.; Kennedy, S. The Genetic Epidemiology of Spontaneous Endometriosis in the Rhesus Monkey. *Ann. N. Y. Acad. Sci.* **2002**, *955*, 233–238. [CrossRef]

248. Zondervan, K.T.; Cardon, L.R. The complex interplay among factors that influence allelic association. *Nat. Rev. Genet.* **2004**, *5*, 89–100. [CrossRef]

249. Hirschhorn, J.N.; Lohmueller, K.; Byrne, E.; Hirschhorn, K. A comprehensive review of genetic association studies. *Genet. Med.* **2002**, *4*, 45–61. [CrossRef]

250. Kruglyak, L.; Lander, E.S. Complete multipoint sib-pair analysis of qualitative and quantitative traits. *Am. J. Hum. Genet.* **1995**, *57*, 439–454.

251. Lander, E.; Kruglyak, L. Genetic dissection of complex traits: Guidelines for interpreting and reporting linkage results. *Nat. Genet.* **1995**, *11*, 241. [CrossRef]

252. Risch, N. Linkage strategies for genetically complex traits. II. The power of affected relative pairs. *Am. J. Hum. Genet.* **1990**, *46*, 229–241.

253. Treloar, S.A.; Wicks, J.; Nyholt, D.R.; Montgomery, G.W.; Bahlo, M.; Smith, V.; Dawson, G.; Mackay, I.J.; Weeks, D.E.; Bennett, S.T.; et al. Genomewide Linkage Study in 1,176 Affected Sister Pair Families Identifies a Significant Susceptibility Locus for Endometriosis on Chromosome 10q26. *Am. J. Hum. Genet.* **2005**, *77*, 365–376. [CrossRef]

254. Miki, Y.; Swensen, J.; Shattuck-Eidens, D.; Futreal, P.A.; Harshman, K.; Tavtigian, S.; Liu, Q.; Cochran, C.; Bennett, L.M.; Ding, W.; et al. A strong candidate for the breast and ovarian cancer susceptibility gene BRCA1. *Science* **1994**, *266*, 66–71. [CrossRef] [PubMed]

255. Wooster, R.; Bignell, G.; Lancaster, J.; Swift, S.; Seal, S.; Mangion, J.; Collins, N.; Gregory, S.; Gumbs, C.; Micklem, G.; et al. Identification of the breast cancer susceptibility gene BRCA2. *Nature* **1995**, *378*, 789. [CrossRef] [PubMed]

256. Zondervan, K.T.; Treloar, S.A.; Lin, J.; Weeks, D.E.; Nyholt, D.R.; Mangion, J.; MacKay, I.J.; Cardon, L.R.; Martin, N.G.; Kennedy, S.H.; et al. Significant evidence of one or more susceptibility loci for endometriosis

with near-Mendelian inheritance on chromosome 7p13–15. *Hum. Reprod.* **2007**, *22*, 717–728. [CrossRef] [PubMed]

257. The International HapMap Consortium A second generation human haplotype map of over 3.1 million SNPs. *Nature* **2007**, *449*, 851–861. [CrossRef]

258. Treloar, S.A.; Zhao, Z.Z.; Le, L.; Zondervan, K.T.; Martin, N.G.; Kennedy, S.; Nyholt, D.R.; Montgomery, G.W. Variants in EMX2 and PTEN do not contribute to risk of endometriosis. *MHR Basic Sci. Reprod. Med.* **2007**, *13*, 587–594. [CrossRef] [PubMed]

259. Daftary, G.S.; Taylor, H.S. EMX2 Gene Expression in the Female Reproductive Tract and Aberrant Expression in the Endometrium of Patients with Endometriosis. *J. Clin. Endocrinol. Metab.* **2004**, *89*, 2390–2396. [CrossRef] [PubMed]

260. Troy, P.J.; Daftary, G.S.; Bagot, C.N.; Taylor, H.S. Transcriptional Repression of Peri-Implantation EMX2 Expression in Mammalian Reproduction by HOXA10. *Mol. Cell. Biol.* **2003**, *23*, 1–13. [CrossRef]

261. Maxwell, G.L.; Risinger, J.I.; Gumbs, C.; Shaw, H.; Bentley, R.C.; Barrett, J.C.; Berchuck, A.; Futreal, P.A. Mutation of the PTEN Tumor Suppressor Gene in Endometrial Hyperplasias. *Cancer Res.* **1998**, *58*, 2500–2503.

262. Easton, D.F.; Pooley, K.A.; Dunning, A.M.; Pharoah, P.D.P.; Thompson, D.; Ballinger, D.G.; Struewing, J.P.; Morrison, J.; Field, H.; Luben, R.; et al. Genome-wide association study identifies novel breast cancer susceptibility loci. *Nature* **2007**, *447*, 1087–1093. [CrossRef]

263. Pollock, P.M.; Gartside, M.G.; Dejeza, L.C.; Powell, M.A.; Mallon, M.A.; Cancer Genome Project; Davies, H.; Mohammadi, M.; Futreal, P.A.; Stratton, M.R.; et al. Frequent activating FGFR2 mutations in endometrial carcinomas parallel germline mutations associated with craniosynostosis and skeletal dysplasia syndromes. *Oncogene* **2007**, *26*, 7158–7162. [CrossRef]

264. Zhao, Z.Z.; Pollock, P.M.; Thomas, S.; Treloar, S.A.; Nyholt, D.R.; Montgomery, G.W. Common variation in the fibroblast growth factor receptor 2 gene is not associated with endometriosis risk. *Hum. Reprod.* **2008**, *23*, 1661–1668. [CrossRef] [PubMed]

265. Zondervan, K.T.; Cardon, L.R. Designing candidate gene and genome-wide case–control association studies. *Nat. Protoc.* **2007**, *2*, 2492–2501. [CrossRef] [PubMed]

266. Zöllner, S.; Pritchard, J.K. Overcoming the Winner's Curse: Estimating Penetrance Parameters from Case-Control Data. *Am. J. Hum. Genet.* **2007**, *80*, 605–615. [CrossRef] [PubMed]

267. Sabeti, P.C.; Varilly, P.; Fry, B.; Lohmueller, J.; Hostetter, E.; Cotsapas, C.; Xie, X.; Byrne, E.H.; McCarroll, S.A.; Gaudet, R.; et al. Genome-wide detection and characterization of positive selection in human populations. *Nature* **2007**, *449*, 913–918. [CrossRef]

268. Uno, S.; Zembutsu, H.; Hirasawa, A.; Takahashi, A.; Kubo, M.; Akahane, T.; Aoki, D.; Kamatani, N.; Hirata, K.; Nakamura, Y. A genome-wide association study identifies genetic variants in the *CDKN2BAS* locus associated with endometriosis in Japanese. *Nat. Genet.* **2010**, *42*, 707–710. [CrossRef]

269. Kondera-Anasz, Z.; Sikora, J.; Mielczarek-Palacz, A.; Jońca, M. Concentrations of interleukin (IL)-1α, IL-1 soluble receptor type II (IL-1 sRII) and IL-1 receptor antagonist (IL-1 Ra) in the peritoneal fluid and serum of infertile women with endometriosis. *Eur. J. Obstet. Gynecol. Reprod. Biol.* **2005**, *123*, 198–203. [CrossRef]

270. Adachi, S.; Tajima, A.; Quan, J.; Haino, K.; Yoshihara, K.; Masuzaki, H.; Katabuchi, H.; Ikuma, K.; Suginami, H.; Nishida, N.; et al. Meta-analysis of genome-wide association scans for genetic susceptibility to endometriosis in Japanese population. *J. Hum. Genet.* **2010**, *55*, 816–821. [CrossRef]

271. Zanatta, A.; Rocha, A.M.; Carvalho, F.M.; Pereira, R.M.A.; Taylor, H.S.; Motta, E.L.A.; Baracat, E.C.; Serafini, P.C. The role of the Hoxa10/HOXA10 gene in the etiology of endometriosis and its related infertility: A review. *J. Assist. Reprod. Genet.* **2010**, *27*, 701–710. [CrossRef]

272. Naillat, F.; Prunskaite-Hyyryläinen, R.; Pietilä, I.; Sormunen, R.; Jokela, T.; Shan, J.; Vainio, S.J. Wnt4/5a signalling coordinates cell adhesion and entry into meiosis during presumptive ovarian follicle development. *Hum. Mol. Genet.* **2010**, *19*, 1539–1550. [CrossRef]

273. Boyer, A.; Lapointe, É.; Zheng, X.; Cowan, R.G.; Li, H.; Quirk, S.M.; DeMayo, F.J.; Richards, J.S.; Boerboom, D. WNT4 is required for normal ovarian follicle development and female fertility. *FASEB J.* **2010**, *24*, 3010–3025. [CrossRef]

274. MacDonald, B.T.; Tamai, K.; He, X. Wnt/β-Catenin Signaling: Components, Mechanisms, and Diseases. *Dev. Cell* **2009**, *17*, 9–26. [CrossRef] [PubMed]

275. Yang, J.; Benyamin, B.; McEvoy, B.P.; Gordon, S.; Henders, A.K.; Nyholt, D.R.; Madden, P.A.; Heath, A.C.; Martin, N.G.; Montgomery, G.W.; et al. Common SNPs explain a large proportion of the heritability for human height. *Nat. Genet.* **2010**, *42*, 565–569. [CrossRef] [PubMed]

276. Painter, J.N.; Anderson, C.A.; Nyholt, D.R.; Macgregor, S.; Lin, J.; Lee, S.H.; Lambert, A.; Zhao, Z.Z.; Roseman, F.; Guo, Q.; et al. Genome-wide association study identifies a locus at 7p15.2 associated with endometriosis. *Nat. Genet.* **2011**, *43*, 51–54. [CrossRef] [PubMed]

277. Bodmer, W.; Bonilla, C. Common and rare variants in multifactorial susceptibility to common diseases. *Nat. Genet.* **2008**, *40*, 695–701. [CrossRef]

278. Gorlov, I.P.; Gorlova, O.Y.; Sunyaev, S.R.; Spitz, M.R.; Amos, C.I. Shifting Paradigm of Association Studies: Value of Rare Single-Nucleotide Polymorphisms. *Am. J. Hum. Genet.* **2008**, *82*, 100–112. [CrossRef]

279. Curtin, K.; Iles, M.M.; Camp, N.J. Identifying Rarer Genetic Variants for Common Complex Diseases: Diseased Versus Neutral Discovery Panels. *Ann. Hum. Genet.* **2009**, *73*, 54–60. [CrossRef]

280. Iles, M.M. What Can Genome-Wide Association Studies Tell Us about the Genetics of Common Disease? *PLOS Genet.* **2008**, *4*, e33. [CrossRef]

281. Mettler, L.; Salmassi, A.; Schollmeyer, T.; Schmutzler, A.G.; Püngel, F.; Jonat, W. Comparison of c-DNA microarray analysis of gene expression between eutopic endometrium and ectopic endometrium (endometriosis). *J. Assist. Reprod. Genet.* **2007**, *24*, 249–258. [CrossRef]

282. Eyster, K.M.; Klinkova, O.; Kennedy, V.; Hansen, K.A. Whole genome deoxyribonucleic acid microarray analysis of gene expression in ectopic versus eutopic endometrium. *Fertil. Steril.* **2007**, *88*, 1505–1533. [CrossRef]

283. Flores, I.; Rivera, E.; Ruiz, L.A.; Santiago, O.I.; Vernon, M.W.; Appleyard, C.B. Molecular profiling of experimental endometriosis identified gene expression patterns in common with human disease. *Fertil. Steril.* **2007**, *87*, 1180–1199. [CrossRef]

284. Hull, M.L.; Escareno, C.R.; Godsland, J.M.; Doig, J.R.; Johnson, C.M.; Phillips, S.C.; Smith, S.K.; Tavaré, S.; Print, C.G.; Charnock-Jones, D.S. Endometrial-Peritoneal Interactions during Endometriotic Lesion Establishment. *Am. J. Pathol.* **2008**, *173*, 700–715. [CrossRef] [PubMed]

285. Zafrakas, M.; Tarlatzis, B.C.; Streichert, T.; Pournaropoulos, F.; Wölfle, U.; Smeets, S.J.; Wittek, B.; Grimbizis, G.; Brakenhoff, R.H.; Pantel, K.; et al. Genome-wide microarray gene expression, array-CGH analysis, and telomerase activity in advanced ovarian endometriosis: A high degree of differentiation rather than malignant potential. *Int. J. Mol. Med.* **2008**, *21*, 335–344. [CrossRef] [PubMed]

286. Pelch, K.E.; Schroder, A.L.; Kimball, P.A.; Sharpe-Timms, K.L.; Davis, J.W.; Nagel, S.C. Aberrant gene expression profile in a mouse model of endometriosis mirrors that observed in women. *Fertil. Steril.* **2010**, *93*, 1615–1627. [CrossRef] [PubMed]

287. Umezawa, M.; Tanaka, N.; Tainaka, H.; Takeda, K.; Ihara, T.; Sugamata, M. Microarray analysis provides insight into the early steps of pathophysiology of mouse endometriosis model induced by autotransplantation of endometrium. *Life Sci.* **2009**, *84*, 832–837. [CrossRef] [PubMed]

288. Bruner-Tran, K.L.; Gnecco, J.; Ding, T.; Glore, D.R.; Pensabene, V.; Osteen, K.G. Exposure to the environmental endocrine disruptor TCDD and human reproductive dysfunction: Translating lessons from murine models. *Reprod. Toxicol. Elmsford N* **2017**, *68*, 59–71. [CrossRef] [PubMed]

289. Morgan, H.D.; Santos, F.; Green, K.; Dean, W.; Reik, W. Epigenetic reprogramming in mammals. *Hum. Mol. Genet.* **2005**, *14*, R47–R58. [CrossRef]

290. Gabory, A.; Attig, L.; Junien, C. Epigenetic mechanisms involved in developmental nutritional programming. *World J. Diabetes* **2011**, *2*, 164–175. [CrossRef]

291. Berger, S.L.; Kouzarides, T.; Shiekhattar, R.; Shilatifard, A. An operational definition of epigenetics. *Genes Dev.* **2009**, *23*, 781–783. [CrossRef]

292. Robertson, K.D. DNA methylation and human disease. *Nat. Rev. Genet.* **2005**, *6*, 597–610. [CrossRef]

293. Robertson, K.D.; Wolffe, A.P. DNA methylation in health and disease. *Nat. Rev. Genet.* **2000**, *1*, 11–19. [CrossRef]

294. Rodenhiser, D.; Mann, M. Epigenetics and human disease: Translating basic biology into clinical applications. *CMAJ Can. Med. Assoc. J. J. Assoc. Medicale Can.* **2006**, *174*, 341–348. [CrossRef] [PubMed]

295. Li, E. Chromatin modification and epigenetic reprogramming in mammalian development. *Nat. Rev. Genet.* **2002**, *3*, 662–673. [CrossRef] [PubMed]

296. Ritchie, W. microRNA Target Prediction. *Methods Mol. Biol. Clifton NJ* **2017**, *1513*, 193–200.

297. Sun, K.; Lai, E.C. Adult-specific functions of animal microRNAs. *Nat. Rev. Genet.* **2013**, *14*, 535–548. [CrossRef]

298. Kurokawa, R.; Rosenfeld, M.G.; Glass, C.K. Transcriptional regulation through noncoding RNAs and epigenetic modifications. *RNA Biol.* **2009**, *6*, 233–236. [CrossRef]

299. Saare, M.; Rekker, K.; Laisk-Podar, T.; Rahmioglu, N.; Zondervan, K.; Salumets, A.; Götte, M.; Peters, M. Challenges in endometriosis miRNA studies - From tissue heterogeneity to disease specific miRNAs. *Biochim. Biophys. Acta Mol. Basis Dis.* **2017**, *1863*, 2282–2292. [CrossRef]

300. Munro, S.K.; Farquhar, C.M.; Mitchell, M.D.; Ponnampalam, A.P. Epigenetic regulation of endometrium during the menstrual cycle. *Mol. Hum. Reprod.* **2010**, *16*, 297–310. [CrossRef]

301. Yamagata, Y.; Asada, H.; Tamura, I.; Lee, L.; Maekawa, R.; Taniguchi, K.; Taketani, T.; Matsuoka, A.; Tamura, H.; Sugino, N. DNA methyltransferase expression in the human endometrium: Down-regulation by progesterone and estrogen. *Hum. Reprod. Oxf. Engl.* **2009**, *24*, 1126–1132. [CrossRef]

302. Krusche, C.A.; Vloet, A.J.; Classen-Linke, I.; von Rango, U.; Beier, H.M.; Alfer, J. Class I histone deacetylase expression in the human cyclic endometrium and endometrial adenocarcinomas. *Hum. Reprod. Oxf. Engl.* **2007**, *22*, 2956–2966. [CrossRef]

303. Sakai, N.; Maruyama, T.; Sakurai, R.; Masuda, H.; Yamamoto, Y.; Shimizu, A.; Kishi, I.; Asada, H.; Yamagoe, S.; Yoshimura, Y. Involvement of histone acetylation in ovarian steroid-induced decidualization of human endometrial stromal cells. *J. Biol. Chem.* **2003**, *278*, 16675–16682. [CrossRef]

304. Uchida, H.; Maruyama, T.; Ohta, K.; Ono, M.; Arase, T.; Kagami, M.; Oda, H.; Kajitani, T.; Asada, H.; Yoshimura, Y. Histone deacetylase inhibitor-induced glycodelin enhances the initial step of implantation. *Hum. Reprod. Oxf. Engl.* **2007**, *22*, 2615–2622. [CrossRef] [PubMed]

305. Uchida, H.; Maruyama, T.; Nagashima, T.; Ono, M.; Masuda, H.; Arase, T.; Sugiura, I.; Onouchi, M.; Kajitani, T.; Asada, H.; et al. Human endometrial cytodifferentiation by histone deacetylase inhibitors. *Hum. Cell* **2006**, *19*, 38–42. [CrossRef] [PubMed]

306. Galliano, D.; Pellicer, A. MicroRNA and implantation. *Fertil. Steril.* **2014**, *101*, 1531–1544. [CrossRef] [PubMed]

307. Hull, M.L.; Nisenblat, V. Tissue and circulating microRNA influence reproductive function in endometrial disease. *Reprod. Biomed. Online* **2013**, *27*, 515–529. [CrossRef]

308. Pan, Q.; Chegini, N. MicroRNA signature and regulatory functions in the endometrium during normal and disease states. *Semin. Reprod. Med.* **2008**, *26*, 479–493. [CrossRef]

309. Kuokkanen, S.; Chen, B.; Ojalvo, L.; Benard, L.; Santoro, N.; Pollard, J.W. Genomic profiling of microRNAs and messenger RNAs reveals hormonal regulation in microRNA expression in human endometrium. *Biol. Reprod.* **2010**, *82*, 791–801. [CrossRef]

310. Lessey, B.A. Fine tuning of endometrial function by estrogen and progesterone through microRNAs. *Biol. Reprod.* **2010**, *82*, 653–655. [CrossRef]

311. Pastorelli, L.M.; Wells, S.; Fray, M.; Smith, A.; Hough, T.; Harfe, B.D.; McManus, M.T.; Smith, L.; Woolf, A.S.; Cheeseman, M.; et al. Genetic analyses reveal a requirement for Dicer1 in the mouse urogenital tract. *Mamm. Genome Off. J. Int. Mamm. Genome Soc.* **2009**, *20*, 140–151. [CrossRef]

312. Hong, X.; Luense, L.J.; McGinnis, L.K.; Nothnick, W.B.; Christenson, L.K. Dicer1 is essential for female fertility and normal development of the female reproductive system. *Endocrinology* **2008**, *149*, 6207–6212. [CrossRef]

313. Koninckx, P.R.; Ussia, A.; Adamyan, L.; Wattiez, A.; Gomel, V.; Martin, D.C. Pathogenesis of endometriosis: The genetic/epigenetic theory. *Fertil. Steril.* **2019**, *111*, 327–340. [CrossRef]

314. Yamagata, Y.; Nishino, K.; Takaki, E.; Sato, S.; Maekawa, R.; Nakai, A.; Sugino, N. Genome-wide DNA methylation profiling in cultured eutopic and ectopic endometrial stromal cells. *PloS ONE* **2014**, *9*, e83612. [CrossRef] [PubMed]

315. Signorile, P.G.; Severino, A.; Santoro, M.; Spyrou, M.; Viceconte, R.; Baldi, A. Methylation analysis of HOXA10 regulatory elements in patients with endometriosis. *BMC Res. Notes* **2018**, *11*. [CrossRef] [PubMed]

316. Wu, Y.; Halverson, G.; Basir, Z.; Strawn, E.; Yan, P.; Guo, S.-W. Aberrant methylation at HOXA10 may be responsible for its aberrant expression in the endometrium of patients with endometriosis. *Am. J. Obstet. Gynecol.* **2005**, *193*, 371–380. [CrossRef] [PubMed]

317. Lee, B.; Du, H.; Taylor, H.S. Experimental Murine Endometriosis Induces DNA Methylation and Altered Gene Expression in Eutopic Endometrium. *Biol. Reprod.* **2009**, *80*, 79–85. [CrossRef]

318. Bromer, J.G.; Wu, J.; Zhou, Y.; Taylor, H.S. Hypermethylation of Homeobox A10 by in Utero Diethylstilbestrol Exposure: An Epigenetic Mechanism for Altered Developmental Programming. *Endocrinology* **2009**, *150*, 3376–3382. [CrossRef]

319. Bromer, J.G.; Zhou, Y.; Taylor, M.B.; Doherty, L.; Taylor, H.S. Bisphenol-A exposure in utero leads to epigenetic alterations in the developmental programming of uterine estrogen response. *FASEB J.* **2010**, *24*, 2273–2280. [CrossRef]

320. Kulp, J.L.; Mamillapalli, R.; Taylor, H.S. Aberrant HOXA10 Methylation in Patients With Common Gynecologic Disorders. *Reprod. Sci.* **2016**, *23*, 455–463. [CrossRef]

321. Wu, Y.; Strawn, E.; Basir, Z.; Halverson, G.; Guo, S.-W. Promoter hypermethylation of progesterone receptor isoform B (PR-B) in endometriosis. *Epigenetics* **2006**, *1*, 106–111. [CrossRef]

322. Attia, G.R.; Zeitoun, K.; Edwards, D.; Johns, A.; Carr, B.R.; Bulun, S.E. Progesterone receptor isoform A but not B is expressed in endometriosis. *J. Clin. Endocrinol. Metab.* **2000**, *85*, 2897–2902. [CrossRef]

323. Nie, J.; Liu, X.; Guo, S.W. Promoter hypermethylation of progesterone receptor isoform B (PR-B) in adenomyosis and its rectification by a histone deacetylase inhibitor and a demethylation agent. *Reprod. Sci. Thousand Oaks Calif* **2010**, *17*, 995–1005.

324. Wu, Y.; Strawn, E.; Basir, Z.; Halverson, G.; Guo, S.-W. Aberrant expression of deoxyribonucleic acid methyltransferases DNMT1, DNMT3A, and DNMT3B in women with endometriosis. *Fertil. Steril.* **2007**, *87*, 24–32. [CrossRef] [PubMed]

325. Dyson, M.T.; Kakinuma, T.; Pavone, M.E.; Monsivais, D.; Navarro, A.; Malpani, S.S.; Ono, M.; Bulun, S.E. Aberrant expression and localization of deoxyribonucleic acid methyltransferase 3B in endometriotic stromal cells. *Fertil. Steril.* **2015**, *104*, 953–963. [CrossRef] [PubMed]

326. Aznaurova, Y.B.; Zhumataev, M.B.; Roberts, T.K.; Aliper, A.M.; Zhavoronkov, A.A. Molecular aspects of development and regulation of endometriosis. *Reprod. Biol. Endocrinol. RBE* **2014**, *12*, 50. [CrossRef] [PubMed]

327. Wu, Y.; Starzinski-Powitz, A.; Guo, S.-W. Trichostatin A, a histone deacetylase inhibitor, attenuates invasiveness and reactivates E-cadherin expression in immortalized endometriotic cells. *Reprod. Sci. Thousand Oaks Calif* **2007**, *14*, 374–382. [CrossRef]

328. KOUKOURA, O.; SIFAKIS, S.; SPANDIDOS, D.A. DNA methylation in endometriosis (Review). *Mol. Med. Rep.* **2016**, *13*, 2939–2948. [CrossRef]

329. Arosh, J.A.; Lee, J.; Starzinski-Powitz, A.; Banu, S.K. Selective inhibition of prostaglandin E2 receptors EP2 and EP4 modulates DNA methylation and histone modification machinery proteins in human endometriotic cells. *Mol. Cell. Endocrinol.* **2015**, *409*, 51–58. [CrossRef]

330. Xue, Q.; Lin, Z.; Yin, P.; Milad, M.P.; Cheng, Y.-H.; Confino, E.; Reierstad, S.; Bulun, S.E. Transcriptional activation of steroidogenic factor-1 by hypomethylation of the 5′ CpG island in endometriosis. *J. Clin. Endocrinol. Metab.* **2007**, *92*, 3261–3267. [CrossRef]

331. Xue, Q.; Lin, Z.; Cheng, Y.-H.; Huang, C.-C.; Marsh, E.; Yin, P.; Milad, M.P.; Confino, E.; Reierstad, S.; Innes, J.; et al. Promoter methylation regulates estrogen receptor 2 in human endometrium and endometriosis. *Biol. Reprod.* **2007**, *77*, 681–687. [CrossRef]

332. Izawa, M.; Taniguchi, F.; Uegaki, T.; Takai, E.; Iwabe, T.; Terakawa, N.; Harada, T. Demethylation of a nonpromoter cytosine-phosphate-guanine island in the aromatase gene may cause the aberrant up-regulation in endometriotic tissues. *Fertil. Steril.* **2011**, *95*, 33–39. [CrossRef]

333. Wang, D.; Chen, Q.; Zhang, C.; Ren, F.; Li, T. DNA hypomethylation of the COX-2 gene promoter is associated with up-regulation of its mRNA expression in eutopic endometrium of endometriosis. *Eur. J. Med. Res.* **2012**, *17*, 12. [CrossRef]

334. Nasu, K.; Kawano, Y.; Kai, K.; Aoyagi, Y.; Abe, W.; Okamoto, M.; Narahara, H. Aberrant histone modification in endometriosis. *Front. Biosci. Landmark Ed.* **2014**, *19*, 1202–1214. [CrossRef] [PubMed]

335. Monteiro, J.B.; Colón-Díaz, M.; García, M.; Gutierrez, S.; Colón, M.; Seto, E.; Laboy, J.; Flores, I. Endometriosis Is Characterized by a Distinct Pattern of Histone 3 and Histone 4 Lysine Modifications. *Reprod. Sci.* **2014**, *21*, 305–318. [CrossRef] [PubMed]

336. Xiaomeng, X.; Ming, Z.; Jiezhi, M.; Xiaoling, F. Aberrant histone acetylation and methylation levels in woman with endometriosis. *Arch. Gynecol. Obstet.* **2013**, *287*, 487–494. [CrossRef]

337. Samartzis, E.P.; Noske, A.; Samartzis, N.; Fink, D.; Imesch, P. The Expression of Histone Deacetylase 1, But Not Other Class I Histone Deacetylases, Is Significantly Increased in Endometriosis. *Reprod. Sci.* **2013**, *20*, 1416–1422. [CrossRef] [PubMed]

338. Kawano, Y.; Nasu, K.; Li, H.; Tsuno, A.; Abe, W.; Takai, N.; Narahara, H. Application of the histone deacetylase inhibitors for the treatment of endometriosis: Histone modifications as pathogenesis and novel therapeutic target. *Hum. Reprod. Oxf. Engl.* **2011**, *26*, 2486–2498. [CrossRef]

339. Imesch, P.; Samartzis, E.P.; Schneider, M.; Fink, D.; Fedier, A. Inhibition of transcription, expression, and secretion of the vascular epithelial growth factor in human epithelial endometriotic cells by romidepsin. *Fertil. Steril.* **2011**, *95*, 1579–1583. [CrossRef] [PubMed]

340. Ayhan, A.; Mao, T.-L.; Seckin, T.; Wu, C.-H.; Guan, B.; Ogawa, H.; Futagami, M.; Mizukami, H.; Yokoyama, Y.; Kurman, R.J.; et al. Loss of ARID1A expression is an early molecular event in tumor progression from ovarian endometriotic cyst to clear cell and endometrioid carcinoma. *Int. J. Gynecol. Cancer Off. J. Int. Gynecol. Cancer Soc.* **2012**, *22*, 1310–1315. [CrossRef]

341. Lowery, W.J.; Schildkraut, J.M.; Akushevich, L.; Bentley, R.; Marks, J.R.; Huntsman, D.; Berchuck, A. Loss of ARID1A-associated Protein Expression Is a Frequent Event in Clear Cell and Endometrioid Ovarian Cancers. *Int. J. Gynecol. Cancer* **2012**, *22*, 9–14. [CrossRef]

342. Chene, G.; Ouellet, V.; Rahimi, K.; Barres, V.; Provencher, D.; Mes-Masson, A.M. The ARID1A pathway in ovarian clear cell and endometrioid carcinoma, contiguous endometriosis, and benign endometriosis. *Int. J. Gynaecol. Obstet. Off. Organ Int. Fed. Gynaecol. Obstet.* **2015**, *130*, 27–30. [CrossRef]

343. Er, T.-K.; Su, Y.-F.; Wu, C.-C.; Chen, C.-C.; Wang, J.; Hsieh, T.-H.; Herreros-Villanueva, M.; Chen, W.-T.; Chen, Y.-T.; Liu, T.-C.; et al. Targeted next-generation sequencing for molecular diagnosis of endometriosis-associated ovarian cancer. *J. Mol. Med. Berl. Ger.* **2016**, *94*, 835–847. [CrossRef]

344. Nothnick, W.B. MicroRNAs and Endometriosis: Distinguishing Drivers from Passengers in Disease Pathogenesis. *Semin. Reprod. Med.* **2017**, *35*, 173–180. [CrossRef] [PubMed]

345. Filigheddu, N.; Gregnanin, I.; Porporato, P.E.; Surico, D.; Perego, B.; Galli, L.; Patrignani, C.; Graziani, A.; Surico, N. Differential Expression of MicroRNAs between Eutopic and Ectopic Endometrium in Ovarian Endometriosis. *J. Biomed. Biotechnol.* **2010**, *2010*. [CrossRef] [PubMed]

346. Burney, R.O.; Hamilton, A.E.; Aghajanova, L.; Vo, K.C.; Nezhat, C.N.; Lessey, B.A.; Giudice, L.C. MicroRNA expression profiling of eutopic secretory endometrium in women with versus without endometriosis. *Mol. Hum. Reprod.* **2009**, *15*, 625–631. [CrossRef] [PubMed]

347. Vasudevan, S.; Tong, Y.; Steitz, J.A. Switching from repression to activation: MicroRNAs can up-regulate translation. *Science* **2007**, *318*, 1931–1934. [CrossRef] [PubMed]

348. Han, A.R.; Lee, T.H.; Kim, S.; Lee, H.Y. Risk factors and biomarkers for the recurrence of ovarian endometrioma: About the immunoreactivity of progesterone receptor isoform B and nuclear factor kappa B. *Gynecol. Endocrinol. Off. J. Int. Soc. Gynecol. Endocrinol.* **2017**, *33*, 70–74. [CrossRef] [PubMed]

349. Wu, Y.; Guo, S.-W. Inhibition of Proliferation of Endometrial Stromal Cells by Trichostatin A, RU486, CDB-2914, N-Acetylcysteine, and ICI 182780. *Gynecol. Obstet. Investig.* **2006**, *62*, 193–205. [CrossRef] [PubMed]

350. Wu, Y.; Guo, S.-W. Histone deacetylase inhibitors trichostatin A and valproic acid induce cell cycle arrest and p21 expression in immortalized human endometrial stromal cells. *Eur. J. Obstet. Gynecol. Reprod. Biol.* **2008**, *137*, 198–203. [CrossRef]

351. Wu, Y.; Guo, S.-W. Suppression of IL-1β-induced COX-2 expression by trichostatin A (TSA) in human endometrial stromal cells. *Eur. J. Obstet. Gynecol. Reprod. Biol.* **2007**, *135*, 88–93. [CrossRef]

352. Wu, Y.; Guo, S.-W. Peroxisome proliferator-activated receptor-gamma and retinoid X receptor agonists synergistically suppress proliferation of immortalized endometrial stromal cells. *Fertil. Steril.* **2009**, *91*, 2142–2147. [CrossRef]

353. Peeters, L.L.H.; Vigne, J.-L.; Tee, M.K.; Zhao, D.; Waite, L.L.; Taylor, R.N. PPARgamma represses VEGF expression in human endometrial cells: Implications for uterine angiogenesis. *Angiogenesis* **2006**, *8*, 373–379. [CrossRef]

354. Ohama, Y.; Harada, T.; Iwabe, T.; Taniguchi, F.; Takenaka, Y.; Terakawa, N. Peroxisome proliferator-activated receptor-γ ligand reduced tumor necrosis factor-α-induced interleukin-8 production and growth in endometriotic stromal cells. *Fertil. Steril.* **2008**, *89*, 311–317. [CrossRef]

355. Lu, Y.; Nie, J.; Liu, X.; Zheng, Y.; Guo, S.-W. Trichostatin A, a histone deacetylase inhibitor, reduces lesion growth and hyperalgesia in experimentally induced endometriosis in mice. *Hum. Reprod. Oxf. Engl.* **2010**, *25*, 1014–1025. [CrossRef] [PubMed]

356. Imesch, P.; Fink, D.; Fedier, A. Romidepsin reduces histone deacetylase activity, induces acetylation of histones, inhibits proliferation, and activates apoptosis in immortalized epithelial endometriotic cells. *Fertil. Steril.* **2010**, *94*, 2838–2842. [CrossRef] [PubMed]

357. Wang, J.; Mahmud, S.A.; Bitterman, P.B.; Huo, Y.; Slungaard, A. Histone Deacetylase Inhibitors Suppress TF-κB-dependent Agonist-driven Tissue Factor Expression in Endothelial Cells and Monocytes. *J. Biol. Chem.* **2007**, *282*, 28408–28418. [CrossRef] [PubMed]

358. Dong, X.-F.; Song, Q.; Li, L.-Z.; Zhao, C.-L.; Wang, L.-Q. Histone deacetylase inhibitor valproic acid inhibits proliferation and induces apoptosis in KM3 cells via downregulating VEGF receptor. *Neuro Endocrinol. Lett.* **2007**, *28*, 775–780.

359. Deroanne, C.F.; Bonjean, K.; Servotte, S.; Devy, L.; Colige, A.; Clausse, N.; Blacher, S.; Verdin, E.; Foidart, J.-M.; Nusgens, B.V.; et al. Histone deacetylases inhibitors as anti-angiogenic agents altering vascular endothelial growth factor signaling. *Oncogene* **2002**, *21*, 427–436. [CrossRef]

360. Lockwood, C.J.; Krikun, G.; Hickey, M.; Huang, S.J.; Schatz, F. Decidualized Human Endometrial Stromal Cells Mediate Hemostasis, Angiogenesis, and Abnormal Uterine Bleeding. *Reprod. Sci. Thousand Oaks Calif* **2009**, *16*, 162–170. [CrossRef]

361. Liu, X.; Guo, S.-W. A pilot study on the off-label use of valproic acid to treat adenomyosis. *Fertil. Steril.* **2008**, *89*, 246–250. [CrossRef]

362. Liu, X.; Yuan, L.; Guo, S.W. Valproic acid as a therapy for adenomyosis: A comparative case series. *Reprod. Sci. Thousand Oaks Calif* **2010**, *17*, 904–912.

363. Liu, M.; Liu, X.; Zhang, Y.; Guo, S.-W. Valproic acid and progestin inhibit lesion growth and reduce hyperalgesia in experimentally induced endometriosis in rats. *Reprod. Sci. Thousand Oaks Calif* **2012**, *19*, 360–373.

364. Barra, F.; Ferrero, S. Epigenetic Drugs in the Treatment of Endometriosis. *Reprod. Sci. Thousand Oaks Calif* **2018**, 1933719118765987. [CrossRef] [PubMed]

Permissions

The contributors of this book come from diverse backgrounds, making this book a truly international effort. This book will bring forth new frontiers with its revolutionizing research information and detailed analysis of the nascent developments around the world.

We would like to thank all the contributing authors for lending their expertise to make the book truly unique. They have played a crucial role in the development of this book. Without their invaluable contributions this book wouldn't have been possible. They have made vital efforts to compile up to date information on the varied aspects of this subject to make this book a valuable addition to the collection of many professionals and students.

This book was conceptualized with the vision of imparting up-to-date information and advanced data in this field. To ensure the same, a matchless editorial board was set up. Every individual on the board went through rigorous rounds of assessment to prove their worth. After which they invested a large part of their time researching and compiling the most relevant data for our readers.

The editorial board has been involved in producing this book since its inception. They have spent rigorous hours researching and exploring the diverse topics which have resulted in the successful publishing of this book. They have passed on their knowledge of decades through this book. To expedite this challenging task, the publisher supported the team at every step. A small team of assistant editors was also appointed to further simplify the editing procedure and attain best results for the readers.

Apart from the editorial board, the designing team has also invested a significant amount of their time in understanding the subject and creating the most relevant covers. They scrutinized every image to scout for the most suitable representation of the subject and create an appropriate cover for the book.

The publishing team has been an ardent support to the editorial, designing and production team. Their endless efforts to recruit the best for this project, has resulted in the accomplishment of this book. They are a veteran in the field of academics and their pool of knowledge is as vast as their experience in printing. Their expertise and guidance has proved useful at every step. Their uncompromising quality standards have made this book an exceptional effort. Their encouragement from time to time has been an inspiration for everyone.

The publisher and the editorial board hope that this book will prove to be a valuable piece of knowledge for researchers, students, practitioners and scholars across the globe.

List of Contributors

Ana M. Sanchez, Luca Pagliardini and Sofia Makieva
Reproductive Sciences Laboratory, Division of Genetics and Cell Biology, IRCCS San Raffaele Scientific Institute, 20132 Milano, Italy

Greta C. Cermisoni, Laura Privitera, Alessandra Alteri, Laura Corti, Elisa Rabellotti and Massimo Candiani
IRCCS San Raffaele Scientific Institute, Obstetrics and Gynecology Unit, 20132 Milano, Italy

Costin Vlad Anastasiu, Marius Alexandru Moga, Andreea Balan, Ioan Scârneciu and Roxana Maria Dragomir
Department of Medical and Surgical Specialties, Faculty of Medicine, Transilvania University of Brasov, 500019 Brasov, Romania

Andrea Elena Neculau
Department of Fundamental, Prophylactic and Clinical Sciences, Faculty of Medicine, University Transilvania Brasov, 500019 Brasov, Romania

Ana-Maria Dull
Regina Maria Hospital, 500091 Brasov, Romania

Liana-Maria Chicea
"Victor Papilian" Medical School, University "Lucian Blaga" of Sibiu, 550024 Sibiu, Romania

Carolina Filipchiuk
Center of Natural and Human Sciences (CCNH), Universidade Federal do ABC, Santo André 09210-580, SP, Brazil

Rubia Beteli, Denise Maria Christofolini and Caio Parente Barbosa
Discipline of Sexual and Reproductive Health and Population Genetics, Department of Collective Health, Faculdade de Medicina do ABC/Centro Universitário Saúde ABC, Santo André 09210-580, Brazil

Tatiana Guida Ponce and Camila Martins Trevisan
Postgraduate Program in Health Sciences, Faculdade de Medicina do ABC/Centro Universitário Saúde ABC, Santo André 09210-580, Brazil

Fernando Luiz Affonso Fonseca
Discipline of Clinical Analysis, Deparment of Pathology, Faculdade de Medicina do ABC/Centro Universitário Saúde ABC, Santo André 09210-580, Brazil

Bianca Bianco
Center of Natural and Human Sciences (CCNH), Universidade Federal do ABC, Santo André 09210-580, SP, Brazil
Discipline of Sexual and Reproductive Health and Population Genetics, Department of Collective Health, Faculdade de Medicina do ABC/Centro Universitário Saúde ABC, Santo André 09210-580, Brazil

Stefano Angioni, Maurizio Nicola D'Alterio and Danilo Deiana
Department of Surgical Science, University of Cagliari, Cittadella Universitaria Blocco I, Asse Didattico Medicina P2, Monserrato, 09042 Cagliari, Italy

Alessandra Coiana
Department of Medical Science and Public Health, University of Cagliari, Laboratory of Genetics and Genomics, Pediatric Hospital Microcitemico "A. Cao", Via Edward Jenner, 09121 Cagliari, Italy

Franco Anni
Department of Medical Science and Public Health, University of Cagliari, Cittadella Universitaria di Monserrato, Asse Didattico E, Monserrato, 09042 Cagliari, Italy

Stefano Gessa
Laboratory of Molecular Genetics, Service of Forensic Medicine, AOU Cagliari, Via Ospedale 54, 09124 Cagliari, Italy

Marco Scioscia, Bruna A. Virgilio, Tommaso Bernardini and Nicola Fattizzi
Department of Obstetrics and Gynecology, Policlinico Hospital, 35031 Abano Terme, PD, Italy

Manuela Neri and Stefano Guerriero
Obstetrics and Gynecology, University of Cagliari, 09124 Cagliari, CA, Italy
Department of Obstetrics and Gynecology, Azienda Ospedaliero Universitaria, Policlinico Universitario Duilio Casula, 09045 Monserrato, CA, Italy

Camila Hernandes, Helen Mendes and Sergio Podgaec
Hospital Israelita Albert Einstein, Av. Albert Einstein 627, Morumbi, São Paulo 05651-901, Brazil

Paola Silveira, Aline Fernanda Rodrigues Sereia, Ana Paula Christoff and Luiz Felipe Valter de Oliveira
BiomeHub, Av. Luiz Boiteux Piazza, 1302, Canasvieiras, Florianópolis 88056-000, Brazil

Jieliang Zhou
Translational 'Omics and Biomarkers group, KK Research Centre, KK Women's and Children's Hospital, Singapore 229899, Singapore

Bernard Su Min Chern and Chee Wai Ku
Division of Obstetrics and Gynaecology, KK Women's and Children's Hospital, Singapore 229899, Singapore
OBGYN-Academic Clinical Program, Duke-NUS Medical School, Singapore 169857, Singapore

Peter Barton-Smith
Department of Obstetrics and Gynaecology, Singapore General Hospital, Singapore 169608, Singapore

Jessie Wai Leng Phoon, Heng Hao Tan and Jerry Kok Yen Chan
OBGYN-Academic Clinical Program, Duke-NUS Medical School, Singapore 169857, Singapore
Department of Reproductive Medicine, KKH, Singapore 229899, Singapore

Tse Yeun Tan and Veronique Viardot-Foucault
Department of Reproductive Medicine, KKH, Singapore 229899, Singapore

Yie Hou Lee
Translational 'Omics and Biomarkers group, KK Research Centre, KK Women's and Children's Hospital, Singapore 229899, Singapore
OBGYN-Academic Clinical Program, Duke-NUS Medical School, Singapore 169857, Singapore

Fabio Barra and Simone Ferrero
Academic Unit of Obstetrics and Gynecology, IRCCS Ospedale Policlinico San Martino, 16132 Genoa, Italy
Department of Neurosciences, Rehabilitation, Ophthalmology, Genetics, Maternal and Child Health (DiNOGMI), University of Genoa, 16132 Genoa, Italy

Ennio Biscaldi
Department of Radiology, Galliera Hospital, 16142, Genoa, Italy

Carolina Scala
Unit of Obstetrics and Gynecology, Gaslini Institute, 16147 Genova, Italy

Valerio Gaetano Vellone and Cesare Stabilini
Department of Surgical and Diagnostic Sciences, IRCCS Ospedale Policlinico San Martino, 16132 Genoa, Italy

Carla Trapero and Mireia Martín-Satué
Departament de Patologia i Terapèutica Experimental, Facultat de Medicina i Ciències de la Salut, Campus Bellvitge, Universitat de Barcelona, 08907 Barcelona, Spain
Oncobell Program, CIBERONC, Institut d'Investigació Biomèdica de Bellvitge (IDIBELL), 08908 Barcelona, Spain

August Vidal
Departament de Patologia i Terapèutica Experimental, Facultat de Medicina i Ciències de la Salut, Campus Bellvitge, Universitat de Barcelona, 08907 Barcelona, Spain
Oncobell Program, CIBERONC, Institut d'Investigació Biomèdica de Bellvitge (IDIBELL), 08908 Barcelona, Spain
Servei d'Anatomia Patològica, Hospital Universitari de Bellvitge, 08907 Barcelona, Spain

Maria Eulàlia Fernández-Montolí and Jordi Ponce
Oncobell Program, CIBERONC, Institut d'Investigació Biomèdica de Bellvitge (IDIBELL), 08908 Barcelona, Spain
Servei de Ginecologia, Hospital Universitari de Bellvitge, 08907 Barcelona, Spain

Buenaventura Coroleu, Francesc Tresserra and Pere Barri
Salud de la Mujer Dexeus, Hospital Universitari Quiron Dexeus, 08028 Barcelona, Spain

Inmaculada Gómez de Aranda
Departament de Patologia i Terapèutica Experimental, Facultat de Medicina i Ciències de la Salut, Campus Bellvitge, Universitat de Barcelona, 08907 Barcelona, Spain

Jean Sévigny
Centre de Recherche du CHU de Québec - Université Laval, Québec City, QC G1V 4G2, Canada
Départment de Microbiologie-Infectiologie et d'Immunologie, Faculté de Médecine, Université Laval, Quebec City, QC G1V 4G2, Canada

Xavier Matias-Guiu
Oncobell Program, CIBERONC, Institut d'Investigació Biomèdica de Bellvitge (IDIBELL), 08908 Barcelona, Spain
Servei d'Anatomia Patològica, Hospital Universitari de Bellvitge, 08907 Barcelona, Spain

Ji Hyun Park and Soohyun Kim
Department of Obstetrics and Gynecology, Gangnam Severance Hospital, Yonsei University College of Medicine, Seoul 06273, Korea

Zeenat Mirza and Umama A. Abdel-dayem
King Fahd Medical Research Center, King Abdulaziz University, Jeddah 21589, Saudi Arabia
Department of Medical Lab Technology, Faculty of Applied Medical Sciences, King Abdulaziz University, Jeddah 21589, Saudi Arabia

Jessica Ottolina, Ludovica Bartiromo, Carolina Dolci, Noemi Salmeri, Matteo Schimberni, Roberta Villanacci and Massimo Candiani
Gynecology/Obstetrics Unit, IRCCS San Raffaele Scientific Institute, 20132 Milan, Italy

Jeong Sook Kim
Department of Obstetrics and Gynecology, University of Ulsan College of Medicine, Ulsan University Hospital, Ulsan 44033, Korea

Young Sik Choi, Bo Hyon Yun, Seok Kyo Seo and Byung Seok Lee
Department of Obstetrics and Gynecology, Severance Hospital, Yonsei University College of Medicine, Seoul 03722, Korea
Institute of Women's Life Medical Science, Yonsei University College of Medicine, Seoul 03722, Korea

Jisun Yun and Jae Hoon Lee
Department of Obstetrics and Gynecology, Severance Hospital, Yonsei University College of Medicine, Seoul 03722, Korea

Joo Hyun Park and SiHyun Cho
Institute of Women's Life Medical Science, Yonsei University College of Medicine, Seoul 03722, Korea
Department of Obstetrics and Gynecology, Gangnam Severance Hospital, Yonsei University College of Medicine, Seoul 06273, Korea

Hyun-Soo Kim
Department of Pathology and Translational Genomics, Samsung Medical Center, Sungkyunkwan University School of Medicine, Seoul 06351, Korea

Cristina Secosan, Ligia Balulescu, Simona Brasoveanu, Oana Balint, Grigoras Dorin and Laurentiu Pirtea
Department of Obstetrics and Gynecology, University of Medicine and Pharmacy "Victor Babeş", 300041 Timişoara, Romania

Paul Pirtea
Department of Ob Gyn and Reproductive Medicine, Hopital Foch—Faculté de Medicine Paris Ouest (UVSQ), 92151 Suresnes, France

Antonio Simone Laganà, Simone Garzon and Fabio Ghezzi
Department of Obstetrics and Gynecology, "Filippo Del Ponte" Hospital, University of Insubria, Piazza Biroldi 1, 21100 Varese, Italy

Martin Götte
Department of Gynecology and Obstetrics, Münster University Hospital, D-48149 Münster, Germany

Paola Viganò
Reproductive Sciences Laboratory, Division of Genetics and Cell Biology, San Raffaele Scientific Institute, Via Olgettina 60, 20136 Milan, Italy
Reproductive Sciences Lab, Division of Genetics and Cell Biology, IRCCS San Raffaele Scientific Institute, 20132 Milan, Italy

Massimo Franchi
Department of Obstetrics and Gynecology, AOUI Verona, University of Verona, Piazzale Aristide Stefani 1, 37126 Verona, Italy

Dan C. Martin
School of Medicine, University of Tennessee Health Science Center, 910 Madison Ave, Memphis, TN 38163, USA
Virginia Commonwealth University, 907 Floyd Ave, Richmond, VA 23284, USA

Index

A

Adenomyomas, 72-73

Adenomyosis, 32, 68, 70-71, 73, 76, 78-80, 102, 119, 121, 123, 145, 157, 168-170, 175, 184, 204, 220, 223, 228, 241, 243

Adenosine Triphosphate, 124-125, 140-141

Angiogenesis, 11, 13-17, 20, 28-30, 35-36, 40-41, 44, 60, 93, 99, 101, 105, 107, 144, 153, 160, 173, 207, 210, 212-214, 220, 222-224, 233-235, 242-243

Angiopoietin, 15, 214, 228

Autoimmune Diseases, 37, 40, 51, 154, 160

B

Blastocysts, 1, 3, 6-7

Blastulation Rate, 1-6

Body Mass Index, 2, 8, 19, 26, 38, 48, 55, 115, 160, 162, 178

Bone Marrow-derived Stem Cells, 12

C

Cadherins, 212, 218, 232

Cell Adhesion Molecules, 14, 100, 233

Cell Fragmentation, 2, 7

Chronic Pelvic Pain, 11-12, 16, 23, 35, 48-49, 56, 68, 80, 143, 177, 192, 198

Confidence Interval, 7-8, 38, 45, 62, 102-103, 116, 159, 161, 173

Cytotoxicity, 15, 99, 101, 187, 209, 230

D

Deep Infiltrating Endometriosis, 6, 17, 30, 49, 65, 78-81, 93-94, 104-107, 110, 119-124, 136, 139, 161, 163-164, 192-193, 198-199, 203, 226

Differential Diagnosis, 68-72, 80-81, 119, 175, 193, 195

Dysmenorrhea, 11, 13, 16, 26, 35, 49, 56, 93, 96, 143, 184, 198, 223

Dyspareunia, 35, 49, 56, 74, 93, 96, 143, 184

E

Embryo Quality, 1-2, 4, 7

Endometrial Cancer, 73, 80, 143, 153-154, 157-158, 196, 198, 215, 217, 230

Endometrial Receptivity, 1, 5, 9, 153, 232

Endometrial Stem Cells, 40, 202-203, 214-215

Endometriosis, 1-6, 8-24, 26-83, 88-112, 114-116, 118-128, 130-131, 133-137, 139-149, 151-166, 168-180, 182-184,187-207, 209-210, 212-243

Endothelial Cells, 16, 40, 51, 126-127, 145, 243

Endothelial Growth Factor, 14-16, 20, 26-27, 30, 34, 50-51, 63, 66, 105, 107, 207-208, 224, 228, 234-235, 243

Enzyme-linked Immunosorbent Assay, 18, 20, 26, 40

Epigenetics, 10, 12, 28, 36, 44, 48, 54-55, 67, 156, 202, 218-220, 223, 236, 239, 241

Epithelial Cells, 43, 47, 126, 128, 130, 132, 135-136, 140, 146, 149, 153-154, 156-157, 205, 220, 227, 229, 233

Eutopic Endometrium, 9, 47, 82-83, 85, 88, 125-126, 133, 136, 140, 144, 153, 157, 172, 177, 179-180, 183, 188, 204-210, 212-215, 217, 219-223, 228, 232, 235, 239, 241

Extracellular Matrix, 14, 153, 183, 210, 212, 224, 234

F

Fallopian Tubes, 6, 73, 88, 94, 102, 135, 143, 205

Fertilization Rate, 1-3, 5-7

Fibrinolysis, 16, 173, 176

Fibrosis, 68-69, 73-74, 153, 157, 159, 173-174, 203

Follicle-stimulating Hormone, 2, 8, 37-38, 47, 218, 225

Follistatin, 17, 25, 30

G

Gene Silencing, 220-222

Genome-wide Association Study, 48, 52, 63-64, 238-239

Glycoproteins, 17, 46, 212

H

Heterogeneity, 6, 46, 66, 80, 94-95, 99-101, 103, 159, 173, 202-203, 216, 224, 240

Histone Deacetylase, 67, 219, 225, 240-243

Histone Modifications, 55, 219, 242

Homeostasis, 40, 53, 211

Hypermethylation, 54, 106, 219-221, 223, 241

I

Immune Cells, 14, 94, 100-101, 209-210

Immunohistochemistry, 40, 43, 124, 138, 180, 185

Immunostaining, 136, 180

In Vitro Fertilization, 1, 7-10

Infertility, 1-2, 4-7, 9, 11, 13, 16, 23, 26-27, 29, 31, 34-35, 37, 41, 49, 68, 93-94, 101-102, 104-105, 107, 124-125, 139, 141, 143, 145, 153-154, 159, 177, 184, 187, 192, 195, 218, 230, 238

Interleukins, 12, 14, 16, 209

Internal Genitalia, 68-72

L

Lymphocytes, 14-15, 29, 40, 162-163, 171, 231

M

Macrophages, 1, 12, 14-16, 28-29, 60, 160, 207, 209-210, 231

Magnetic Resonance Imaging, 77, 79-80, 110, 121-123, 192, 199

Matrix Metalloproteinases, 14, 24, 34, 188, 212, 224, 233-234

Methylation, 54-55, 61, 99, 188, 208, 219-223, 230, 239-242

Migration Inhibitory Factor, 12, 14, 25, 34

N

Natural Killer Cells, 15, 29, 107, 209, 224

Negative Predictive Value, 39, 114, 116

Next-generation Sequencing, 48, 52-53, 63, 67, 242

O

Odds Ratio, 7-8, 45, 57-59, 62, 159, 166

Organogenesis, 12, 40, 204, 220

Ovarian Cyst, 6, 172, 174

Ovarian Endometrioma, 17, 31-32, 55, 93-94, 105, 139, 161, 163-164, 170-171, 242

Oxidative Stress, 14, 19, 28, 31, 40, 51-52, 67, 104, 106-107, 209

P

Pathogenesis, 14, 20, 27-29, 36, 40-47, 50, 52, 55, 61, 65-66, 78, 81-83, 89-90, 94, 104-105, 107, 136, 141, 144, 152-155, 157-158, 174, 177-178, 183, 191, 198, 202-203, 207-208, 213, 215-217, 219-220, 222, 225-229, 232-235, 240, 242

Peptides, 19, 21, 23, 136

Peripheral Blood, 18, 22, 25, 30-31, 33-41, 160, 173

Peritoneal Endometriosis, 17, 28, 53, 89, 93-94, 104, 107-108, 126, 128, 137, 140, 142, 153, 155, 161, 163-164, 174, 226, 228, 235

Peritoneal Fluid, 1, 12, 14-15, 17, 29-31, 34, 51, 82-83, 88-89, 91, 93-94, 96-98, 104-107, 159, 174, 205, 209, 212-213, 217, 227, 230-234, 238

Polymerase Chain Reaction, 40, 49, 63, 184

Positive Predictive Value, 24, 39, 114, 116

Progesterone Receptor, 47, 50, 63, 65-66, 94, 104, 157-158, 208, 224, 230, 241-242

Proteoglycans, 212, 233

Proteomics, 11-13, 21, 25-26, 34, 142

Purinergic Signaling, 124-125, 133, 137, 139

R

Reactive Oxygen Species, 14, 19, 27, 29, 51, 100, 215

S

Serum Substitute Supplement, 7

Sex Hormones, 49, 53, 216

Single Nucleotide Polymorphisms, 45, 48-49, 52-53, 62, 217, 225

Standard Deviation, 2-3, 8, 137, 161

Steroidogenesis, 19, 49, 159, 175, 218

Survivin, 35-36, 40-41, 43-44

T

Transvaginal Ultrasonography, 42, 78, 80, 109-110, 112, 116-117, 122-123

Tumor Necrosis Factor-alpha, 12, 18, 66

U

Urinary Biomarkers, 11, 23

V

Vascular Endothelial Growth Factor, 14-16, 27, 30, 34, 50-51, 63, 66, 105, 107, 207-208, 224, 228, 234-235, 243

Vascularization, 16, 72-74, 76, 214, 231

Visual Analogue Scale, 49, 56, 114, 178